Which Country Has the World's Best Health Care?

Which Country Has the World's Best Health Care?

EZEKIEL J. EMANUEL

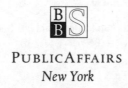

PublicAffairs
New York

PublicAffairs
Hachette Book Group
1290 Avenue of the Americas, New York, NY 10104
www.publicaffairsbooks.com
@Public_Affairs

Printed in the United States of America
First Edition: June 2020

Published by PublicAffairs, an imprint of Perseus Books, LLC, a subsidiary of Hachette Book Group, Inc. The PublicAffairs name and logo is a trademark of the Hachette Book Group.

The Hachette Speakers Bureau provides a wide range of authors for speaking events. To find out more, go to www.hachettespeakersbureau.com or call (866) 376-6591.

The publisher is not responsible for websites (or their content) that are not owned by the publisher.

Editorial production by Christine Marra, Marrathon Production Services, www.marrathoneditorial.org

Print book interior design by Jane Raese

Library of Congress Cataloging-in-Publication Data has been applied for.
ISBN 978-1-5417-9773-4 (hardcover), ISBN 978-1-5417-9772-7 (ebook)

LSC-C

Printing 4, 2021

DISCLAIMER

All the countries covered in this book have dynamic health care systems. They are frequently—even constantly—modifying their health care systems. Occasionally this is by a major piece of legislation, but more frequently it is by new regulations or other arrangements. Furthermore, many of the nongovernmental actors in a country—the insurance companies, the physicians, the hospitals, and others—are taking action. For instance, insurance companies merge or cease functioning.

In addition, the countries studied in this book tabulate and report data in substantially different ways. For instance, official statistics regarding drug costs vary widely. In some cases, validated drug spending is reported only as retail pharmacy sales. In other cases, official drug spending statistics include drugs administered in hospitals. Other governments only report the cost of drugs the government subsidizes.

Finally, some of my sources disagreed about how some aspects of the health care system operate or should be described. For instance, there is disagreement about whether to consider long-term care financing as part of the health care budget. These differences are a function of both professional judgment and the particular history of each country's health care system.

The consequence of these issues is that accuracy is a matter of direction and degree. I have done my best to report all facts using 2017 data and to make the data as comparable as possible, so that the overall picture conveyed is as close to reality as it can be. I apologize if I have missed any changes in these health care systems since the writing of this book. Nevertheless, the overall structures and tendencies I report are valid and, I hope, helpful to the reader.

CONTENTS

Introduction 1

1 United States 18

2 Canada 55

3 United Kingdom 83

4 Norway 115

5 France 143

6 Germany 169

7 Netherlands 197

8 Switzerland 229

9 Australia 261

10 Taiwan 300

11 China 324

12 Who's the Best? 351

13 Conclusion 385

Coda: Coronavirus and the Performance
of Health Care Systems 406

Acknowledgments 412

Glossary of Acronyms 415

Recommended Reading 422

Index 432

About the Author 453

INTRODUCTION

Why Search for the World's Best Health Care System?

"Which country has the world's best health care system?"

I get this question at almost every speech I give. Most of the time the question comes from someone who wants to know which country the United States should model itself after to create the world's best system here at home. But sometimes I wonder whether I'm really being asked a question about medical tourism—whether the questioner wants to know which country they should go to if they need to get some medical service, such as dental care, a hip replacement, or cataract surgery.

This is the type of question I usually love.

I rank everything. I rank the 10 best meals I've ever had (#1 Alinea in Chicago, #2 Tanja Grandits in Basel, and #3 OCD in Tel-Aviv). I rank chocolates (#1 Askinosie, #2 Dick Taylor of California, and #3 Fruition of New York). I rank Alpine cheeses (#1 is a tie between Alpha Tolman and Alp Blossom). I rank colleges. I rank academic departments of bioethics and health policy that compete with my own. I rank the meals I cook, the races I run, the bike rides I take, the speeches I give.

I should love ranking health systems. But I don't. When asked, I answer, "That is a terrible question." You cannot just take the world's "best" system, whether it is the Dutch or Swiss or Norwegian or Australian one, and plunk it down in the United States and think we will get better health care. Health care is path dependent. We have built up numerous institutions over decades that constrain and limit our ability

1

to change the system. And each country prioritizes different values that color which policy options they adopt. Some of these systems, like Norway, provide free insurance with no co-pays for children and people who need a lot of health care. Others, like the United States, emphasize making patients have more "skin in the game." Some emphasize hospital-based care, others want more care in the home. Some, anticipating the aging of the population, have proactively instituted mandatory long-term care insurance. Others prioritize more comprehensive, free care for children. Still others are more passive, waiting for a crisis to stimulate policy changes.

Consider where the US system is now. About half of all Americans get their coverage through employer-sponsored insurance, with employers "paying" most of the premium as a pre-tax fringe benefit. (I use "paying" ironically because the money really comes from reduced worker wages. Although economists believe and can prove that, no one else seems to accept the idea.) The majority of other Americans are covered by 2 government-financed programs: Medicare and Medicaid. Nearly 5,000 private community hospitals and hundreds of thousands of privately employed physicians deliver care. Insurers organize these hospitals and physicians into preferred networks and adjust co-payments to encourage patients to stay in network. We have built up extensive networks of private home health care agencies and home hospices, commercial dialysis centers, ambulatory surgical centers, and skilled nursing facilities. Myriad governmental bodies—from state insurance commissioners and physician and nurse licensure boards to the federal Food and Drug Administration (FDA) and the Federal Trade Commission—regulate various components of the system. Private organizations, such as the Joint Commission and boards of medical and surgical specialties, help ensure quality of care. All these institutions— the way they are paid, how they deliver care, and what they regulate— shape how the system operates and constrain what reforms can be instituted.

Other countries lack many of these core features. Norway doesn't have a fragmented insurance market with employer-sponsored insurance, a separate government program for the elderly, and another one with different benefits for low-income individuals. Switzerland has an individual mandate to buy insurance—but not a tax exclusion to help people pay for it. Germany has employer-sponsored insurance; it also has no tax exclusion, but employer and employee contributions go to a single agency that then pays the insurance companies a uniform premium. Similarly, Germany has almost no health care provider networks or financial incentives to stay in network. We cannot eliminate preexisting institutional structures to become like the Norwegian or Swiss or German systems overnight—or even over decades. One of the reasons the Clinton health care reform proposal in the early 1990s failed was because it tried to change too much of that preexisting institutional structure in one go. Insurers, some of which were threatened with extinction, fought back. These organizations would do the same today if we tried to adopt foreign health care systems.

Another reason I dislike this ranking system is that I have read many different rankings of health care systems—none of which agree. The granddaddy of rankings is the World Health Organization (WHO)'s *World Health Report 2000*, which ranked the health care systems of 191 countries. France won, followed by Italy, with the United States coming in a distant 37th. Many people still cite this ranking, implying it is the definitive criterion of system success. But there are reasons not to take it seriously. First, it was published nearly 20 years ago and has not been updated. Second, it focused on 5 broad categories of care and weighted them haphazardly. Third, its methodologies have been roundly criticized as favoring certain countries—notably France. But most importantly, it doesn't pass the common-sense test. The idea that the health care systems of Oman or Greece or Portugal or Colombia or Cyprus are all ranked higher than the United States might be believable, but they are all ranked higher than Germany, Canada, Australia, and Denmark as well.

Those results should raise more than a few skeptical eyebrows. Indeed, it led 2 British health economists to wryly observe that there was a "significant relationship between a country's FIFA [soccer] ranking and its ranking by the WHO. Taken at face value, the statistical analysis suggests that, if the national football [soccer] team does well, the WHO score improves." The WHO's authors' use of fancy equations and colored graphs to justify the rankings does not make the results seem more plausible; it only conjures up Mark Twain's comment that "there are three kinds of lies: lies, damned lies, and statistics."

Nevertheless, the WHO report opened the floodgates. Many groups have since gotten into the ranking game. A group of French academics identified 9 different rankings of health care systems. Not surprisingly, the rankings don't agree on what measures matter and which countries are the best. The Health Consumer Powerhouse, which only ranks European countries, concludes that the top 4 are the Netherlands, Switzerland, Denmark, and Norway. Legatum has a wholly different result: (1) Luxembourg, (2) Singapore, (3) Switzerland, (5) Netherlands, (13) Norway, and (23) Denmark. Bloomberg looks only at efficiency and finds the top European country is Italy (3), with France (8) and the UK (10) close behind. All surpass the Scandinavian countries, Germany, and Switzerland—countries with much better reputations for efficiency. Public surveys about the quality of their country's health care system produce yet another set of rankings, with Denmark at the top, followed by Sweden, Canada, and the UK. Switzerland, Germany, and Norway are not in the top 10. Do their systems perform less well? Or are these countries' cultures less conducive to appreciating their own institutions?

Ranking these rankings, as it were—different results with different "top" countries—is head spinning and confusing. It is hard to know which country is the best—or even good. Interestingly, there is only one thing these rankings seem to agree on: the United States does not rank in the top 10 in any of them.

Moreover, none of these rankings seem to answer the question that patients are often really asking: Where can I get the best health care for my condition? There are few rankings of countries by treatment for certain ailments; those rankings that exist are often superficial. For example, the United States is often purported to be the best place for cancer care, but if that care is unaffordable, the high quality is not doing anyone any good. A patient dealing with chronic illness might look at the WHO rankings and think they ought to move to France, but they may not realize that although France finances chronic care well, the delivery is not on par with countries like the Netherlands or even care for chronic illnesses in parts of the United States where new chronic care coordination techniques are being pioneered. Those who need long-term care might think Taiwan is a cheap place to get it, but Germany or the Netherlands would serve them better. Anyone whose children need a lot of health care would do best in Norway, where children's health insurance is basically free. And low-income individuals are well covered by the German system, which requires no cost-sharing for people below a certain income threshold.

So which country has the world's best health care system?

When answering this question at a talk, I would say that no one can know what the real rankings are and that I do not spend much time thinking about other countries' health care systems because they cannot help us reform the dysfunctional American system.

I have repeated these points for years. But the question keeps coming up. Clearly, I have not satisfied my audiences. And after a while, repeating the "path dependence" answer and the problem of the numerous rankings began to feel hollow to me too.

One day I stopped dismissing the question. I realized I was wrong. I was not being curious—just dismissive. So a few years ago I began to seriously consider what we can learn from a comparative study of the health systems of other, high-income countries.

As it turns out, thinking about other health care systems can be extremely valuable—who knew? Even though path dependence prevents the United States from adopting another country's health care system *in toto*, there are *some* lessons to learn by studying these systems. Although the question posed by my audiences may not be the best one, there is a point to seriously pondering what we can learn from other systems, even if we cannot rank or mimic them. There are at least 4 lessons that a comprehensive comparative study of other health care systems can elucidate.

The first lesson is that no health care system is perfect or even performing in the A+ or A range. (There I go with a ranking!) Although other countries may be doing better than the United States (not a high bar), all high-income countries' health care systems face significant challenges. Even the countries that regularly get high scores by the various rankings have serious problems and face difficulties in addressing them. For instance, Germany has an oversupply of hospital beds and a rigid separation of hospital-based physicians and ambulatory care (outpatient) physicians, making care coordination a real challenge. Eliminating hospital beds is extremely difficult, but maintaining them is inefficient, expensive, and exacerbates the country's nursing shortage. In Norway the federal government finances hospital care, while local governments largely finance outpatient care. This means local governments have little incentive to encourage—and may even discourage—less expensive care at home or in outpatient settings. Despite being ranked number 1 by the WHO, France continues to struggle with treating patients with chronic illnesses. As I delineate in this book, other countries face similar challenges. These problems are not the ordinary ones of any large organization serving millions of people—problems of administrative efficiency and bureaucratic coordination—but rather fundamental financial and structural problems, problems that are typically among the most pressing domestic issues facing governments. And confronting them will require painful choices and trade-offs. Consequently, learning from the challenges that confront other health care systems can help us understand the challenges of our own system and help us imagine potential solutions.

A 2nd lesson—and a corollary to the first one—is this: a comparative study of health care systems reveals common problems in high-income countries as well as which ones are particular to one or a few systems. The commonalities suggest that these issues are not unique to the United States' financing and delivery systems but instead arise from several factors, such as the aging of the population. No country has yet figured out a sustainable, efficient way to address mental health care, to completely contain the rising costs of chronic conditions, or to eliminate low-value care.

Conversely, challenges present only in the American system or in just a few systems suggest that they arise from some particular organizational or structural factors. Many other countries have a budget for health care that limits total spending. Neither the United States nor Switzerland does, and they have the highest per capita health care spending, which continues to grow at high rates. The United States' tendency to solve a problem by layering on another system—such as Medicaid for the poor, Children's Health Insurance Program (CHIP) for children, and the exchanges for the uninsured above a certain income—is problematic. The American system is an order of magnitude more complex and difficult for patients to navigate than any other health care system I studied. Yes, all countries struggle with high drug prices, but the United States does not regulate drug prices and is an outlier in drug spending—but not because we are hypochondriacs using a lot of medications. Some other countries have some form of national long-term care insurance. Many countries, including the United States, have been unable to institute this policy and are facing challenges financing long-term care. This distinction between common challenges and unique issues allows us to focus attention more carefully on what might be the source of a particular problem or set of problems.

A 3rd lesson is the realization that there is probably no "best" health care system in the world. This is true of any ranking project. Despite my tendency to rank restaurant meals, there probably is no single-best restaurant. You can tell a good one from a bad one and a great one from a good one. But not the best overall. One restaurant might be more innovative at desserts or at the aesthetics of presentations or at combining different flavors, textures, and temperatures. It may be possible to compare in more focused domains—for example, desserts or wine pairings—but not in overall performance. Similarly, there are various dimensions on which to evaluate health care systems, and systems perform differently on those dimensions. One country's health care system might be outstanding at choice—allowing consumers to use whatever services they desire without a gatekeeper—but might not excel at getting value for money or quality of care. A system that excels at getting value for money spent might not excel at simplicity or innovation. And one that excels at innovation might not provide the highest quality care.

Fundamentally, so much of health care is value driven. Value arguments are often conflated with "better" or "worse" care. For instance, there are multiple ways to provide insurance to an entire population, be it through a single public payer or a comprehensive network of private insurers. Each strategy has strengths and weaknesses, but both *can* be "good"—or "bad."

This means the real question is not "Which country has the world's best health care system?" but rather something closer to "Which country has the health care system that allows the most consumer choice?" or "Which country has the most innovative health care system?" or "Which country best addresses the needs of chronically ill patients?" We need to define the particular dimension we are going to compare countries on.

Indeed, one of the insights I gleaned from this comparative study is that even the US health care system, which does not perform well—let alone the best—on many dimensions, is best in at least one domain: innovation. And I am not speaking only about innovation in drugs or devices or surgical procedures, but also innovation in payment to hospitals and physicians and how to deliver care. In the 1970s and early 1980s the United States pioneered the DRG—Diagnosis Related Group—payment formula for hospitals, and almost all other countries have since adopted, adapted, and revised it. In the last few years Switzerland has become one of the latest countries to do so. Today, the United States is pioneering many new risk-based payment methods, such as bundled payments and capitation with bonuses for quality and reducing total cost of care. As before, other countries are interested in how that innovation is going and considering whether to adopt some of these payment methods. Even a system with many problems can still excel along some dimensions, providing lessons for other countries.

This leads us to the 4th lesson: comparing systems and seeing which ones excel at which dimensions and how they do it can help inform the design of particular reforms in other countries. Countries' health care systems cannot be imported wholesale—what one commentator called "lift and shift"—but understanding how one country solves a problem or fails to solve a problem may inform other countries facing a similar problem. Reforms of particular aspects of another country's health care system can be adapted. US policymakers can learn something from countries that operate health insurance exchanges similar to the American state-based exchanges. We can learn from other countries about how to incentivize the provision of home-based, long-term care. We can learn from other countries about the advantages and disadvantages of the different approaches to regulating drug prices. The United States can learn what makes strong primary care gatekeeper models work effectively and what their limitations are.

THIS BOOK ASSESSES the health systems of the United States and 10 other countries: Australia, Canada, China, France, Germany, the Netherlands, Norway, Switzerland, Taiwan, and the United Kingdom. I chose these countries for several reasons. First, I wanted to study different kinds of financing and delivery systems. The United Kingdom has the traditional socialized health care system in which most financing is public and most of the hospitals and physicians are government owned and operated. Canada and France have state financing but predominantly private delivery systems. Germany has mandatory payroll deductions for health care, but the financing flows through private insurance companies—called sickness funds—that pay privately employed physicians and hospitals. Switzerland has a mandate that all people purchase private health insurance. The major Swiss hospitals are public, but there are many private hospitals, and physicians are private.

Second, I selected countries that many people are familiar with from the American health care debates, adding a few that people may be unfamiliar with so as to enrich future discussions. Canada and Britain are often invoked in debates about health reform. Yet their health systems are both poorly understood and frequently mischaracterized. Including them allows us to clarify their history, financing, and delivery system structures. Conversely, the French, Australian, Taiwanese, and Chinese systems are rarely—if ever—cited in debates about health policy. Few Americans—even health policy experts—know much about their evolution, how they are financed, and their care delivery systems' structure. Although language barriers may explain ignorance of the French, Taiwanese, and Chinese systems, including them allows us to expand the discussion of alternatives and lessons to be learned.

Third, I selected countries that might have plausible claims to being ideal systems—or at least best along some critical dimensions—for the United States to emulate. Since the WHO's 2000 ranking, many people believe France is the best. Many conservative commentators tout the Swiss system. American liberals regularly look at the Scandinavian countries, such as Norway, as offering excellent models that the United States should emulate. People who experience the Taiwanese system often sing its praises. Some leading American health policy experts like the Dutch system because of its emphasis on regulated competition and a strong gatekeeper role for primary care physicians. The Chinese system is notable for high coverage rates in an enormous population. All the while the Canadian system, frequently denounced as "socialized medicine" by conservative commentators, may ironically be the most similar system to American health care abroad.

To compare the various health care systems thoroughly and to determine "the best" along the various dimensions, I have described all systems along the same 8 topics: (1) history, (2) coverage, (3) financing, (4) payment, (5) the delivery of care, (6) prescription drug regulation, (7) human resources, and (8) future challenges. In a later chapter I compare the countries on their performance based on different dimensions organized by these 8 topics, such as most consumer friendly, most choice of providers, innovation, generosity of coverage, and equality of care.

BEFORE I DELVE into the details of each health care system, I will delineate 7 major challenges that are common to every system. These challenges manifest in different ways in each system, and therefore solutions may not be generalizable. But it is useful to consider the commonalities as we proceed through each country.

One common problem facing all high-income countries is cost pressure. Spending just under 18% of GDP on health care makes the United States a very expensive outlier. Nevertheless, all countries face health care cost pressures and anticipate growing crises with their aging populations and the introduction of new technologies. Citizens demand ever more care, yet they strenuously object to higher taxes and premiums to pay for it. Thus, all governments of high-income countries are wrestling with how to satisfy—and perhaps adjust—public expectations and demands while reining in future health care cost growth.

A 2nd and particular manifestation of the cost pressure is the high and rising cost of drugs. Again, the United States is an outlier—with just over 4% of the world's population, we account for about half of the world's drug spending. Other countries regulate drug prices. Nevertheless, all countries find rising drug costs burdensome. These drug cost pressures will escalate with the growing prevalence of chronic illness as well as new specialty drugs and cell and gene therapies with 6- or 7-figure prices. All countries are looking for ways to moderate future drug cost increases.

A 3rd common challenge relates to reducing the inefficiency in the provision of care as well as the unnecessary care in the system. In 2009 the US National Academy of Medicine estimated that the United States wasted over $140 billion on the inefficient delivery of health care services and provided over $200 billion in unnecessary services that, moreover, did not improve patients' health.

These problems of inefficiency and unnecessary care are not unique to the United States. For instance, many policymakers in Germany believe that unnecessary admissions drive the country's high hospitalization rate. In general, the substantial differences between the United States and European countries on cost do not exist exclusively because other countries provide care more efficiently or have lower use of services; quite the contrary: many have greater use of hospitals and drugs. Many experts believe these countries have substantial rates of unnecessary care.

A 4th challenge is the coordination of care for patients with chronic illnesses. Coordination between hospitals and outpatient health care providers is necessary for comprehensive care of patients with chronic illnesses. Yet the long-standing financial, administrative, and other divisions between hospitals and ambulatory care physicians in most countries impede this coordination. Chronic care coordination requires health care providers to be proactive and initiate frequent interactions with patients. Such proactive care systems are not well developed anywhere. The challenge is thus to develop and deploy at scale the right structures that provide coordinated outpatient chronic care for millions.

A 5th and related challenge is the mismatch between health care delivery institutions and the population's chronic health care needs. The existing health care institutions have evolved over the last 100 years largely to respond to infections, trauma, and other acute illnesses. Hospitals have come to dominate all health care systems in high-income countries and consume approximately a quarter to a third of health care spending in almost all countries. Yet today's most serious health problems are those of chronic illness—congestive heart failure, chronic obstructive pulmonary disease, diabetes, asthma, hypertension, stroke, cancer, and inflammatory conditions. Episodic interventions in acute care hospitals do not lead to optimal management of lifelong conditions. All health care systems are trying to modify or shift away from these institutions, but doing so is difficult. Citizens are often enamored of their local hospitals and mightily fight downsizing or closing them. The common challenge in high-income countries is how to match 21st-century health needs for chronic care with anachronistic but well-entrenched, hospital-based models for the delivery of care.

A 6th challenge in every country is the provision of mental health care. For over 100 years mental health had been stigmatized largely because there was no recognized understanding of its biological basis. One consequence was the segregation of mental health care services from somatic care ones: they had different hospitals, different medical records, and different financing mechanisms. This may have been useful once, but not in the 21st century.

We now understand that mental health conditions are widespread and costly, even if they are less visible than physical ones. In the United States mental health care is the 4th most expensive health care service area. A large proportion of patients with chronic conditions also experience comorbid depression, anxiety, and other mental health conditions that dramatically increase their use of all health care services. Integrating mental health care into somatic care is another challenge facing every country, although it is not always fully appreciated even by policymakers.

Finally, all countries face the challenge of how to provide long-term care and how to pay for it. In every country hundreds of thousands—if not millions—of older people are living longer and require custodial care in addition to medical care. Institutional care in nursing homes is extremely expensive on a per-person basis. However, many older people do not have family to provide appropriate personal care. A few countries, such as Germany and the Netherlands, have instituted universal long-term care insurance. While universal long-term care insurance provides a financing mechanism, it does not necessarily make the costs manageable or create an effective delivery infrastructure.

These 7 challenges are common to all high-income countries. Importantly, they will become more intense and pressing because of 2 inevitable mega-trends: the aging population and the development of expensive health care technologies. These changes will increase (1) the number of people with (multiple) chronic conditions, (2) the need for more chronic care coordination, and (3) the demand for long-term care. This in turn will increase use of drugs and medical services. And all of this will intensify cost and access pressures.

THIS EFFORT TO compare different health care systems is not the first such attempt. In addition to the various rankings, there are books and academic articles. In 2009 T. R. Reid, a renowned *Washington Post* correspondent and *Frontline* TV reporter, published *The Healing of America: A Global Quest for Better, Cheaper, and Fairer Health Care*. It was a lighthearted exploration of 10 different systems for treatment of his bum shoulder. It is a fun and accessible read, but the subjective comparisons are not systematic. Plus, by looking at the problem through the lens of one medical condition, it ignores many key elements of health care systems, such as drug coverage, mental health care, care for chronic illnesses, and long-term care.

The European Observatory on Health Systems and Policies produces a more rigorous series, *Health Systems in Transition* (HiT). These are comprehensive books—upward of 150 pages each—that exhaustively outline the technical aspects of many countries' health systems. They are written from the viewpoint of the particular country's domestic policy experts and are directed toward other academics and policymakers. They are excellent as references, but they are not comparative. The reader must draw comparisons after reading thousands of pages about several countries. In addition, they are published episodically over years, so they may not address recent changes. They are thus of little interest to health care workers, citizens, students, policymakers, or journalists who want to understand multiple different systems efficiently—and accessibly.

The Commonwealth Fund publishes excellent profiles of many countries written by experts from each country using a question-and-answer format. Unlike the *Health Systems in Transition* (HiT) series, they are manageable in length and updated periodically. There are obvious areas of overlap with this book—both use a standard framework for each country that includes analyses of coverage, financing, and the delivery of care. Yet there are several important differences between the Commonwealth Fund's country profiles and ours.

First, because of the importance of path dependence, this book stresses the different systems' histories. Current structures and arrangements result from the past policy decisions that, in turn, reflect each country's politics and culture. Considering history challenges us to think harder about how we might adopt another country's practices.

Second, there are important differences in emphasis. For example, the Commonwealth Fund profiles have a substantial focus on electronic health records (EHRs); this book does not. Instead, because of the importance of global drug costs, this book has a much greater focus on drug price regulation. In addition, *Which Country Has the World's Best Health Care?* is written by a team of outsiders that visited the countries, not insiders. My team did not assume cultural knowledge that a nonresident would lack. I hope the descriptions of each country are accessible to readers unfamiliar with a particular country's system.

Finally, there is a difference in how I assess the countries. The Commonwealth Fund compares countries on quantitative measures, frequently from the Organisation for Economic Co-operation and Development (OECD), and on surveys of citizens asking, for instance, about experiencing a medical, medication, or lab error or gaps in hospital discharge planning. These are important. But I chose to take a qualitative tack.

Quantitative assessments are today's ascendant way of thinking. Experts often repeat the phrase, "if you can't measure it, you can't manage or improve it." This perspective is often attributed to the guru of quality improvement, W. Edwards Deming. After World War II he helped revive Japanese industry by introducing statistical process control in manufacturing, uniform product quality, the removal of waste in production, and especially the Plan-Do-Study-Act cycle. Deming rejected the myopia behind the attempt to measure everything. While he was an engineer, statistician, and management consultant, he argued that those things that are measured are managed. However, he emphasized that this is different from believing that if you cannot measure it, you cannot manage it. He recognized that the philosophy of "if you can't measure it, you can't manage it" is a costly myth—and a wrong one too. Trying to run a business based only on numbers was, he believed, one of the 7 deadly sins of management. For some important things we don't have data. Some important metrics cannot be measured, like judgment and corporate culture. According to Deming, we still need to manage and improve those things we cannot measure.

I have also learned that quantitative measures often entail qualitative judgments. What might seem to be similarly titled categories are different, rendering cross-country comparisons less accurate and useful. For example, there is no international standard on where to differentiate social and health services, so comparing spending on long-term care is rarely apples to apples. Some countries, like the Netherlands, consider elderly custodial care delivered at home or in residential homes to be part of health care spending. Others, like Australia, classify most long-term care as a social welfare service. Both countries pay for long-term care through government-run programs, but only one counts that money as a health care expenditure.

Drug spending is also difficult to compare. In some countries the drug spending reported is that in retail pharmacies, while others include all drug spending both in retail pharmacies and in hospitals, physician offices, and other settings. In addition, what drugs are sold and measured in the retail pharmacy category in some countries might be counted in hospital drug costs in others. For instance, Humira, the world's best-selling drug, is categorized in the Netherlands in hospital spending, but in other countries it is placed in retail pharmacy spending. This makes international comparisons on "retail drug spending" indirect as well as inaccurate.

Furthermore, the complicated payment systems for drugs in all countries—including consumer rebates, secret price negotiations, and dozens of other innovations—make getting accurate, comparative data on drug costs nearly impossible. Total invoice level (i.e., manufacturer revenue) pharmaceutical spending rarely matches the sum of government-reported retail and nonretail drug spending. Prescriptions and other measures of utilization vary across countries, and over-the-counter medicines and drugs not covered by insurance are often not counted. In an effort to get clarity, I reached out to IQVIA—the leading industry consultancy that produces detailed drug spending reports for the United States and other countries. They provided generous, detailed data on drug spending and costs, but their data didn't match canonical OECD or government figures. Their staff were very clear: the numbers had to be taken with heaping grains of salt.

Similarly, in some countries, such as Norway, specialists are paid through hospitals and budgeted accordingly. In many other countries, though, specialists run their own offices and are classed under physician and ambulatory care services. There is no one right way to quantify these kinds of activities. But emphasizing quantitative comparisons across different countries that ultimately measure different things can be more deceptive than illuminating.

As I assessed countries, I realized that most of the important dimensions may not have comparable data between countries or may not necessarily be amenable to quantification. For instance, one important dimension is patient choice of providers. This seems more amenable to a qualitative assessment. The case is similar with innovating care delivery and with having a thorough, transparent process for determining drug prices. Hence, I have opted not for a score or number but for qualitative assessments along 19 different qualitative dimensions organized into 8 topics. In chapter 12 I will discuss the "winners" on these qualitative dimensions. One implication is that different countries excel at different dimensions.

THIS BOOK BEGAN as a way to answer questions posed by American audiences and find insights for reforming the American health care system. Along the way, though, I learned that these lessons are not just relevant for the United States; they can also help policymakers imagine different ways to improve their individual country's health care system. All countries are experiencing problems—and searching for solutions. A book outlining the way other countries organize health care can help non-American policymakers address challenges.

As Dr. Stephan Hofmeister, one of the physician heads of the German National Association of Statutory Health Insurance Physicians (Kassenärztliche Bundesvereinigung [KBV]), which is the equivalent of the American Medical Association (AMA), noted,

> [Comparing] health care systems throughout the world is very important to our daily work. Politicians around the world tend to compare their respective systems with those in other countries. Most of the time these comparisons seem to be apples-to-pears that ignore substantial differences in basic structures of those countries. In order to avoid short sighted policies with potential for long-term backlash on the functioning of the health care system, we have increased our efforts to exchange knowledge with health care experts in other countries to help implement truly sustainable reforms.

I learned that many citizens and policy leaders have no holistic understanding of their own health care system. *World's Best Health Care* should also serve as a resource for citizens and people who work in health care. It will educate them about how their own country's system works and how it compares on specific dimensions to other countries.

This was most clearly demonstrated in Norway. No one—including many of the country's leading health policy experts—could offer a succinct history of the system, how it came into being, and the key pieces of legislation that helped it evolve into its current structure. They could not even offer an article that summarized the history. Many noted that a brief summary of the country's system would be an invaluable resource for Norwegian medical, nursing, public health, and health administration students. Educators knew that few students or practitioners would read the 160-page book, *Norway, Health System Review*, produced by the European Observatory, but they might read a 15-page summary of the system, especially if it compared Norway to other countries.

A 3rd audience for this book is health policy–focused journalists and politicians. They often have little knowledge of health care before they are assigned a beat or committee seat in a legislative chamber. When they compare their own health care system to another country's, they often have little knowledge of the structure of the other country's financing or delivery system. The summaries in this book can provide a good comparative reference for them to quickly learn about the complexities of health care and potential ways of addressing current challenges.

The book can also help patients who might be thinking about getting treatments abroad—the medical tourists—when selecting different countries.

I HOPE THIS BOOK satisfies my audiences' curiosity—a curiosity I learned to embrace. I hope it helps students in health care fields and practitioners understand their work's international context. I also hope it can help policymakers in the United States and other countries as they confront the difficult choices about how to reform their own health systems. Maybe they can learn how to adapt some of the good policies found in other countries and avoid repeating others' mistakes.

CHAPTER ONE

UNITED STATES

Mrs. Wilkes gave birth to a bouncing 10-pound baby at full term. When his circumcision would not stop bleeding, a hematologist was called and diagnosed the healthy-looking baby boy with hemophilia. He was transferred to the neonatal intensive care unit (NICU) and infused with clotting factor. After a day of observation the baby was discharged.

Despite having health insurance, Mrs. Wilkes was billed $50,000 for the one night in the NICU—not including the hematologist who came and generously infused the clotting factor at no charge for both her time and the drug.

Ironically, Mrs. Wilkes made sure both her OB-GYN and the hospital were in network. But to her surprise, the hospital had subcontracted out the NICU to a 3rd party that refused to sign a contract with the insurer and, thus, was out of network—and able to charge whatever it wanted directly to the patient.

A dedicated and generous hematologist. Quick access to clotting factor. A system of in-network and out-of-network coverage that is impossible to navigate. Hidden and outrageously high prices for hospital care. Exorbitant patient out-of-pocket costs. In a few days, Mrs. Wilkes experienced many—though not all—of the evils of American health care . . . and this is with "good insurance."

HISTORY

In 19th-century America, hospitals and physicians were not highly regarded.

Benjamin Rush, the father of psychiatry and signer of the Declaration of Independence, called hospitals the "sinks of human life." Physicians were called snake oil salesmen. Change ensued at the end of the 19th century when scientific advances began making medical care safe and effective. Ether and subsequent anesthetics, initially demonstrated in 1846, allowed for painless, longer, and more careful surgeries. Germ theory, bacterial staining, and aseptic techniques reduced hospital-acquired infections, making surgery, recovery, and hospital stays safer. X-rays allowed for more accurate diagnoses. Consequently, middle-class Americans stopped fearing hospitals and began using them in larger numbers in the early 20th century.

In 1910, the Flexner Report on medical education led to the closure of many proprietary medical schools, replaced by university-affiliated medical schools modeled on those at Johns Hopkins, Case Western Reserve, and the University of Michigan. Instructors were no longer community practitioners earning side money but now full-time academic professors. The Report also ushered in a new curriculum composed of 2 years of preclinical scientific training and 2 years of clinical rotations in hospital wards. These changes drastically improved physicians' quality and social standing, though the changes decreased the number of students from lower-income and rural communities.

Employers made the earliest attempts to provide health care or insurance in America. Many of these early plans consisted of employers hiring company doctors to care for rural workers, such as lumberjacks, who could not otherwise access medical services. In some cities unions created sickness funds to provide health benefits for their members. Physicians in rural locations also experimented with prepaid group practices.

But none of these efforts led to widespread health insurance coverage. This changed in 1929 in Dallas, Texas. Because of the Great Depression, hospital occupancy rates declined. To increase bed occupancy, Baylor University Hospital made a deal with Dallas schoolteachers. Baylor offered up to 21 days of hospital care per year for an annual premium of $6 per teacher. This arrangement succeeded and spread to other locales. It also evolved. Contracts were not with just one hospital but rather gave potential patients free choice among any hospital in a city. This nascent health insurance arrangement was further cata-lyzed because states permitted such plans to be tax-exempt charitable organizations, allowing them to circumvent many of the traditional in-surance regulations, particularly the need to have substantial financial reserves. These hospital-focused plans adopted the Blue Cross symbol.

For a long time physicians were hostile to health insurance for phy-sician services, worrying that insurance companies would threaten their clinical autonomy. Simultaneously, they worried that Blue Cross plans might begin to include hospital-based physicians in their in-surance, taking business away from those in private practice. Ulti-mately, resistance to health insurance for physician services eroded because of the need to preempt Blue Cross plans and the persistent financial stress of the Great Depression. In 1939, the California Med-ical Association created an insurance product covering physician of-fice visits, house calls, and physicians' in-hospital services. Physicians controlled the insurance company, and it enshrined a patient's right to choose their physician. The patient was to pay the physician and get reimbursed by the insurance company without any financial in-termediary. This physician-focused model spread, and it often called upon state Blue Cross plans for management assistance and expertise. These physician-focused insurance companies became known as Blue Shield. Eventually the Blue Cross and Blue Shield plans merged. They were state-based because health insurance was regulated in the United States at the state level. They embodied key values: they were not for profit and sold community-rated policies that charged all people the same premium (regardless of health status) to cover as many people as possible at affordable rates.

In 1943, the first bill to create a national social insurance model for health coverage was introduced to Congress. After his unexpected victory in 1948, President Harry S. Truman also pushed for enacting government-provided universal health insurance. Primarily because of AMA opposition and worries about socialism at the start of the Cold War, the House and Senate did not vote on his proposal.

In the 1940s and 1950s, the US government enacted policies that accelerated the spread of employer-focused health insurance. First, in 1943 the US government enacted wage and price controls but exempted health insurance, allowing employers to provide coverage valued up to 5% of workers' wages without violating the wage controls. Then in 1954, to encourage the further dissemination of employer-sponsored insurance, Congress enacted the tax exclusion, excluding an employer's contribution toward health insurance premiums from an employee's income and payroll taxes. This made a nontaxed dollar in health insurance more valuable than a taxed dollar in cash wages.

In 2019, this tax exemption amounted to nearly $300 billion per year and remains the largest single tax exemption in the United States. This spurred employers to cover more workers with richer health insurance offerings. Also, Congress passed the Hill-Burton Act in 1946, which provided federal funds to community hospitals for constructing and expanding facilities. It is estimated that through the 1970s the federal government paid one-third the cost of the country's hospital construction and expansion.

Something became obvious in the 1950s, though: an employer-based system excluded retired, self-employed, and unemployed Americans from health insurance. In 1957, the first bill to provide coverage to seniors—Medicare—was introduced. But it took until 1964 and Lyndon Johnson's landslide election victory for Medicare, government payment of care for the elderly, and Medicaid, government payment for some of the poor, to finally be enacted. The federal government's generous payments to hospitals under Medicare further facilitated hospital expansion.

There were additional efforts to improve the US health insurance system—most notably in the early 1970s under President Nixon and in the early 1990s under President Clinton. Neither succeeded.

However, during these decades the health care system became increasingly costly and complex, with the addition of many new technologies and services, ranging from MRI scanners, new drugs, and laparoscopic surgical procedures to hospice, home care, and skilled nursing facilities. After adjusting for inflation, the annual cost of health care increased from $1,832 per capita in 1970 to $11,172 per capita in 2018.

Finally, in March 2010, President Obama and the congressional Democrats passed the Affordable Care Act (ACA), achieving what had eluded politicians for decades: a structure for universal coverage. Rather than enacting a social insurance model, the ACA expanded

Medicaid to cover lower-income individuals and established insurance exchanges with an individual and employer mandate as well as income-linked subsidies for Americans earning up to $100,000. It also instituted policies to change payment structures and to achieve significant cost savings. This basic structure has remained in place despite the repeal of the individual mandate under President Trump.

COVERAGE

The American health care system is a patchwork of different insurance arrangements that is very confusing to navigate. The system has 4 main components and myriad smaller programs to provide health insurance to 290 million citizens, leaving approximately 28 to 30 million Americans without coverage.

The largest part of the system is employer-sponsored insurance. Employers either buy insurance for their employees and their families or are self-insured and have an insurance company, such as United-Health or a state Blue Cross Blue Shield plan, paying claims and administering the plan. In 2017, employer-sponsored insurance covered about half of all Americans.

Second, Medicare covers all Americans aged 65 and older as well as permanently disabled Americans under 65. Medicare is composed of 4 programs covering different overlapping groups of people.

The original—what is called traditional Medicare—is Part A (hospital care) and Part B (physician and other ambulatory care services). The federal government's Centers for Medicare and Medicaid Services (CMS) administers it. Elderly Americans and those who are disabled and have contributed taxes to Medicare (or are a relative of someone who has) get Part A, but people need to sign up and pay a premium to receive Part B benefits.

Enacted in 1997, Part C—or Medicare Advantage—allows Medicare beneficiaries to select a private insurer or a health care plan associated with a delivery system for health insurance rather than traditional Medicare (Parts A and B). In 2003, Part D, Medicare's drug benefit program, was passed. Private pharmacy insurance plans administer

Figure 1. Health Care Coverage* (United States)

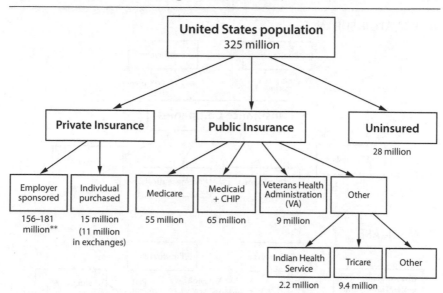

*Some individuals have more than one type of insurance. For instance, some veterans have VA health care and Medicare, and some elderly are "dual eligible" being poor and eligible for both Medicare and Medicaid.

**Data varies depending upon method of study.

it. Medicare beneficiaries must pay a modest premium if they want the drug coverage. In 2017, Medicare covered about 18% of the population—58 million Americans, composed of about 49 million elderly and nearly 9 million disabled. About 20 million (34%) have Part C, and 43 million (76%) have Part D.

Third, Medicaid provides coverage to lower-income Americans as well as the blind and disabled. The original Medicaid program was limited to the "deserving poor"—specifically, poor children, pregnant women, poor elderly, and the disabled. Each state administers traditional Medicaid, and they determine the qualifying level of income for coverage; sometimes it is as low as 25% of the poverty line for able-bodied adults.

Traditional Medicaid exists in the 14 states that have not expanded Medicaid. However, for states that expanded Medicaid under the ACA, eligibility changed. It is no longer limited to the deserving poor with

Figure 2. Financing Health Care (United States)

A. PRIVATE INSURANCE

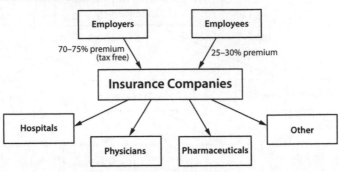

B. MEDICARE

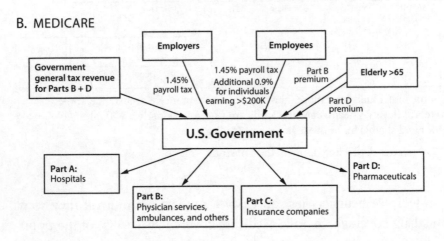

C. MEDICAID AND CHIP

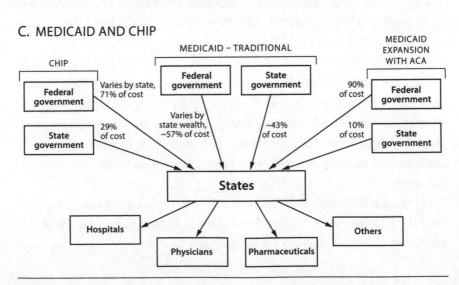

state-determined income thresholds. Instead, all people with incomes under 138% of the federal poverty line ($16,643 for an individual and $33,948 for a family of 4 in 2017) can receive Medicaid.

Another layer of the American health care system, the Children's Health Insurance Program (CHIP), provides health coverage for children whose parents earn too much to qualify for Medicaid but whose private health insurance does not allow them to get the children insured. In 2017, Medicaid and CHIP together covered just over 19% of the population (62 million people); of that, about 9 million were children in the CHIP program. Notably, Americans who qualify for both Medicare and Medicaid—as old and poor—receive additional payments and are referred to as "dual eligible."

Fourth, individuals under 65 who otherwise do not have employer-sponsored insurance or earn too much for Medicaid buy their own health insurance. They can purchase insurance from insurance companies either through the insurance exchanges the ACA created or directly through insurance companies. If Americans purchase through the exchanges, they are eligible for income-linked subsidies to offset premium costs. Overall, about 7% of the population (22 million people) buy their own insurance, with about 11 million buying on the insurance exchanges and with over 8 million receiving subsidies.

Finally, there are myriad special insurance programs for special groups that cover other Americans. There is the Indian Health Service (IHS) for Native Americans, Department of Veterans Affairs (VA) health care, Tricare for the military, and other programs.

A SIGNIFICANT PORTION of the population moves between insurance programs each year and, thus, might have multiple types of insurance during any given year. Experts call this "churn." For instance, it is common for someone to be unemployed and have Medicaid, then to find a job with employer-sponsored insurance. Similarly, older veterans may have veterans' health coverage and Medicare simultaneously. One measure of this churn is that between one-quarter and one-third of the people who get insurance through the exchanges set up by the ACA are new each year.

There is yet another layer of complexity for health insurance. The ACA required dental and vision care be provided to children under the age of 19. However, for adults, dental and vision care are not part of traditional health insurance and need to be purchased separately with additional premiums. Employers often offer dental and vision insurance. Medicare does not cover dental care, although some of the Medicare Advantage plans cover it. In Medicaid dental care is covered for children, but coverage for adults varies between states. Preventive care, such as cleanings, has no deductibles and co-pays, while for more expensive treatments, such as crowns, insurance may cover only 50% of the cost.

About 10% of the population, or about 28 to 30 million Americans, lacked health insurance in 2017. The highest percentage of people without health insurance are those between the ages of 20 and 40. Overall, about 75 million Americans lack dental coverage altogether, and about 63 million lack any type of vision insurance.

FINANCING

In 2017, the United States spent 17.9% of its GDP—about $3.5 trillion—on health care, accounting for nearly $11,000 per person. Overall, 45.2% of health care is publicly financed. Private business paid for 19.9% of total health spending; the federal government, 28.3%; state and local governments, 16.9%; individuals, 28.1%; and other private sources, 6.7%.

Employer-Sponsored Insurance

Employers arrange for—or, in technical terms, "sponsor"—health insurance for their employees. In 2018, employer-sponsored health insurance cost $6,690 per individual and $18,764 for a family. On average, employees pay out of pocket 18% of the premium for individual plans and 31% for family plans. But the extent of services covered by insurance and the amount employees pay for in premiums vary significantly among employers. On average, the insurance provided by smaller employers is less generous and is accompanied by higher employee payments. In addition, there are out-of-pocket costs for deductibles, co-payments, and uncovered services.

Both economic theory and empirical data indicate that the employer contributions are, to some extent, taken from wages—that is, if the employer did not offer health insurance, the amount the employer contributes would, over time, go back into employees' cash wages. Finally, employees pay no taxes on the employer's contribution to their premiums; this is called the health insurance tax exclusion.

Medicare

The federal government finances and administers Medicare. But each of the 4 parts is financed differently.

Part A for hospital costs is financed by a mandatory payroll tax of 1.45% of employee wages paid for by employers, plus 1.45% paid for by employees. For well-off individuals and families there is a Medicare surtax, an additional 0.9% for earnings over $125,000 for individuals or over $250,000 for couples. All workers pay this tax, including those under age 65, those with other forms of insurance coverage, and those not eligible for the program.

Part B for physician services is financed by income-linked premiums assessed on individuals who elect coverage (covering around 25% of costs) and general federal revenue (covering the remaining 75%). For most elderly who earn under $85,000, the premium in 2018 was about $130 per month.

Part C—Medicare Advantage—is financed by the federal government and flows through private health plans. The private insurance companies can charge enrollees additional premiums, but they can also offer additional services such as dental care.

Part D, the drug benefit, is financed similarly to Part B, with only those who elect coverage paying premiums.

Medicaid

The federal and state governments jointly finance and administer Medicaid. The federal government pays states a fixed percentage of total costs, known as the Federal Medicaid Assistance Percentage (FMAP), for traditional Medicaid; the money comes from general revenues. On average for the traditional Medicaid part, the federal government pays 57%, but how much it pays each state depends on that state's economic status. For example, Mississippi, the poorest state, receives 76%, while the richest 14 states receive only 50% of the costs. The percentage the federal government pays differs for the ACA expansion. For states that expanded Medicaid, the federal government now pays 90% of the cost for newly insured people. Similarly, the federal government pays over 90% of the cost of CHIP; states pay the remainder. In many states Medicaid is the single largest part of the state budget, ahead of even primary and secondary education.

Individual Insurance Plans

Individuals who are either self-employed or whose employer does not offer insurance and who earn too much for Medicaid can purchase health insurance on their own. They can do so either through the ACA's insurance exchanges or directly from an insurance company. They pay for these insurance policies out of pocket. If they earn between 100% and 400% of the federal poverty line (between $24,600 and $98,400 for a family of 4 in 2017) and purchase in the insurance exchanges, they can receive income-linked subsidies for their premium payment. The subsidies come from general federal tax revenue. However, individuals get no preferred tax treatment for their purchase of health insurance. About 8 million people buying insurance on the exchanges receive subsidies.

For lower-income individuals and families who purchase insurance on the exchanges—those earning less than 250% of the poverty line ($61,500 for a family of 4 in 2017)—the federal government used to offer cost-sharing subsidies to insurance companies to cover deductibles and co-pays. Although President Trump suspended payment of these cost-sharing subsidies, insurers nonetheless still need to provide them. To compensate for this added cost, insurers have increased the premiums on the exchanges.

Overall, in 2017 individual purchase of insurance constituted approximately $90 billion, and the federal government subsidized $34 billion.

Cost Control

Health care costs in the United States have increased substantially from $1.86 trillion in 2000 (in 2017 dollars) to $3.5 trillion in 2017—or roughly from $6,580 per capita in 2000 to $10,700 in 2017. There have been many cost-control initiatives. One of the more promising initiatives began in 2012 when Massachusetts established the Health Policy Commission to define a limit on health care cost growth based on growth in the state's GDP and aging of the population. Despite being mostly voluntary and lacking legal enforcement powers—mainly the power to shame institutions contributing to high cost growth—this approach has been somewhat successful. Massachusetts has had below-average health care cost growth for 7 years; it even reduced private health care spending. Several other states have adopted this cost-control approach as well.

Long-Term Care

Long-term care in the United States is both in high demand and very expensive. It is estimated that in the coming decades about one-half to two-thirds of elderly Americans will need some form of long-term care. But the median annual cost of a private room in a nursing home is over $90,000, the cost for an assisted-living facility is over $45,000 per year, and for a home health assistant is about $50,000 per year.

Yet there is no comprehensive long-term care insurance program in the United States. The ACA had a provision for voluntary long-term care insurance—the Community Living Assistance Services and Supports Act (CLASS Act) of 2010. Because it was voluntary, though, it was deemed fiscally unsustainable and was repealed.

Existing long-term care arrangements are largely funded in 3 ways. One is through voluntary insurance usually purchased as a fringe benefit through employers or other groups. Surprisingly, sales of these plans are declining sharply just when the need is increasing. Only 12 insurers exist, and only about 0.5% of employers offer such long-term insurance. Typically employees must pay the full amount of the insurance; as a result, fewer than 10% of employees offered long-term insurance buy it and few Americans have such insurance.

The 2nd main funding mechanism for long-term care is through Medicaid, the federal-state program to provide health care coverage for lower-income Americans. Medicare pays for only 100 days of skilled nursing care per illness. This care must be triggered by a 3-day hospitalization and be related to the illness that caused the hospitalization. Medicare does not pay for custodial care. Conversely, Medicaid helps lower-income individuals pay for long-term care. This care includes both nursing homes and custodial services to help people stay in their own homes, such as bathing, feeding, and housecleaning. Overall Medicaid pays $72 billion for long-term care, including $55 billion for nursing homes. This covers 62% of nursing home residents and 50% of all long-term care costs in the United States.

PAYMENT

Payments to Hospitals
Hospital payments in the United States consume over $1.1 trillion, or about 33% of total national health care spending.

Hospital payment in the United States is complex. Since the early 1980s hospitals have been paid largely—but not exclusively—based on Diagnosis Related Groups (DRGs). Importantly, the monetary value of a DRG is not uniform among all the different private insurers and government payers.

DRGs are fixed, prospective payments designed to reflect the resources used to treat a typical patient with a specific condition. There is a base case DRG—a hypothetical single condition. This DRG incorporates operating and capital expenses and is adjusted based on regional variations in labor costs. It is then modified by a weighting factor to reflect the patient's specific clinical condition. This basic component is then further modified to incorporate the patient's other health problems or secondary diagnoses, whether there were complications during hospitalization, and several other adjustments (discussed below). This current system is now called the Medicare Severity Diagnosis Related Groups System (MS-DRG). There are over 750 MS-DRGs, ranging from pancreas transplants to pleural effusions without major complications.

Importantly, the DRG is supposed to cover all the direct hospital costs associated with a diagnosis. It excludes physician services provided in the hospital, such as radiologists reading images or anesthesiologists administering anesthesia. These physician services are billed separately. It also excludes payments for outpatient care, even if it is incurred at the hospital.

Figure 3. Payment to Hospitals (United States)

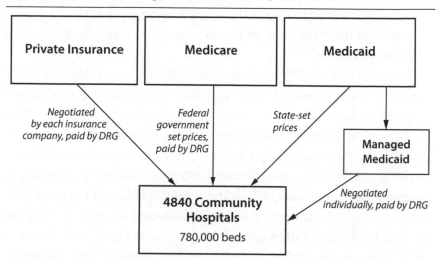

DRGs provide a classification of services and goods for payment. But the amount hospitals are actually paid varies depending on who is paying. Typically, private insurers pay the highest rates, Medicare rates are in the middle, and Medicaid has the lowest payment rates.

The absolute highest DRG rate is called the *charge master rate*. This is a rate made up by American hospitals, a kind of "retail" price. Typically, it is exorbitant. No one except foreign nationals who come to the United States for care, the uninsured, or patients whose insurance has no contract with the hospital pay this rate. Medicare is a price setter and sets a rate for each DRG: the federal government establishes the price it will pay, and hospitals must take that rate or opt out of the programs entirely—there are no negotiations, although there is lobbying of Congress to get rates adjusted. Medicare adjusts the base DRG rate in 3 ways. First, there are various special payments for rural and other hospitals. Second, the federal government makes Disproportionate Share Hospital (DSH, pronounced "dish") payments to hospitals to partially pay for the uncompensated care the hospitals provide. Finally, hospitals that train residents receive direct graduate medical education (GME) payments to pay for the residents' salaries and the physician teachers. They also receive indirect medical education (IME) payments to pay patient costs associated with teaching—namely, the additional resources residents are assumed to use in caring for patients.

Medicaid payments are set by states and are typically lower than Medicare payments.

The situation is different for private insurance. While Medicare is a price setter, private insurers negotiate their rates with individual hospitals or hospital systems. The rates are typically multiples of the Medicare rate. To really complicate matters, each insurer has a different DRG rate with each hospital. For instance, a hospital might receive 1.8 times the Medicare rate for cardiac bypass surgery from a health insurance company. But the hospital can have different rates with different private insurers, so another *private* insurer might pay 2.2 times the Medicare rate for the same cardiac bypass surgery *at the same hospital*. These commercial rates depend on hospitals' relative bargaining power with the insurers as well as the number of patients each insurer typically sends to the hospital. On average it is estimated that in 2017 private insurers paid hospitals about 2.4 times the Medicare rate for DRGs.

There is an exception to this complexity in hospital payment: Maryland. In the 1970s Maryland adopted an all-payer rate setting that is used in other countries such as France, Germany, and the Netherlands. An independent state commission defines *one* price for hospitals regardless of whether Medicare, Medicaid, or private insurers are paying the hospital. The result has been below-average hospital cost increases. In 2014, Maryland adopted another payment change to limit increases in per capita hospital spending to historical averages (3.58%) or 0.5% below national increases—whichever is lower.

Payments to Ambulatory or Office-Based Physicians

Overall, physician services accounted for about 20% of total health care spending in 2017—just under $700 billion.

American physicians are largely paid on a fee-for-service basis, but an increasing amount of payments are shifting to what is called alternative payment models (APMs) such as capitation, bundled payments, and global budgets. Fee-for-service uses the relative value unit (RVU) system that Medicare introduced in the late 1980s. RVUs are supposed to create a common metric to compare the human and other resources

Figure 4. Payment to Physicians (United States)

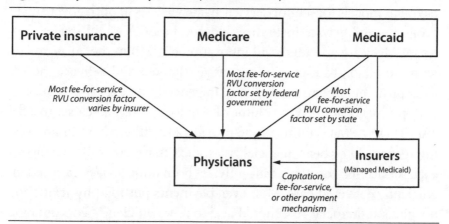

needed to provide a specific physician service. They are composed of 3 components: (1) physician work, based on time, skill, and intensity; (2) practice expenses, including nonphysician labor, building costs, and supplies; and (3) malpractice premiums. These 3 components are adjusted to reflect geographic variation in the cost of living so as to arrive at a total RVU for each medical service specified by a CPT code. A CPT code defines a specific medical, service, surgical, or diagnostic procedure that is rendered to a patient and to be reimbursed. On average the physician work accounts for 44% of total RVU value, malpractice 3%, and practice expenses 53%. Then a conversion factor is applied that turns the RVU into a dollar amount to be paid to the doctor.

To understand the RVU system, we can compare a moderate office visit with a laparoscopic gallbladder removal. The office visit has an RVU of 2.18 and the gallbladder removal 18.81—this covers only the physician component, not the hospital payment for the surgical procedure. In 2017, Medicare's conversion factor for one RVU was $35.89. Private insurers usually use higher conversion factors. For one private insurer, an office visit conversion factor pays $55.64 for one RVU, while the conversion for the gallbladder surgery is $76.82 for one RVU. Compared to an office visit, the gallbladder surgery is deemed to involve 8 times more time, skill, and practice expenses, but it is also paid at an almost 40% higher rate for each RVU. In general, physicians' medical work is devalued compared to surgical work.

The ACA spurred significant experimentation with replacement payment models for fee-for-service: namely APMs in both government programs and private insurance. Indeed, the ACA established a Center for Medicare and Medicaid Innovation (CMMI) in the government, with $10 billion to invest in innovative payment and delivery models to improve quality and lower cost. In general, the experimentation is with payments not tied to volume of activity but instead closer to a flat rate. These APMs require all the providers to either share in any savings generated or bear financial risk for excessive costs. By paying for each service, fee-for-service incentivizes both unnecessary care and inefficiently delivered care. Moreover, payments putting physicians and hospitals at financial risk should lead to more efficiency, coordination of care, and delivery of appropriate and higher quality care.

One form of APMs is called *bundled payments*, a single payment that covers all services related to one type of service over a specified period of time. Typically, for surgical and many medical bundled payments, the initiation of the payment occurs with the procedure itself. For a few medical bundled payments, such as those for cancer, the payment is initiated by a specific treatment option, such as the start of chemotherapy. For instance, payment for a hip replacement historically involved separate payments to (1) the hospital for the operating room, (2) the recovery room and hospital bed, and (3) the orthopedic surgeon for the surgery itself. Separate payments were also made to the anesthesiologist, skilled nursing facilities (if used), physical therapist for rehabilitation, and any other services, such as a visit to the emergency room after discharge for post-op issues. Bundled payments combine these separate payments into one fee for all services associated with a hip replacement up to 90 days after the procedure. The bundle is sometimes thought of as a "super DRG." Increasingly, if actual costs for a patient are above the single fee, the physicians and hospitals assume the financial loss. Classic bundles incentivize efficiency and reducing prices of inputs but do not decrease the frequency of use.

In the United States, capitation—in which a physician is paid a fixed fee to care for a patient for a specified period, typically a year—goes back to the early 20th century. The AMA had long opposed it, but it grew rapidly in the 1990s, although it was never a dominant payment method and was typically limited to health maintenance organizations

(HMOs). Recently interest in it has been renewed, with insurers moving primary care physicians to capitation, paying a per-member-per-month (PMPM) fee that can be adjusted for a patient's risk. Accountable Care Organizations (ACOs) are new organizations that are paid similarly to capitation. They care for a population of patients and are responsible for their total cost of care. Most ACOs have been paid under a system that limits their financial risk for overspending but rewards them for some of the savings. There is, however, increasing pressure to require "two-sided risk"—that is, for both savings from a predetermined benchmark of cost and for financial costs if total patient costs exceed that benchmark. In Medicare ACOs must take care of at least 5,000 Medicare patients.

In 2017, about one-third of payments were some kind of APM, but in only 12.5% of payments were providers at downside risk. Although thousands of American hospitals and physicians are now involved in bundled payment, capitation, and ACO payment changes, the level of savings has been limited. In general, bundles have largely focused on procedures and oncology care. When applied to surgical procedures, they seem to generate some cost savings and stable or moderately improved quality of care, but when applied to medical conditions, bundles do not seem to produce savings. Nonetheless, experimentation in alternative payments is expanding because of the strong belief that moving off fee-for-service is necessary in order to sustainably improve the health care system's performance.

Payments for Long-Term Care

Open-ended, private, long-term care plans no longer exist in the United States.

Existing long-term insurance plans help pay for a limited time of services or a specified dollar amount, and they pay a fixed daily fee that the patient—or their family—can use. A typical plan might pay $260 per day for nursing home or assisted-living facilities or $195 per day for home- or community-based care, up to a maximum of $300,000. These plans usually pay once a patient needs help with 2 activities of daily living, such as eating and bathing.

Medicare covers 100% of the initial 20-day stay in a skilled nursing facility. Patients are then responsible for $167 per day for days 21 through 100, with Medicare covering the rest. After 100 days patients cover all the costs of the skilled nursing facility.

Most long-term care is paid for by Medicaid. But to limit access there are restrictive and complex rules. To receive Medicaid payment, patients must meet 2 requirements: they must (1) have low assets and (2) require assistance with personal care such as bathing, dressing, and feeding. Additionally, a person must have no more than $2,000 in assets (excluding a car and a home if its value is below $552,000). In the past, middle-class Americans tried to transfer their assets to their children to qualify for Medicaid's long-term care funding. This loophole has largely been closed because the law requires a "look back" of 5 years to be sure such transfers have not occurred and requires that the elderly person get a fair value in return for any transfer of assets.

Preventive Medicine

Private, ambulatory physicians provide most primary prevention services such as immunizations and cancer-screening tests. Medicare, Medicaid, private insurers, and other payers pay for them. A major change included in the ACA was that preventive services are provided without requiring patients to pay deductibles or co-pays, thus eliminating financial barriers to using these services.

Public health education campaigns are largely the domain of public health agencies at the federal and state levels, such as the CDC.

DELIVERY OF HEALTH CARE SERVICES

Care is delivered largely through private hospitals and physicians. However, there remain some critical public hospitals and public clinics, such as the Federally Qualified Health Clinics (FQHCs). In addition, the VA is a fully socialized medical care system—with the federal government owning hospitals and clinics, employing physicians and other health care personnel, and buying and dispensing drugs and other medical services. The ACA initiated an era of experimentation focused on changing how health care services are delivered so as to improve quality and reduce costs.

Table 1. Historical Trends in Hospitals, Hospital Beds, and Hospital
Admissions, United States, 1980–2017

	1980	2017
Population	227 million	325 million
Community hospitals	5830	4840
Community hospital beds	988,000	780,000
Beds per 1,000 population	4.3	2.4
Hospital admissions	36.1 million	33.4 million
Admissions per 1,000 population	159	103
Length of stay	7.6 days	5.4 days

Hospital Care

In 2017, there were about 4,840 community hospitals in the United States, with approximately 780,000 beds for about 325 million people, yielding 2.4 beds per 1,000 people. About 59% of hospitals are nongovernmental and not for profit; 21% are for profit, and 20% are owned by state and local governments. In 2017, there were about 33.4 million hospital admissions. Trends show that the number of hospitals, hospital beds, hospitalizations, and lengths of stay have substantially declined since 1980, when the US population was 227 million (Table 1).

In the United States there has been growing consolidation in the delivery system. Some has been *horizontal* consolidation, with hospitals buying other hospitals. This leads to increased geographical catchment areas as well as increased bargaining power with private insurers to increase the hospital payment rates. Some has been *vertical* consolidation, with hospitals employing physician groups and owning other aspects of care, such as ambulatory surgical centers and home health care agencies. In 2017, about two-thirds of hospitals were part of a larger health system. Similarly, the percentage of office-based physicians working in practices owned by a hospital has increased from 30% in 2010 to about 50% in 2017.

The impact of such consolidation has been hotly debated. The American Hospital Association claims consolidation decreases costs through scale and efficiencies as well as through a decline in prices for services. However, most independent research shows that consolidation typically leads to higher prices for physician services, drugs, laboratory tests, and other services and also suggests either no improvement or a decline in quality because of a lack of competition.

Once a patient is admitted to the hospital, hospital-based physicians—also called *hospitalists*—often take over their care from the primary care or even specialist physician. These hospitalists' incentives may be different from those of the primary care physician. In particular, they may have a financial incentive to order many tests or to rapidly discharge patients to reduce the hospital length of stay and, thus, costs.

Hospitals in the United States face multiple layers of regulation. There is accreditation by nongovernmental bodies such as the Joint Commission. Accreditation is often required to receive governmental payments through Medicare and Medicaid. Hospitals are also required to report data on quality and are graded accordingly. Similarly, the federal government gave them financial incentives to implement electronic health records and, in return, comply with regulations on the "meaningful use" of the electronic health data. Hospitals complain about excessive regulation and, especially, the costs associated with the need for reporting on their quality.

Increasingly, hospitals are evaluated and reimbursed for their quality. Hospital Compare has been a long-standing project to provide the public with information on hospital performance on quality measures. In 2016, the Overall Hospital Quality "star rating" system was introduced. It ranks hospitals based on 57 quality measures, including patient experience, using 1 to 5 stars (5 stars being the best) to make ratings of hospital quality easily understandable to the public.

As part of the quality measurement, beginning October 2012, the ACA had Medicare penalize hospitals for a high 30-day readmission rate on certain conditions (such as acute myocardial infarction and chronic obstructive pulmonary disease [COPD] exacerbation). The penalty is based on an excessive predicted-to-expected rate of readmission given the patient population. The penalty is capped at 3% of Medicare payments. This has incentivized some important revisions in care, especially having hospitals engage in improving post-hospital discharge arrangements. There has been some debate on whether this increased patient mortality. Most studies suggest a 3% decline in readmissions, with no increase in mortality. Beginning in October 2014 Medicare penalized hospitals that rank in the bottom 25% for high rates of hospital-acquired conditions, such as catheter-associated urinary tract infections, central line–associated infections, surgical site infections, C. difficile infections, falls, and medication errors.

There has been significant experimentation in using home health agencies and visiting nurses to care for patients in their own home instead of admitting them to the hospital. The aim is to avert hospitalization's high costs. One type of experiment is Hospital at Home. Most of these experiments involve patients with conditions such as exacerbation of congestive heart failure or community-acquired pneumonia. The early results suggest equal or improved outcomes: faster recoveries, similar readmission rates, higher patient satisfaction, and lower costs. Similarly, many procedures traditionally performed in a hospital, such as hip and knee replacements, are being done in ambulatory surgical centers with follow-up physical therapy and rehabilitation performed at home. Again, the results suggest equal or improved quality and with lower costs. Many experts expect more care services to shift out of the hospital in the future.

Ambulatory (Outpatient) Care

In the United States there are approximately 850,000 physicians in active patient care. Many others are in administration or research or they work for various health care and non–health care companies but do not care for patients. Primary care physicians have about 2,000 patients in their panel. About 60% of primary care physicians see 20 or fewer patients per day and about 3,500 patients per year. Specialists tend to see about 2,700 patients per year. Only 18% of American physicians remain in solo practice, with about 60% of physicians working in group practices or for hospitals.

There are extensive ambulatory care facilities in the United States: over 6,000 ambulatory surgery centers, with a combined annual revenue of $40 billion, and just over 13,000 ambulatory imaging centers, with an annual revenue of $19 billion. There are just under 12,000 Medicare-certified home health care agencies, and home health care consumes about $100 billion in expenditures. There are about 4,000 freestanding dialysis centers that care for just under 500,000 patients.

Medicare, the predominant payer for dialysis in the United States, spends over $35 billion per year on it.

There is extensive use of networks and selective contracting with physicians. The most restrictive networks involve closed-panel HMOs, like Kaiser Permanente, which pays only for care in the limited number of physicians who are formally part of the HMO or those contracted for highly specialized services, such as bone marrow transplants. These organizations can deploy care pathways for specific conditions, create a distinctive medical culture, and better manage patients. About 16% of privately insured Americans are in HMOs. An increasing number of Medicare and Medicaid patients are in HMOs through Medicare Advantage (Part C) or Medicaid Managed Care plans.

In 2017, about half of privately insured patients got coverage through preferred provider organizations (PPOs). PPOs offer a network of physicians—in-network—in which patient costs are lower because the insurer has negotiated lower reimbursement rates. Patients can still see out-of-network physicians or hospitals, but they have to pay higher deductibles and co-payments. There is a growing trend toward more narrow networks that steer patients only to physicians who are judged to be efficient and low cost. This restricts physicians' referral patterns but is attractive because it seems to lower costs and may improve quality.

The American delivery system is in the midst of tremendous innovation and experimentation. One major focus is the integration of wireless technologies that allow telemedicine visits as well as continuous patient monitoring. These experiments are early and have yet to yield major successes. Another focus has been on better coordination of care for patients with chronic illness. About 85% of all health care costs are for patients with chronic conditions. Having multiple specialists caring for patients or delivering services during an acute hospital admission is not optimal care for lifelong chronic conditions. Numerous health systems, especially those with financial incentives to control the total cost of care, have pioneered ways to coordinate care for chronically ill patients so as to avert exacerbations of health problems requiring more intensive—and expensive—services. Typically these care coordination arrangements entail embedding chronic care coordinators in primary care or specialty practices. These coordinators are then entrusted with educating patients about disease self-management and proactively reaching out to patients to ensure they are properly monitoring their conditions and taking their medications. They also work to ensure the patients are getting their care in the optimal setting—that is, going to the physician's office instead of an emergency room if a problem arises. If the patients are admitted to hospitals, care coordinators work to quickly discharge them to lower-cost settings such as home with the necessary home care arrangements.

Experimentation with these innovations has revealed that integrating them into care processes is neither simple nor quick. Nevertheless, over the last decade many medical groups in different parts of the country have adopted these innovations successfully and reduced the rate of emergency room use and hospitalization, improved quality, and lowered costs. The big challenge is to scale successful programs that have been developed by individual systems to physician practices throughout the country.

Mental Health Care

Like many other countries, since the 1950s and especially the 1960s the United States has undergone a process of deinstitutionalization for patients with mental illness. Since 1955 the number of inpatient psychiatric beds has declined 97%. Between 2005 and 2010 the number of state psychiatric beds dropped 14%, and since 2010 it dropped another 13% to fewer than 38,000 beds for 325 million people.

Community-based care has not adequately filled the void. There are only 28,000 psychiatrists in the United States. The number is declining, as most are over 55 and beginning to retire. There are about 100,000 psychologists and about 125,000 mental health and substance abuse social workers. Projections show a significant growth in the demand for all types of mental health providers over the next decade. Indeed, the rising opioid and substance abuse problems in the United States has further exacerbated the need for mental health providers. One consequence is that only about half of all adults with serious mental health needs actually receive services. Another consequence is that many patients with mental illnesses now end up in prison; in fact, 21% of prisoners in the United States have one or more mental health diagnoses.

There has been a growing appreciation for the role of depression and anxiety in the management of patients with chronic illnesses, such as diabetes and cancer. Studies have shown that about 25% to 33% of patients with chronic illness or those admitted to a hospital for medical reasons or surgical procedures have comorbid depression and anxiety. Having comorbid mental health conditions substantially increases health care costs, often by 60% to 70%.

New efforts are being made to routinely screen patients for depression and anxiety and rapidly link them to mental health care. Some of the new models of care involve routinely screening patients in the hospital and office setting and embedding mental health providers in primary and specialty care offices to support these patients. In addition, start-up companies are trying to address the demand through linking patients with mental health providers online to improve access and regularly assess patients to track their improvement and the mental health providers' performance.

Long-Term Care
There are about 50 million Americans 65 years and older. Over the next 2 decades this number will grow by 50%.

There is a high demand for long-term care but limited supply. Approximately 1.5 million Americans receive long-term care in nursing homes; this number has been declining. In addition, there are 1 million Americans in assisted-living facilities, and this number has been rising. Another 300,000 elderly Americans receive care in adult day care centers. Others receive care from home health care agencies and hospices. Consequently, the majority of Americans who need assistance with long-term care needs receive care from their family or informal care networks.

Most long-term care providers in the United States, including nursing homes and residential care communities, are for-profit organizations, although there are many religious and community-based facilities that are not for profit. Compared to hospitals, the nursing home industry is loosely regulated. However, like with hospitals, Medicare introduced a Nursing Home Compare website that ranks nursing homes with stars based on staffing ratios and different clinical and physical measures.

Preventive Medicine

Ambulatory physicians provide most individually focused primary preventive activities, such as immunizations and cancer screening. Increasingly, physicians are being evaluated—and sometimes provided bonus payments—based on providing these services. Immunization rates for children have increased. In 2010, 69% of children received all 7 recommended pediatric vaccines by age 3; today it is over 77%. Similarly, since 2010 flu vaccinations have also increased among children, but rates among adults fluctuate. There is a slight decrease among women getting Pap smears and mammograms, but there are significant increases among adults getting colon cancer and other screenings.

PHARMACEUTICAL COVERAGE AND PRICE CONTROLS

Pharmaceutical Market

The United States accounts for by far the largest portion of the nearly $1 trillion worldwide annual pharmaceutical spending. It spends just under $500 billion on drugs per year, constituting approximately 17% of US health care spending. A total of 10% of health care spending is for purchases of drugs in retail pharmacies, and the other 7% is for drugs administered in hospitals, nursing homes, or physicians' offices. This amounts to over $1,400 per capita for prescription drugs, more than twice the per capita spending in most European countries. This high spending for drugs is a result of high drug prices, not high drug use by Americans.

Approximately 90% of all prescriptions written in the United States are for generic drugs, but they account for only 26% of drug costs. This represents a significant increase in the use of generics since Medicare began paying for drugs in 2006; their use is significantly higher in the United States than in almost any other developed countries.

Coverage Determination

In the United States, new drugs are granted patents for 20 years from discovery. Pharmaceutical manufacturers then must demonstrate safety and effectiveness through clinical trials, which takes an average of 8 years. In approving drugs, the FDA is not supposed to consider anticipated drug costs or cost effectiveness. Once a pharmaceutical is proven safe and effective, the FDA grants marketing exclusivity, which extends for 7 years for orphan drugs and 5 years for new chemical entities. A drug approved for adults and then tested on children for its safety and efficacy gets 6 additional months of marketing exclusivity.

Shortly before a drug comes off patent, generic drug manufacturers can submit an abbreviated new drug application to the FDA, requesting to market generic copies of brand-name drugs. These generics must fulfill certain criteria, including showing they have the same active ingredient, the same strength and route of administration, and manufacturing systems that meet the same rigorous standards.

There is no governmental drug coverage policy for the whole country and no national formulary. Both in private insurance and Medicare, pharmacy benefit management companies (PBMs) create formularies and negotiate prices with pharmaceutical companies. PBMs create formularies that include or exclude drugs. Typically payers must pay for an FDA-approved drug except when there are multiple drugs in the same class, such as the multiple statins to lower cholesterol, when they can choose which one to cover, usually based upon the lowest negotiated price. Thus, a specific drug may be covered by one PBM but, if there are competitors, not covered by a different PBM. In Medicare every PBM must cover all drugs for 6 specific conditions: immunosuppressants, antidepressants, antipsychotics, anticonvulsants, HIV/AIDS, and cancer drugs.

Price Regulation

Whereas the US government grants monopolies to pharmaceutical companies through patents and marketing exclusivity, there is no national price regulation for drugs. Pharmaceutical companies set prices for brand-name drugs. PBMs then negotiate based on those prices and typically get price reductions or rebates when there are competitors in the same class or when they include a group of the company's drugs on their formulary. Nevertheless, because PBMs represent fragmented purchasing power compared to national negotiations, their price reductions are limited. On average, generics are about 5% the price of brand-name pharmaceuticals.

Figure 5. Regulation of Pharmaceutical Prices (United States)

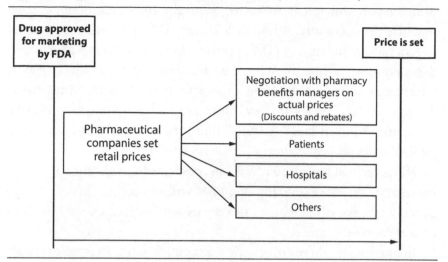

The VA cares for about 9 million military veterans; about 5 million of them use its pharmacy. In 2017, it spent about $7 billion per year on drugs. In 1997, the VA created a national formulary that was made public and—by law—gets a minimum discount of 24% off the average manufacturer's price sold outside the federal government. It can also negotiate even lower prices if possible. Typically, the VA prices are estimated to be about half of what non-federal drug purchasers pay.

Medicaid spends over $35 billion on drugs per year. The price Medicaid pays is complex. Compared to prices paid by private insurance companies, drug manufacturers are legally required to pay state Medicaid programs' rebates for the drug prescribed. The rebate level is determined by either a 23.1% discount from the average manufacturer's price or the best price (i.e., the lowest price paid by any PBM), whichever is lowest.

Regulation of Physician Prescriptions
There are 3 important practices codified in law that govern physician prescriptions.

American physicians can prescribe drugs for the FDA-approved indication, but they can also prescribe drugs for nonapproved indications—so-called off-label use. Sometimes this prescribing is to reduce costs. For instance, Avastin, which the FDA approved for the treatment of metastatic cancers, is also effective in the treatment of age-related macular degeneration, although it is not FDA approved for macular degeneration. Lucentis is FDA approved for the treatment of macular degeneration. Although Avastin and Lucentis are equally effective, Lucentis is considerably more expensive than Avastin. Thus, using Avastin off-label saves money. More typically, physicians prescribe medications for off-label use when there are no other treatments for a patient's condition and they want "to try something."

However, just because a physician prescribes a medication does not mean an insurance company or a PBM will pay for it. This can be especially true for off-label uses of very expensive medications, such as cancer chemotherapies.

In many states there are generic substitution laws. These allow pharmacists to substitute generic drugs for a brand-name drug if a generic exists, is bioequivalent, and of the same dosage if the physician has not marked that the brand-name drug must be dispensed. The main justification of these laws is to save patients money for therapeutically equivalent drugs.

Finally, certain drugs—especially cancer chemotherapies, injectable anti-inflammatory drugs, and others—are not sold through pharmacies. Instead, physicians purchase them, administer them in the clinic or office, and are paid by insurance companies. This is called the *buy-and-bill* system. Since 2003, Medicare has paid based on the average wholesale price of the drug plus 6% for an administrative fee. This payment formula incentivizes the use of more expensive drugs when there are clinically equivalent options because the 6% fee is higher on expensive drugs. Research indicates that physicians respond to this incentive and use more expensive drugs to generate higher payments. There have been multiple attempts to change this buy-and-bill system, but it remains in place.

Prices Paid by Patients

Patients with private insurance and Medicare have tiered co-payments. A typical tiered structure has 4 or 5 tiers, with co-payments rising as drugs become more expensive (Table 2). What drugs are in each tier depends on the insurer or PBM and what drugs they have negotiated

Table 2. Typical Tiered Pharmacy Benefits Plan (United States)

Tier	Type of drugs	Typical drug	Patient payment per prescription
1	Generic drug	Generic lipid-lowering agent—Simvastatin	$10
2	Preferred brand-name drug (on formulary and that the PBM negotiated lower prices on)	Brand-name lipid-lowering agent—Crestor	$35
3	Nonpreferred brand-name drugs (not on formulary and the PBM has not negotiated a special price on)	Nonformulary brand-name lipid-lowering agent—Livalo	$70
4	Specialty drugs	Repatha—PCSK-9 lipid-lowering agent	25% coinsurance

good prices on, put on the company formulary, and designated as "preferred." The consequence is that for some drugs patient co-pays can be quite high. For instance, for many cancer chemotherapies the total price for the insurer could be $10,000 per month, with the patient responsible for $1,000 or even $2,000 per month. But for generic drugs the co-pay can be small and sometimes free.

Outpatient prescription drugs are covered on Medicaid with nominal co-pays for any drug. Typically co-pays range from $0.50 to $3 per prescription. Similarly, there are low co-pays for patients in the Department of Veterans Affairs—$5 for generic drugs. But many types of veteran patients, such as those with low incomes or a service-related disability, are eligible for free prescription drugs.

HUMAN RESOURCES

Physicians

There are approximately 850,000 active physicians for 325 million Americans, or 2.6 physicians per 1,000 people, which is below the international average. Of these physicians, about 45% are primary care physicians, although in the United States pediatricians and internal medicine physicians are considered primary care providers, whereas in many other countries they are deemed specialists. As in most countries, there is a geographic maldistribution of physicians. In Massachusetts there are 3.5 active physicians delivering care for every 1,000 people, while in a rural state like Oklahoma it is 1.9 physicians per 1,000 people. Over a third of physicians are women, and about 45% are over 55 and approaching retirement age. As in other countries, the proportion of female physicians is increasing, as women make up over 50% of medical school enrollment.

About 25% of all US physicians are foreign trained—that is, their medical degrees come from non-US medical schools. Foreign physicians typically need to do their residencies in the United States to obtain a license.

Historically, American physicians were self-employed in small groups, what is often colloquially referred to as "onesies and twosies." More recently there has been consolidation, with growth both in larger physician groups and hospitals' employment of physicians. Today there are about 230,000 physician practices, with 40% or fewer having 4 or fewer physicians. Similarly, the rate of physicians being employed by other organizations rather than self-employed has increased rapidly: in 1983 76% of physicians owned their own practice, but by 2016 that number had declined to 47%.

Physician salaries in the United States are high. The precise amount paid is hard to determine because different survey samples produce different results. On average American physicians make $299,000, with primary care physicians making an average of $223,000 and specialists $329,000. Pediatricians and pediatric specialists are among the lowest earners. Among the highest-paid physicians are orthopedic surgeons, who earn nearly $500,000, and cardiologists, who earn an average of $450,000. Physicians who own their own practices make more than those employed by larger organizations. Physicians in less populated areas also tend to earn more. For instance, the highest-paid physicians work in North Dakota.

There are 154 medical schools (and 36 doctor of osteopathy schools) in the country, which produce just under 20,000 medical graduates and 6,500 doctors of osteopathy each year. Many of the leading medical schools are private. Many, but not all, states also have one or more state-financed medical schools. Tuition at private medical schools is approximately $65,000 per year, but it is lower at state medical schools. Most students borrow money to pay for medical school, with the average medical student graduating with over $190,000 in debt, while only 15% of medical students graduate with no debt.

Is there a physician shortage? The answer is hotly debated. Relying on current patterns of delivering care, the Association of American Medical Colleges argues that there is a big deficit and that the country will need an additional 120,000 physicians by 2030. But others argue that redesigning care, using more nurse practitioners, and using new technologies—telephonic or text- and video-based patient interactions—can ensure that all patients get timely care.

A major concern is physician burnout. Just under one-third of American physicians report being depressed or disengaged with caring for their patients. Much of this is thought to be a result of the increased use of EHRs, the loss of autonomy accompanying the need to follow guidelines and specified pathways, the need to report more data for quality assessments, and increases in other administrative demands.

Nurses
There are approximately 4 million nurses in the United States, or 12.5 per 1,000 people. Of those, approximately 3.4 million are registered nurses (RNs), and the remaining are licensed practical nurses (LPNs). About 60% work in hospitals. There are 250,000 nurse practitioners (NPs) in the United States, with most working in outpatient primary care offices seeing patients. On average, RNs earn $68,000 per year, while NPs earn over $105,000 per year.

There is growing use of NPs that provide services previously restricted to only physicians, such as routine primary care visits, ordering diagnostic tests and cancer screenings, and writing prescriptions. States determine NPs' scope of practice and how much physician oversight there must be. NPs are active in rural areas for primary care services and often work in organized systems for specialty care as well. Their use varies by how much responsibility they can assume in states.

One thing that is not debated: there is a shortage of nurses. The government estimates that the United States will need 1 million more nurses by 2024. There are 674 baccalaureate nursing programs in the

United States. Nevertheless, one major reason for the nursing shortage is a dearth of nursing faculty. The ACA has attempted to increase incentives for nursing faculty, without much success in solving the nursing shortage.

CHALLENGES

The US health care system underperforms in many ways. It is very complex, more so than that of any other country in the world. And it has a strange combination of being lean—with fewer physicians, hospital admissions, and other services than almost any country—while having bloated costs. Yet it is tremendously innovative—not just in developing new drugs and devices but also in trying to improve how care is delivered and paid for. This means that there are significant challenges facing the American health care system over the next 10 years alongside tremendous experimentation and innovation.

The first and one of the biggest challenges remains excessive cost. Since the passage of the ACA in 2010, health care expenditures have actually moderated and remained below 18% of GDP. But 18% of GDP is still substantially higher than the 2nd-highest country and almost double the OECD average. In 2017, health care expenditures were approximately $10,700 per capita. Surprisingly, the United States does not use more of the most expensive services than OECD countries do, such as hospitalizations or visits to a doctor, although it does use more expensive technologies, such as MRIs and expensive drugs.

The big reason for the higher expenditures in the United States is the higher prices paid for health services. The United States has significantly higher prices for most parts of the health care system, from physician and nurse salaries and hospital bed days to imaging tests and device and drug costs. There is, thus, a growing focus on reducing prices to reduce costs. There are some successful experiments with reducing prices. For instance, Medicare introduced a competitive bidding process for durable medical equipment, such as home oxygen, walkers, and electric wheelchairs, that reduced prices. Similarly, some private payers have introduced reference pricing—paying a fixed fee for specific services such as colonoscopies and cataract surgeries, and having patients pay the difference if they choose to get their care at a higher-priced facility. Finally, others are focusing on "steering" patients to lower-cost but higher-quality providers, especially specialists and hospitals. This would save money while improving care quality. The challenge is whether these and other experiments can be successfully expanded across the country, and to other medical goods and services, and whether they can reduce total cost of care.

In addition, there are efforts to reduce overuse of unnecessary services and the use of expensive services, such as proton beam radiation, when lower-cost services provide the same clinical benefits. There are related efforts to increase the use of optimal care, such as cancer screenings, medication adherence, and other measures, to reduce the use of more intensive services. Many such efforts are being tried, and some have succeeded. Whether other experiments can succeed and whether successful efforts to control costs can be scaled across the system is the big challenge facing the US health care system.

A related challenge is the exorbitant price of drugs. New cancer drugs routinely cost in excess of $120,000 per year. Similarly, anti-inflammatory drugs are also expensive. On average, drug prices in the United States are 56% higher than in European countries and constitute the single-largest cost category, explaining higher US health care costs compared to European countries. Indeed, bringing per capita US drug spending down to the per capita spending of the 2nd-most expensive country would save about $150 billion per year (or 5% of total health care expenditures). The most popular proposal is for the federal government to negotiate Medicare drug prices with pharmaceutical manufacturers. New legislation would need to establish the details for this proposal, but the public sentiment is in favor of drug price regulation. The challenge is to determine whether a political coalition can be forged to enact this or any other law to meaningfully reduce drug prices.

A 3rd challenge growing out of the problem of high cost relates to transforming how American physicians and hospitals are paid to move away from fee-for-service and to alternative payment models or more value-based payments. Historically, the United States pioneered payment reforms such as introducing the DRG method of paying hospitals, which is now widely used in most developed countries. Many experts believe the only way to ensure sustained cost control is by changing how physicians and hospitals deliver care so it is more cost conscious, encourages lower-cost tests and treatments, increases efficiency, and decreases unnecessary services. These experts also believe that a necessary prerequisite for this transformation in the delivery of care is changing how physicians and hospitals are paid. Over the last decade there has been substantial experimentation in the United States with APMs—capitation, ACOs, bundled payments, and global budgets. Over the next decade the challenge will be to identify a set of APMs and other interventions that reliably improve quality of care and reduce the total cost of care, and then to scale them throughout the system.

A 4th challenge remains: coverage. The ACA substantially reduced the uninsurance rate from about 18% to about 10%. But that means that 28 to 30 million Americans still lack health insurance. Policies introduced by the Trump administration, including eliminating the mandate, are likely to increase the number of uninsured, while increasing the number of states expanding Medicaid might decrease that number. Nevertheless, there is agreement that policies are needed to increase coverage. Working within the current system, the probable key changes are to move as close to auto-enrollment as possible. This involves a number of technical changes. The top 3 changes are: (1) changing income eligibility rules in the exchanges so that they are like Medicaid and rely on the most recent monthly income, (2) removing the barrier of precluding people from getting subsidies who have an offer of employer-sponsored insurance, and (3) increasing subsidies for low-income people so there are more plans available with zero premium payments needed.

A 5th challenge is the complexity of the system, which average Americans struggle to navigate. The complexity of insurance—with numerous deductible and co-pay levels, changing physician and hospital networks, and complex bills—is enormously time consuming and confusing even to well-educated patients. Some of this complexity arises from the different ways people get insurance, some is related to employers seeking their own special networks of physicians and benefits, and some is an attempt to reduce costs. But it is becoming something patients resent and may even be counterproductive if patients cannot act rationally.

There are a number of ways to reduce complexity, including simplifying eligibility rules for government programs or standardizing the number of insurance options. An under-the-radar way would be to move from annual open enrollment to enrollments that last for 2 or 3 years, thus reducing movement between programs, reducing administrative costs, and allowing more continuity of care.

A 6th challenge is electronic health records. Before the ACA, Congress passed the Recovery Act, which included financial incentives for physicians and hospitals to adopt EHRs. It worked . . . to a point: almost all practices adopted EHRs. But it failed in other ways, producing 3 significant problems. Physicians resent the screens and argue that completing them takes substantial time, time away from engaging meaningfully with patients. Additionally, EHR vendors have not opened up their products to make the clinical data easily accessible. Consequently, when a patient shows up at a hospital or other facility, their medical record with their physician or from a previous hospital stay at another facility cannot be accessed, so the efficiency gain has not materialized. Finally, getting data out of the EHR has been hampered in large measure because they were developed for billing. The most important clinical data are not in structured format but rather in unstructured ones—the words in provider notes—that are not easily accessible. Various workarounds are being tried, such as scribes to liberate physicians from screens. But the challenge is to realize free flow of data that would improve care.

A 7th challenge is physician burnout, namely the depression or disengagement hampering patient care. How to effectively combat burnout is unclear and worrisome. One key way would be to reduce the hassle factors related to administration and prior authorization as well as the burdens of the EHRs.

An 8th challenge is the nursing shortage. To address the problem, the United States has largely used nurses trained in other countries. The United States will need 1 million additional nurses in the next 5 years. Whether this gap can be filled by immigrants or by task-shifting nursing roles to non-nurse providers is unclear.

Finally, there is a long-term care crisis looming. Between now and 2060 the number of Americans over 65 is expected to double to around 100 million. There is no mandatory long-term care insurance; indeed, the proportion of Americans with long-term care insurance is actually declining. If it was hard to get universal health insurance enacted in the United States, there is probably no chance to get young people to pay for long-term care for the elderly when they are worried about educational debt, buying a house, and paying for childcare and skeptical that such programs will exist when they age. Unlike other issues, such as drug prices, long-term care is not on the political agenda in the United States. The challenge is how to address it in a fiscally sound manner before it becomes a crisis.

THE US HEALTH CARE SYSTEM has substantial challenges. It is underperforming on almost every measure—coverage, quality, and cost. It is more complex than any other health system, with more uninsured people and substantially higher costs. Yet the major reason for optimism about the US health care system is that it is innovative. The government and insurers are trying new payment models to improve quality and to lower costs. Venture capitalists are backing hundreds if not thousands of new companies entering the market to try novel approaches to addressing challenges, especially in areas that were previously deemed unimportant, such as primary care, mental health care, end-of-life care, and hospital efficiency. And providers are engaged in transforming their delivery of care. So much activity gives hope that some, if not all, of these challenges can be ameliorated in the decade ahead.

CHAPTER TWO

CANADA

To many conservatives in the United States, the Canadian health care system—also called Medicare—represents the perils of "socialized medicine," rife with prolonged wait times and disgruntled physicians. Conversely, to many liberal Americans, it is the standard for sensible single-payer health care reform.

Paradoxically, there is no one Canadian health care system. Although united by 5 common principles, there are in reality 13 separate provincial and territorial Medicare programs that incorporate a diverse array of unique programs and financing mechanisms to provide care to their residents. As explained by Dr. John Lavis, "There are times Canadian provinces' [health care systems] resemble another country far more than a neighboring province."

Canadian Medicare constitutes a true single-payer system with an almost exclusively private delivery system. It also offers patients free choice of physician and no referral necessary for specialist care. There also are absolutely no deductibles or co-pays for CT or MRI scans, a physician visit, or any other service deemed "medically essential." Yet there are serious problems, the most conspicuous of which is the absence of universal drug coverage in Canada. While the majority of Canadians have some kind of coverage for outpatient drugs through a hodge-podge of plans funded by provinces and employers, many Canadians, especially low-income citizens, totally lack drug coverage or have very inadequate coverage. As one Canadian physician complained, "I have patients who take their pills every other day, or who take them for a few weeks and then have to wait until the check comes in to fill [their prescriptions] again."

Although the vast majority of Canadians support expanding Medicare to include drugs, the total cost and lobbying by the pharmaceutical industry has prevented legislation from passing. All the while many Canadians face a dilemma that is eerily similar to that found in the United States: patients failing to fill their prescriptions, taking smaller doses than their physicians ordered, or foraging for food and cutting back on heat and other necessities of life to pay for pills.

HISTORY

The origins of Canada's health system lie in the rural prairies of Saskatchewan and Alberta, away from the bright city lights of Toronto, Montreal, or Vancouver. In these sparsely populated provinces citizens were spread thin, and doctors were a rare sight. In 1916, the provincial government of Saskatchewan passed the Rural Municipality Act to secure reliable medical care for remote populations. This act permitted local communities to hire physicians on contract. Given the region's small population, this was one of the only ways to attract physicians with adequate compensation. This was highly atypical: the majority of basic health systems pay physicians a fee-for-service on the individual level rather than as a prepayment or guaranteed salary on a community level. The provincial governments also established multiple community hospitals. By 1930, Saskatchewan had 30 such rural hospitals. To finance these hospitals, the province charged residents a capitated rate of $1.21 USD ($1.60 CA) per year. In 1947, the Saskatchewan government passed the Hospitalization Act, which provided universal hospital coverage for all citizens, and over the next 2 years the federal government subsidized this program. Beginning in 1950, Alberta and British Columbia adopted similar models for hospital care.

After seeing the successes of these early programs, the federal government passed the Hospital Insurance and Diagnostic Services (HIDS) Act in 1957. It offered matching funds to any provincial health plan that provided citizens with coverage for hospital care and diagnostic procedures. Over the next several years, provinces across Canada adopted their own health plans. By 1962, all provinces had instituted coverage for hospital services.

In 1962, Saskatchewan again pushed the envelope by including coverage for physician services in its insurance plan. The Canadian debate
was similar to that in other countries: physicians did not want to hand
over billing control and potentially lose professional autonomy, while
the government sought more uniform coverage and better negotiating
power.

A prolonged physician strike intended to repeal Medicare finally
ended the impasse by turning public opinion against physicians. As with
hospital coverage, over the next several years other provinces adopted
their own plans covering physician services. Then, in 1966, through the
passage of the Medical Care Act (MCA), the federal government again
offered matching funds to any province offering a program that covered
physician services. By 1972, all provinces also covered physician services.

Two decades later, in 1984, these 2 separate bills—the HIDS Act,
covering hospital care, and the MCA, covering physician services—
were unified through the passage of the Canada Health Act (CHA). This
bill provided universal health care coverage for all medically necessary
procedures and codified the 5 guiding principles of the Canadian health
system: (1) universality, (2) accessibility, (3) public administration, (4)
comprehensiveness, and (5) portability.

The universality and accessibility provisions guaranteed universal
health coverage to all citizens without any cost sharing at the point
of service for all services deemed medically necessary. The public administration provision locked provincial governments in as the insurance providers and stymied the rise of a 2-tiered insurance market by
prohibiting private insurers from covering any services covered under
Medicare. All plans were required to be comprehensive—to cover all
medically necessary services—and to be portable between provinces.
Notably, at the time, pharmaceutical spending was only a fraction of
what it is today, so it was not covered.

What is perhaps most remarkable about the CHA, however, is how
much it omits. Beyond outlining the 5 guiding principles to which
provinces must adhere in order to receive federal funding, the CHA
leaves everything else to the provinces and territories. This has led to a
highly decentralized system—there truly is no single Canadian health
care system; rather, there are 13 distinct systems united by common
values. But *how* they realize these values differs sharply.

Since the passage of the CHA, the Canadian system has been remarkably stable compared to other nations. On the federal level especially, the CHA's tenets continue to define the Canadian health care system's organizing principles. On the provincial level, a great deal of experimentation, gradual expansion of health benefits, and a gradual—albeit growing—trend toward centralization have characterized the last few decades.

COVERAGE

Canada is a country of 37 million people. It has achieved truly universal health coverage through a 2-layered system: (1) mandatory basic health insurance provided by a diverse system of provincially administered public insurance programs and (2) a network of voluntary supplemental health insurance provided by private companies.

There are also a handful of federally administered programs that care for special populations, including the First Nations and members of the Canadian Armed Forces.

Coverage Model
All Canadian citizens enroll in one of the 13 provincial or territorial statutory health insurance plans, collectively referred to as Medicare. In accordance with the CHA of 1984, these plans are required to provide all "medically necessary services." This includes all medically necessary hospital care, physician services, diagnostic tests, and inpatient pharmaceuticals. It is ultimately up to the province or territory to define the package, as there is no required list of procedures and interventions that must be covered. All services deemed medically necessary by provinces are both universal and completely free at the point of care. There are no co-payments, no coinsurance, and no balance billing.

What is considered to be medically necessary, however, is quite sparse.

Dental care, vision care, long-term care, ambulance services, and even outpatient pharmaceuticals are not uniformly covered by every province. In fact, Canada is the only developed country with a universal health plan that does *not* cover outpatient pharmaceuticals, though it is

Figure 1. Health Care Coverage (Canada)

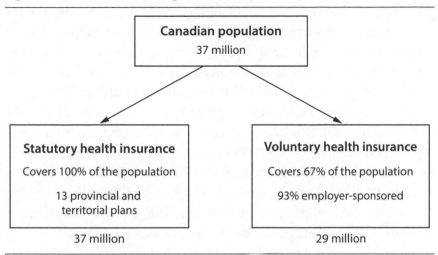

not for lack of trying. In the early 1960s, when provinces were expanding from only hospital coverage to physician services, pharmaceutical
coverage seemed a natural next step. Including prescription drugs in
health plans had significant support, such as a strong recommendation from a national committee known as the 1964 Hall Commission.
But the federal government was ultimately scared off by the potential
cost and restricted its offer of matching funds to only include physician
services.

At the time, pharmaceutical spending was a fraction of what it is
today. It also was not seen as essential. In the mid-1990s, the debate was
revived when the National Forum on Health, an advisory body formed
by the prime minister, made a strong recommendation for a national
prescription drug plan. Ultimately an economic slowdown stifled it.
As a result, the Canadian health system now relies on a patchwork of
provincial plans, population-specific federal plans, private supplemental insurance plans, and out-of-pocket payments to cover outpatient
pharmaceuticals and other services not deemed medically necessary.

Each province also has its own additional health benefit programs;
these are typically needs based, target select populations, and have
some element of cost sharing. For example, in Ontario outpatient
pharmaceuticals are covered for all persons aged 65 and older through
the Ontario Health Insurance Program's (OHIP) Ontario Drug Benefit

(ODB). The disabled population enrolled in Ontario's Disability Support Program and the poor population enrolled in Ontario Works are also eligible for this benefit. All persons aged 25 and younger without private coverage are insured through OHIP+. Those with significant drug expenditures can apply for needs-based coverage through the Trillium Drug Program (TDP). However, there is little uniformity between these programs. OHIP+ for persons under 25 has no deductible or coinsurance, ODB for the disabled, poor, and elderly has no deductible but does have a $1.52 USD ($2.00 CA) co-payment per prescription for low-income households or a $75.80 USD ($100 CA) deductible with a $4.63 USD ($6.11 CA) co-payment for high-income households, while TDP for the medically burdened with high drug costs has a deductible equal to around 3% of household income without coinsurance.

Quebec also has a publicly administered plan, the Public Drug Insurance Plan (PDIP), but only offers it to persons aged 65 and older and those younger than 65 who lack access to a private pharmaceutical plan. Quebec couples this with an individual mandate requiring all persons younger than 65 who *can* purchase a private plan through their employer, professional association, or spouse to do so. Quebec's PDIP has monthly premiums ranging from $0 to $480.10 USD ($0 to $636 CA), depending on income, a $16.45 USD ($21.75 CA) deductible, 0% to 37% coinsurance, depending on income, and monthly and annual caps of $70.38 USD ($93.08 CA) or $844.62 USD ($1,117 CA).

The federal government also offers coverage for additional fringe benefits to special populations, including the Inuit and First Nations. These benefits vary, but they generally include outpatient prescription drugs and some dental and vision coverage.

AS A RESULT of the patchwork pharmaceutical, dental, and vision coverage, over two-thirds of Canadians purchase private supplemental health insurance plans. These plans are almost exclusively provided through employers (93%). While there are some individual plans, they are not subsidized either directly or through the tax system. Historically these plans have been prohibited from competing with Medicare by offering duplicative benefits. But in a landmark decision, *Chaoulli v. Quebec* in 2005, the Canadian Supreme Court ruled that Quebec's statute prohibiting private insurers from covering Medicare-covered services was unconstitutional.

Since 2005, little movement has occurred in the market, and these plans continue to be largely complementary. These plans, moreover, are *not* used to increase access to desired physicians. They are typically used to decrease wait times for diagnostic procedures and elective surgeries. Several provinces and territories have enacted additional legislation to discourage these plans by, for example, prohibiting physicians from accepting both supplemental insurance and Medicare.

Households bear the remainder of costs. These out-of-pocket costs represent 14% of total spending, or $669 USD ($882 CA) per person, mostly for prescription drugs (21%), long-term care (22%), dental care (16%), vision care (9%), and over-the-counter medications (10%). While balance billing continues to be almost nonexistent, doctors in some provinces are allowed to charge annual fees for non-Medicare services, such as doctors' notes and over-the-phone refills.

FINANCING

Canada spends $193 billion USD ($254 billion CA) per year on health care, equal to 11.3% of its GDP, or about $4,800 USD ($6,400 CA) per person. This is relatively high compared to other developed countries, but it is far below the United States and Switzerland. Staying true to the CHA, Canada maintains a federalist funding scheme for Medicare: the national government provides an annual payment to provinces in exchange for their adherence to the 5 core principles. The supplemental market is almost exclusively financed through private, employer-sponsored health companies.

Provincial and Territorial Health Insurance Plans: Canadian Medicare
Medicare finances around 70% of total health care spending and is funded jointly by individual provinces and the federal government through a highly progressive system of taxation.

Provinces pay for roughly three-fourths of Medicare costs, covering all essential health benefits and any additional special benefit

Figure 2. Financing Health Care: Medicare (Canada)

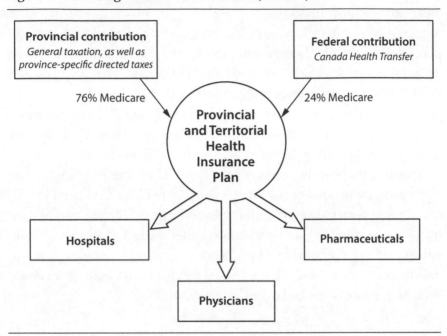

programs. The vast majority of provincial funds comes from general taxation, although some provinces have developed a variety of special funding mechanisms. For instance, in Quebec there are surcharges on each household's regular income tax, and any individual who registers for their public pharmaceutical coverage is subject to an additional monthly premium. In Ontario, there is a dedicated Ontario Health Premium that can be as much as $682 USD ($900 CA) per year for households making more than $15,159 USD ($20,000 CA) annually. In British Columbia, a fixed monthly premium supplements general tax funding—although it's waived for low-income households.

The federal government pays for roughly one-quarter of Medicare costs through a fixed annual block grant known as the Canada Health Transfer (CHT). Originally the federal government paid half of the costs each province incurred while providing hospital and physician services. This was an annual shared-cost transfer. In 1977, however, the provinces and federal government agreed to change this arrangement. The provinces took the amount they were paying (half of all costs) and converted half of it into a permanent tax transfer and the other half into

an annual cash transfer. The permanent tax transfer took taxable revenue from the federal domain and gave it to provinces, while the annual
cash transfer was indexed to economic growth. The federal government favored this approach because its annual contribution was now
fixed and not tied to fluctuating rates of health care expenditure, while
provinces favored this because the tax transfer was projected to bring
in more revenue than the previous shared-cost transfer, especially for
the economically advantaged—and politically powerful—provinces of
Ontario and Quebec.

Since that decision was made, this arrangement has been quite favorable to the provinces. Whereas the annual cash allocation—the
CHT—represents only 24% of Medicare expenses, the net value of that
24% cash transfer plus the additional tax transfer far exceeds 50% of
Medicare costs. Still, as Dr. Gregory Marchildon, chair of health policy
at the University of Toronto, explains, "provinces have conveniently
forgotten the tax transfer, and because it's such a complicated argument, it's hard for the public to appreciate."

Although the Canada Health Transfer is similar in many ways to the
United States' Federal Medicaid Assistance Percentage (FMAP) annual
grants to states to finance Medicaid, there are several key differences.
First, the CHT is calculated strictly based on a per capita basis, without
adjustments for different levels of economic prosperity at the provincial
level. Second, the CHT rate increases at a standard rate each year set by
law regardless of whether health costs increase more or less than the
standard. And finally, the CHT amount is not used as a stimulus during
economic downturns as the FMAP is routinely used in the United States.

Supplemental Insurance

The supplemental insurance market pays $21 billion USD ($28 billion
CA) per year, or around 12% of total health spending. Premiums collected by private insurance companies fund it. As of 2016, there were
133 private health insurance companies, 80% of which were for profit.
The vast majority of these plans (95%) are offered through employers
or unions, and premiums are tax exempt in all provinces except Quebec. Companies tend to cover the premium when offered as a benefit.

The private, supplemental insurance market is loosely regulated. As
Dr. Marchildon says,

Provincial governments are responsible for regulating the market, but there's not a lot of control in the traditional sense because these services—outpatient pharmaceuticals, dental, and vision—are not considered life or death. So, it's up to the employers dealing with their unions to decide exactly what and how deep and broad coverage should be. It's like the US market, except the stakes are not too high.

This has led to a largely self-regulated market that does, technically, allow for exclusions based on preexisting conditions, age, gender, and geography, although these practices are rare and, culturally speaking, nonstarters. Maximum payout limits are also not uncommon among private insurers. For instance, some private plans limit the total amount of drug coverage an employer may purchase for its employees to around $15,000 USD per beneficiary.

Long-Term Care
Long-term care in Canada accounts for just under 10% of total health care spending, or $15 USD billion ($20 billion CA) annually. Like pharmaceuticals, long-term care coverage is provided through a patchwork of provincial plans, special federal programs, and out-of-pocket costs. Unlike pharmaceuticals, though, the private insurance market is underdeveloped and pushes a significant share of costs to patients as out-of-pocket payments.

Long-term medical services, including devices and nursing services, are largely covered through provincial health plans. Not surprisingly, these plans' generosity varies between provinces. Some are means tested; others are not. Additionally, *what* is covered varies by province. In Ontario all physician services are covered through the provincial Medicare program, known as OHIP, while nursing and support services are covered through the Local Health Integration Network (LHIN) without cost sharing to all eligible citizens.

Long-term housing services, such as board for nursing homes or assisted-living facilities, are generally left for patients to pay out of pocket, although safety-net programs exist in many provinces. However, these safety nets' quality is also highly variable, and out-of-pocket caps in some provinces exceed $22,740 USD ($30,000 CA) per year. In

Ontario, patients are charged a standard housing fee of around $1,345 USD ($1,775 CA) per month for a shared room, $1,630 USD ($2,150 CA) for a semiprivate room, or $1,933 USD ($2,550 CA) for a private room. Subsidies are available for those unable to afford these rates, and daily rates of around $29 USD ($38 CA) are possible for short stays. In Quebec, rates are set significantly lower: $866 USD ($1,142 CA) per month for a shared room, $1,164 USD ($1,536 CA) for a semiprivate room, and $1,392 USD ($1,837 CA) for a private room.

Payment for long-term care remains a contentious issue in Canada. Prominent think tanks and policymakers have made several calls to include coverage under Medicare. Recently one provincial party promised to incorporate long-term coverage in Medicare, but this was ultimately not implemented due to resistance around funding. Although the private market could potentially fill this void, a lack of regulations prohibiting exclusions based on preexisting conditions hinders this option.

Public Health
Public health represents 1% to 3% of total health care spending and is funded through a variety of federal and provincial sources. Preventive services such as vaccines and cancer-screening tests for individuals are considered essential and are covered in full by Medicare in all provinces. Screening rates for breast, cervical, and colon cancer are all higher than the average for developed countries, as are childhood vaccinations and rates for seasonal flu shots.

PAYMENT

Payment in Canada is considerably more variable than in many other developed nations due to the decentralized provincial model. Although the majority of hospitals are reimbursed through global budgets, there has been some recent movement toward activity-based payments in several provinces. Also, most physicians are paid on a fee-for-service basis by Medicare or private insurance, but physician services in a variety of settings—notably primary care—are beginning to transition to alternative payment models such as capitation.

Figure 3. Payment to Hospitals (Canada)

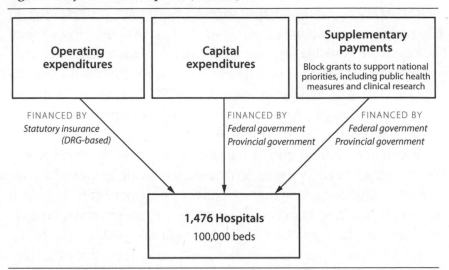

Operating expenditures	Capital expenditures	**Supplementary payments** Block grants to support national priorities, including public health measures and clinical research
FINANCED BY *Statutory insurance* *(DRG-based)*	FINANCED BY *Federal government* *Provincial government*	FINANCED BY *Federal government* *Provincial government*

1,476 Hospitals
100,000 beds

Payment to Hospitals

Global budgets negotiated by provincial governments primarily cover inpatient services, although several provinces have begun experimenting with activity-based payments.

Funding for inpatient services generally flows from provincial ministries of health to provincial or regional health authorities before being allocated to individual hospitals and other facilities. Provinces collect taxes and designate funds to sub-provincial regional health authorities as a mix of unrestricted block grants (traditionally on a per capita basis) and targeted line-item funding tied to specific policies. Regional health authorities then divvy up their funding to specific hospitals, long-term care facilities, and other community-based providers. Importantly, although significant sums of money continue to flow through these regional agencies, much of these funds are constrained. For instance, in Ontario 36% of public funding is tied to hospital funding.

Lately there has been movement toward greater centralization. Alberta dissolved its regional health authorities in 2009 and established a single, province-wide authority referred to as the Alberta Health Services. Ontario consolidated its 14 LHINs into a single agency, Health Ontario. By contrast, Quebec still maintains 22 territorial health authorities.

Regardless of the exact funding route, the majority of hospital payments in all provinces remains global budgets. In this arrangement, the funding for each hospital is based on historical spending with annual adjustments that consider inflation and the growing cost of medical care. Hospital funding is not adjusted for the number of patients, complexity of procedures, or quality of care provided. It also does not incentivize improvements in efficiency or outcomes. Given Canada's high-profile struggles with wait times for elective procedures, such arguably archaic payment mechanisms have come under intense scrutiny. However, as described by Dr. Allan Detsky, global budgets have stuck around because they can be appealing from both cost-control and predictability perspectives:

> Global budgeting is successful at one main thing: capping costs. If you're the Ministry of Finance, you love global budget because you look at last year's budget and increase it by a certain percent . . . this system works to control costs and anything that you do for volume-based reimbursement goes away from predictable funding and opens the door to the same problems as fee-for-service.

There has been *some* progress: a handful of provinces have incorporated elements of activity-based payment, in which hospitals are paid for services that they complete rather than a fixed annual budget. In 2010, British Columbia became the first province to tie 20% of its hospital payments to activity. Since then both Alberta and Ontario have also introduced elements of activity-based payments. The Ontario system ties roughly 30% of hospital payments to activity through its Quality-Based Procedure program. This program pays hospitals a fixed amount for each patient they provide care for, provided the patient has one of 10 targeted conditions. These include a mix of common surgical and medical conditions, such as major lower extremity joint replacement, stroke, pneumonia, and congestive heart failure exacerbation. There have also been several pilot programs toward bundled payments for entire episodes of care. The largest of these, known as the Integrated Comprehensive Care Project in Ontario, was launched in 2013 and offers bundles for both surgical and medical procedures.

Figure 4. Payment to Ambulatory Physicians (Canada)

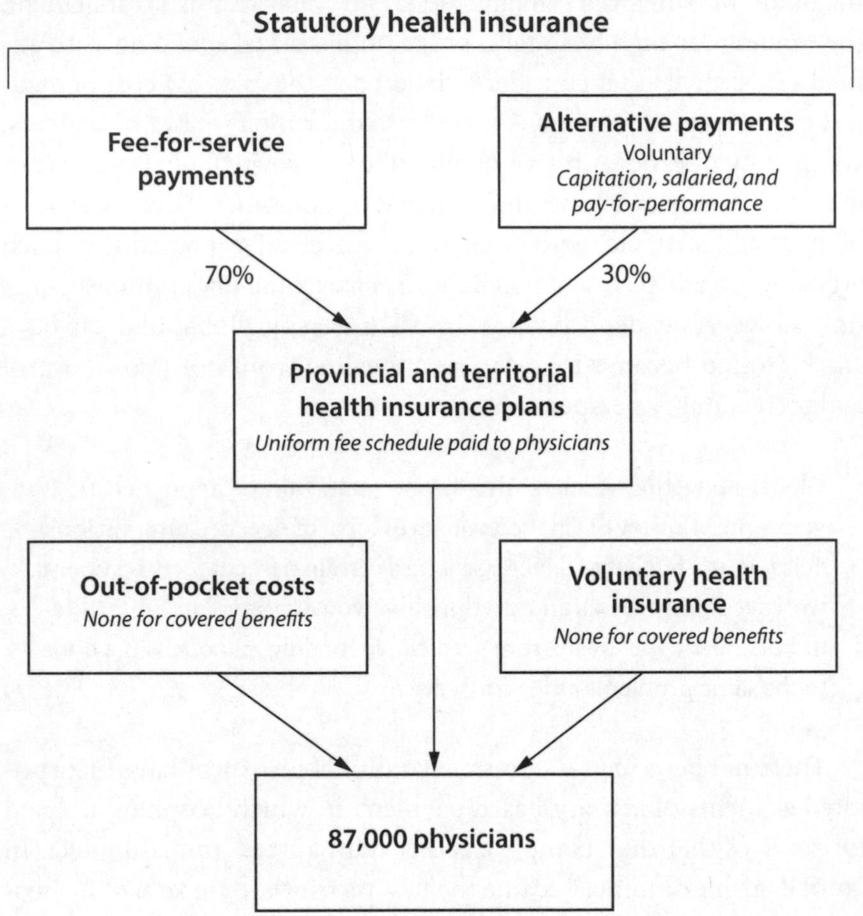

Statutory health insurance

Fee-for-service payments	**Alternative payments** Voluntary *Capitation, salaried, and pay-for-performance*

70%   30%

Provincial and territorial health insurance plans
Uniform fee schedule paid to physicians

Out-of-pocket costs *None for covered benefits*	**Voluntary health insurance** *None for covered benefits*

87,000 physicians

Payment to Physicians

Reimbursement is highly variable among provinces. However, fee-for-service remains the dominant form of payment for physician services, accounting for roughly 70% of physician payment. There are also a variety of alternative payment models, including capitation, salaried wages, and performance-based payments.

Variability is high because both provincial ministries of health and individual group practices have the right to negotiate their own contracts. Each provincial ministry of health not only publishes its own fee schedule but can also offer physicians myriad alternative payment arrangements. At the moment these alternative payment models are all voluntary. Simultaneously, individual physicians are privately employed and can either accept the fee schedule or attempt to negotiate their own payment arrangement.

Canadian fee-for-service is similar to other nations' fee-for-service except that individual provinces are tasked with negotiating their own fee schedule with the appropriate professional society. And if the 2 parties fail to agree to terms, provinces have the right to unilaterally set prices. For instance, every few years in Ontario the Ministry of Health and Ontario Medical Association negotiate a new Physician Services Agreement that establishes a fee schedule. Although the fee schedules in Canada tend to be somewhat simpler than those in the United States, there are variations in classification and amount paid, making comparisons between provinces challenging.

As for alternative payment models, the most recent wave of interest dates back to the early 2000s, when Ontario introduced a wide-scale capitation model for primary care services. The program offered capitated payments with incentives for primary care physicians to form group practices and, among other things, offer reliable access to after-hours care. Although the program was intended to be mandatory, this was politically unfeasible. Consequently, it was rolled out with voluntary enrollment. Not surprisingly, adverse selection occurred, and only providers without many medically complicated patients enrolled. As Dr. Detsky explained,

> Nothing's been successful . . . to have political agreement it had to be voluntary. But then any physician can figure out their own work-to-pay ratio. If you only saw young healthy people, you'd go for [the capitation model]. If you saw medically complicated patients, you'd pass [and keep fee-for-service].

Still, there remains significant interest and experimentation, especially for primary care reimbursement. Ontario is trying 8 different alternative payment models for primary care physicians alone. Moving specialists away from fee-for-service remains a challenge, but there have been some early pilot studies with bundled payments.

Payments for Long-Term Care

Long-term care is paid through a mix of traditional mechanisms. Medical services are generally paid directly as fee-for-service under Medicare, while housing, accommodation, and custodial services are generally paid at a fixed daily rate. The federal government supports in-kind home care through its Compassionate Care Benefit, which allows for 6 weeks of paid leave for all workers who have a family member in their last 6 months of life.

Payments for Complementary and Alternative Medicine

As the majority of complementary and alternative medicine services are not deemed medically essential, Medicare does not reimburse these services, and few provinces include them in their benefits packages. This means the majority of complementary services and alternative medicines are paid for either by private insurance or individual out-of-pocket costs.

Preventive Medicine

Most vaccines and recommended screening tests are paid for by Medicare on a fee-for-service basis without coinsurance.

DELIVERY OF HEALTH CARE SERVICES

While Canadian health care is largely publicly financed, the provision of care remains almost exclusively private. Almost all medical practitioners are self-employed, and the majority of hospitals are private and not for profit. Given this high degree of autonomy, fragmentation of care remains a major issue.

Hospital Care

Canada has 1,476 hospitals, with a total of around 100,000 beds for 37 million people, equal to 2.7 hospital beds per 1,000 inhabitants. Similar to other countries, there has been a steady decline in the number of hospital beds in Canada since the 1990s.

The vast majority of acute care hospitals (95%) are private, not for profit. These hospitals also provide the vast majority of medically essential services covered under Medicare. Most are run by regional boards appointed by provincial health authorities, although many have private boards that operate under contract with provincial health authorities. Many solicit charitable donations to fund capital expenditures, but their operating expenses are paid for almost exclusively through the provincial governments. Hence, hospitals and provincial ministries of health are intimately tied together.

The remaining handful of hospitals are private and for profit. These for-profit hospitals are not legally allowed to provide services covered under Medicare and several provinces have statutes prohibiting physicians from working simultaneously at for-profit and not-for-profit hospitals; their role remains minimal and focused on services not covered under Medicare.

Ambulatory (Outpatient) Care

Outpatient care is centered on primary care physicians, who serve as care coordinators and relatively strong gatekeepers. At a rate of 7.7 annual consultations per person per year, Canadians visit physicians slightly more than other developed countries and nearly twice as much as patients in the United States. Similarly, Canadian physicians see on average around 3,100 patients per year, around 15 patients per day for a 200-day work year. Almost all physicians are privately employed, including hospitalists.

Primary care physicians are the first point of contact for the majority of patients, and primary care physicians are tasked with coordinating their care. The majority operate in small-group practices; fewer than one in 6 remain true solo practitioners. They are paid fee-for-service, although several provinces have begun to incentivize the formation of integrated care networks, each with its own name: in Alberta these are known as Primary Care Networks; in Quebec, Family Medicine Groups; in Manitoba, Physician Integrated Networks; and in Ontario, either Family Health Groups, Family Health Networks, or Family Health Organizations. All of these programs incentivize integration of care between physicians and other nonphysician providers by using mixed payment models.

Despite these promising strides toward more integrated primary care, fragmentation remains a huge problem. According to David

Rudoler, assistant professor at the University of Ontario Institute of Technology,

> Everywhere fragmentation is the rule and it's a major issue we're deal-ing with. At least in Ontario, physicians run independent practices and are private business owners, so the vast majority of primary care is delivered by independent, privately-owned physician practices. There is very little in terms of accountability to the provincial government or regional bodies. Although that has changed in the last couple years with Family Health Teams, there has been little attempt to integrate community services with other sectors of the health care system. For the vast majority, little has changed.

Medical and surgical specialists are even more independent. Almost all are privately self-employed, and each specialty is largely self-regu-lated through their own professional societies. The majority (65%) work primarily out of hospitals, while only 24% work out of an office or clinic. They are free to open a new practice anywhere they would like, and pro-vincial governments have almost no authority to regulate specialists.

Although access to specialists generally requires a referral from a primary care physician, referrals last for 2 years, and primary care phy-sicians have no direct financial incentive to consider total cost of care. Referral networks are mostly organic, forming from personal relation-ships and geographic proximity. (Outcomes data at the individual level is difficult to obtain, and even if it were available, there is no specific incentive to guide patients to higher-value providers.) Moreover, once a patient has a referral, they are "in" the system, and specialists are al-lowed to refer them to other specialists.

From a patient's perspective, the Canadian system is quite attractive. Except for queues for some elective procedures, Canadians are allowed to visit any primary care physician in any province without any cost sharing. They can also see any specialist for whom they have a referral without any cost sharing.

Mental Health Care
Like other developed countries, since the 1980s Canada has undergone a process of deinstitutionalization for mental health services. The ma-

jority of mental health care is now provided on an outpatient basis. However, there is a strong division between physician-provided mental health care and therapist- or social worker–provided mental health care.

Physician-provided mental health care is considered essential and is, therefore, covered by all provincial Medicare plans. Non-physician-led mental health care is not covered by Medicare plans. Therefore, payment for therapists, social workers, and occupational therapists is left to provincial plans, private health insurance plans, or out-of-pocket costs.

A recent but growing innovation is for family care networks to employ in-house mental health professionals. In Ontario, Family Health Organizations can apply for funding to incorporate a psychologist for their patients, and physicians who roster a patient with a known severe mental illness can receive a one-time bonus payment. Coordination for patients with mental health services is poor. It is not uncommon for these patients to become lost in the system.

Long-Term Care
Compared to other countries, Canada has a high percentage of inpatient beds dedicated to long-term care (20%, compared to the OECD average of 13%). But, with its aging population, there remains concern over a bed shortage. Long-term care is not guaranteed under the CHA, and both private and public institutions provide long-term care. The prevalence of each varies by province, with some provinces, such as British Columbia, having the majority being private and not for profit, while others, such as Ontario, having mostly private, for-profit, long-term care facilities. Of the 636 long-term care homes and 117 hospital-based continuing care facilities in Ontario, 51% are private and for profit, 27% are public, and 22% are private and not for profit.

Preventive Medicine
Privately employed ambulatory physicians typically perform screenings and immunizations, although citizens can also receive some vaccines directly through regional health agencies. Both the provincial and national governments spearhead their own campaigns to improve public health, including largely successful campaigns to increase screening rates for breast cancer and colon cancer.

PHARMACEUTICAL COVERAGE AND PRICE CONTROLS

Pharmaceutical Market

Canada is the world's 9th largest pharmaceutical market, with around $30.2 billion USD ($39.8 billion CA) in annual sales. This translates to 16% of total health care expenditures, or $823 USD ($1,086 CA) per person. This is the 3rd-highest per capita spending in the world, and it's rising rapidly—around 4% per year.

Coverage Determination

For a new medication to be approved, it must first be determined to be safe and effective by the Health Products and Food Branch (HPFB) of Health Canada, analogous to the United States' FDA within the Department of Health and Human Services.

First, pharmaceutical companies submit a New Drug Submission (NDS) to the HPFB that contains the scientific data to support use of a medication for a specific aim. The application is referred to the proper directorate—either Therapeutic Products or Biologics and Genetic Therapies—and then to the appropriate bureau for review. For instance, a novel statin would be referred to the Therapeutic Products director and be reviewed by the Bureau of Cardiology, Allergy, and Neurologic Sciences. The bureau assesses the safety and efficacy of the new medication as well as the quality of data behind it. It also has the ability to review the new product's proposed packaging and labeling. However, the committee does *not* look at the medication's economic impact. Unlike the FDA, this process occurs behind closed doors; there are no standard public hearings.

If the HPFB committee determines that a drug's benefits outweigh its risks, it issues a Notification of Compliance (NOC) and a Drug Identification Number (DIN) that allows for sale of the medication. If the committee determines that the benefits do not outweigh the risks, the medication is not legally allowed to be prescribed. This process takes, on average, one year to complete.

Price Regulation of Branded Medicines

After HPFB determines the medication to be safe and effective, a 3-step process sets the prescription drug's prices. First, the Patented Med-

Figure 5. Regulation of Pharmaceutical Prices (Canada)

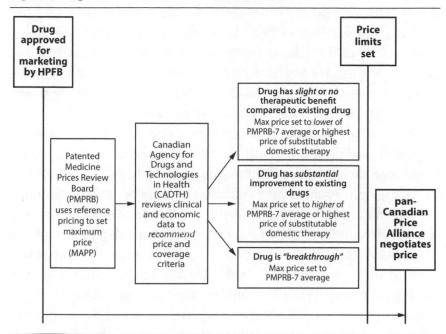

icines Prices Review Board (PMPRB) sets a maximum national sales price using reference pricing. Second, the Canadian Agency for Drugs and Technologies in Health (CADTH) assesses the medication's cost effectiveness and publishes a report, the Common Drug Review (CDR). Finally, public drug plans—provincial, territorial, and federal—negotiate the final confidential sales price with pharmaceutical companies through the pan-Canadian Pharmaceutical Alliance (pCPA).

The Patented Medicines Prices Review Board (PMPRB) begins by classifying the benefit of the new medicine into one of 4 categories: breakthrough, substantial improvement, moderate improvement, or slight or no improvement. Breakthrough medications are truly innovative products without competitors in the same therapeutic category. The degree of improvement for drugs with competitors is based on a holistic review that includes improved outcomes and reductions in adverse events.

The PMPRB then compares the proposed factory price to (1) what other nations pay for the same drug and (2) what Canadian provinces pay for therapeutically similar drugs. By statute, the PMPRB compares the proposed price to that paid by a group of 7 nations, referred to as the PMPRB-7: France, Germany, Italy, Sweden, Switzerland, UK, and the United States. The PMPRB also compares the proposed price to what is being charged domestically for other medications in the same therapeutic class. For instance, if another statin is introduced, its proposed price would be compared to what is being charged domestically for atorvastatin, rosuvastatin, and all other statins.

The PMPRB concludes its analysis by calculating a maximum average potential price (MAPP), above which the proposed price would be deemed excessive. For breakthrough medications, MAPP is set as the average price paid in the 7 comparator countries. For medications with substantial improvement, MAPP is set as the *higher* of either the average price in PMPRB-7 or the highest price paid domestically for substitutable therapy. And for medications with slight or no improvement, MAPP is set as the *lower* of either the average price in PMPRB-7 or the highest price paid domestically for substitutable therapy. If the introductory price is deemed excessive, pharmaceutical companies can either voluntarily reduce the price or appeal. This is rare, however, because pharmaceutical companies can calculate the MAPP themselves and set their factory price to just under this ceiling.

In August 2019, Canada amended the Patented Medicines Regulations to remove the United States and Switzerland from the PMPRB's basket of countries used for reference pricing, beginning in July of 2020. The amendments also will allow the PMPRB to consider the actual market price of medicines in Canada—as opposed to only the proposed factory price—as well as whether the price of a drug actually reflects its value for patients.

Once the PMPRB gives its maximum price, the CADTH takes over. It conducts a national cost-effective analysis, known as the Common Drug Review (CDR). In this report, the CADTH reviews the clinical and economic data behind the medication and compiles a Clinical Report and a Pharmacoeconomic Report, with nonbinding pricing and coverage recommendations to the provincial and territorial governments.

The final sales price is set through negotiations between provincial Medicare plans or private insurers and pharmaceutical companies. Although provinces have traditionally negotiated individually with pharmaceutical companies, since 2010 all provinces except Quebec have been in the pCPA to negotiate jointly. Quebec, the one exception, has a "most-preferred" clause that only allows pharmaceutical companies to sell them medications at the lowest price offered anywhere in Canada. While they are not technically part of the agreement, then, they de facto benefit from the negotiations.

For branded medications, the pCPA negotiates rates with pharmaceutical companies individually. By combining all provinces' buying power, the pCPA has lowered branded pharmaceutical prices and decreased price variation between provinces. Given the concentration of Canada's populations in several provinces (nearly two-thirds live in Ontario and Quebec alone), this has been especially beneficial to the smaller provinces and territories.

For generic medications, the pCPA uses a tiered pricing framework based on the number of generic manufacturers on the market. If a new generic is the only one on the market, its price is set at 75% of the brand listing. Once a 2nd generic is introduced, the price of *both* decreases to 50% of the brand price. Upon entry of a 3rd generic, the prices all decrease to either 25% for oral solid medications (pills) or 35% for nonoral medications (liquid oral, inhalers, etc.). Since its creation the pCPA has lowered generic drug prices by over 50%.

Private insurance plans are free to negotiate their own rates for branded and generic medications. However, as described by one expert I spoke with, "They're more generous and usually just accept whatever price is offered."

While recent reforms, including the CDR and pCPA, have been widely acknowledged as successful in increasing uniformity and reducing prices, the PMPRB is highly controversial. In particular the PMPRB-7 includes some of the highest-paying countries and—until the 2020 reform—included the 2 highest paying countries of all, the United States and Switzerland. The reason is intimately tied to history. Before 1987 Canada kept pharmaceutical drug prices exceptionally low through a practice known as *compulsory licensing*: the government allowed for domestic generic production of branded pharmaceuticals *immediately* after approval in exchange for a 4% royalty to the patent holder.

Not surprisingly, this was unpopular with trading partners that had significant pharmaceutical interests. The North American Free Trade

Agreement (NAFTA) ended the practice and replaced it with the external reference pricing through the PMPRB. The PMPRB-7 were then selected not as a way to control costs but as part of a *quid pro quo* in an effort to attract pharmaceutical R&D investment in Canada. As described by one Canadian professor,

> At that time, pharmaceutical brand companies were mostly subsidiaries of European or US drug companies like Pfizer or AstraZeneca. Those companies essentially said, "Canada, we're going to substantially increase our R&D footprint. But if you want to be in the club with the US, UK, Germany, Sweden, and France, you're going to have to allow higher prices." The conservative government at the time believed that this was a good tradeoff. In the House of Commons debate, [Prime Minister] Mulroney said, "Let's not lose out on the biotechnology revolution" and make this a Silicon Valley in the north. So domestic drug prices were set to be in line with drug prices in countries that had substantial pharmaceutical R&D sectors.

In the years since, there have been multiple reforms suggested, including switching the reference countries to lower-cost nations, including Spain and South Korea, and using cost-effective analysis. None were successful until the 2020 reforms were passed to shift reference pricing from the highest paying to more comparable countries.

Regulation of Physician Prescriptions

While physicians are free to prescribe any drug approved for sale by Health Canada to any patient for any indication they see fit, professional and financial regulations restrict prescribing. First, just because a physician prescribes a medication does not mean Medicare or private insurers will reimburse its purchase. Medications must be on a formulary to be reimbursed, and public plans have the power to either not list or specify reimbursement criteria for certain prescription drugs. Off-label prescribing is allowed, but reimbursement is variable. In some cases, patients may need to pay out of pocket.

Second, pharmacists can freely substitute generics without physician consent. For instance, if a physician prescribes a branded antihypertensive while a generic equivalent is available, pharmacies can—and do—switch to the cheaper generic alternative. Not only is the pharmacy incentivized financially to do this by pocketing the difference, but so are patients; provincial Medicare plans will not pay for more than the cost of the generic. In fact, in Ontario the only way a physician can prevent automatic substitution is filling out a special form outlining the clinical rationale for the branded drug and a subsequent form reporting adverse events from the generic. These policies have helped Canadian generics capture a 70% market share by volume, almost as high as the United States' exceptional share.

Prices Paid by Patients

Outpatient medications as well as over-the-counter medications are covered through a mix of provincial plans (45%), private plans (35%), and out-of-pocket costs (20%). These represent a large and growing share of health expenditures and remain a challenge for Canadian policymakers.

All inpatient pharmaceuticals are completely covered without co-payment through Medicare. Patients are also not responsible for any sales taxes on these.

HUMAN RESOURCES

Physicians

There are nearly 90,000 practicing physicians in Canada. This represents 2.4 practicing physicians per 1,000 inhabitants, lower than the OECD average of 3.5 per 1,000 people. About 42% of physicians are women, and just over a quarter received their medical training outside of Canada. Nearly half (47%) are generalists, significantly higher than the OECD average of 30%. The vast majority are privately employed, even those who are employed in hospitals.

Canadian physicians are well compensated. As of 2016, the average income was $193,000 USD ($225,207 CAD) for a primary care physician, $276,000 USD ($364,959 CAD) for a medical specialist, and $347,000 USD ($458,843 CAD) for a surgeon. The highest compensated specialists, ophthalmologists, earned $539,000 USD ($712,728 CAD), while the average among all physicians was $256,000 USD ($338,513 CAD).

As with other developed countries, Canada faces a serious maldistribution of physicians. Whereas 19% of Canadians live in rural areas, only 14% of primary care physicians and 2% of specialists live in rural areas. Especially in the northern territories and rural areas of the southern provinces, it has been hard to recruit physicians to move and impossible to force them to do so, given their status as independent, privately employed practitioners. Although provinces have attempted to attract physicians by offering higher compensation in the form of capitated payments, guaranteed salaries, higher fee-for-service rates, and lump-sum bonuses, little progress has been made. Some provinces, such as Saskatchewan, have begun to rely heavily on foreign medical graduates, while others have empowered nurse practitioners to set up supervised practices in these areas.

There are 17 medical schools in Canada that together train around 2,300 physicians each year. Provincial governments set the number of training spots available each year (*numerus clausus*). Prior to entering medical school, applicants generally must complete at least 2 years of higher education. The majority of medical schools last 4 years, although 2 offer 3-year tracks, and they are structured similarly to the US system of 2 years of preclinical classroom work and 2 years of clinical training. Graduating students apply through a match process identical to that in the United States and enter residency for anywhere between 2 (family medicine) and 6 years. Medical school costs students around $11,400 USD ($15,000 CA) per year, although it varies significantly by province.

Nurses
As of 2015, Canada had 9.5 nurses per 1,000 inhabitants, in line with comparable countries. As in most other countries, there remains a concern of an impending nursing shortage.

Going back to 1967, Canada has a long history of advanced practice nurses. The Canadian government recognizes 2 forms of advanced practice nurses: nurse practitioners and clinical nurse specialists. Nurse practitioners directly manage patients and specialize in a field of medicine, similar to the United States. Clinical nurse specialists also specialize in a subfield and assist in developing nursing guidelines. Both require graduate degrees.

Registered nurses in Canada make an average of $54,000 USD ($71,405 CAD) per year, less than the average wage for US nurses. By contrast, advanced practice nurses can earn up to $120,000 USD ($158,768 CAD) per year. Becoming a nurse in Canada is similar to becoming a nurse in the United States and requires a bachelor's degree.

CHALLENGES

There is much to like about the Canadian health care system. Patients have truly universal coverage, with free choice of doctor, direct access to specialists, and no cost sharing for necessary medical services. Physicians have high wages, professional autonomy, and a relatively efficient billing system. And although costs are high, they are far from the highest, while providing high-quality care with no cost sharing.

Still, there remain several key challenges.

The most glaring deficit in Canadian Medicare programs is their lack of universal coverage for pharmaceuticals. Canada remains the only developed country to not include outpatient pharmaceutical coverage in its statutory plan. While well intentioned, provincial plans offer a porous safety net that lets select populations fall through while only marginally helping others in need. Given Canada's lack of cost sharing for any other medically necessary services, this omission is striking and problematic. Efforts to remedy the situation have consistently failed.

Pharmaceutical pricing also remains tied to a reference pricing mechanism intended as an incentive for pharmaceutical companies to invest in Canada that failed. Although external reference pricing has been used successfully in other countries, such as Norway and Taiwan, tying pharmaceutical prices to 7 of the *most expensive* countries in the world seems unjustifiable. The creation of the pCPA and CDR to aggregate all provincial buying power to increase the leverage in price negotiations are strong steps in the right direction, and the 2020 reforms have eliminated the 2 highest paying countries. Only time will tell whether the set of 11 countries selected will satisfactorily curb pharmaceutical spending. The potential for stronger central regulation of pricing is also palpable. With growing pharmaceutical expenditures across all developed nations, the pressure for further reform will only continue to gain steam.

Third, Canada's health system remains largely fragmented as a result of its provincial model and strongly independent physicians. Primary care physicians' strong role and their incorporation into interprofessional practice is a strong step in the right direction, but networks remain underdeveloped. Continued experimentation with alternative payment models for primary care providers—and specialists—will eventually have more success and lead to a higher quality of chronic care management.

Fourth, the hesitancy to transition to activity-based payments for hospitals has helped perpetuate significant wait times for many elective procedures. Although wait times in Canada are often overblown by conservative commentators and media in the US, they do exist and can be a problem. Broader adoption of activity-based payments and quality-based incentives could help improve hospital efficiency, decrease wait times, and, potentially, improve quality.

Finally, as with other countries, Canada's health system has yet to figure out how best to finance long-term care for its citizens and for patients with mental illness.

CHAPTER THREE

UNITED KINGDOM

A 1948 leaflet entitled "Your New National Health Service" informed the British public that on July 5, the National Health Service (NHS) "will provide you with all medical, dental, and nursing care. Everyone—rich or poor, man, woman or child—can use it or any part of it. There are no charges, except for a few special items. There are no insurance qualifications. But it is not a 'charity.' You are all paying for it, mainly as taxpayers, and it will relieve your money worries in times of illness."

Over the last 70 years, this pledge has largely been honored. The NHS has certainly faced its fair share of challenges: most recently, growing shortages of physicians, nurses, and other health care personnel; the deteriorating condition of its hospitals and other facilities; the failure of a seamless system-wide introduction of electronic records in hospitals; disagreements about how much to pay for drugs and other new technologies; and a lack of funding for long-term care.

Despite these and other controversies, the NHS retains widespread public support and pride. Indeed, NHS doctors and nurses dancing in hospital beds were featured in the celebrations of the 2012 London Olympics. The British public wants to improve the system by investing more funds rather than scrapping the government system altogether and expanding the private sector.

Reviled as the epitome of inefficient "big government" health care by some and praised as a model of egalitarian care delivery by others—perhaps no other health care system in the world has been as exhaustively studied and debated as that of the United Kingdom. Much of the discussion about the NHS today rehashes old arguments. However, as more and more countries *consider shifting toward universal coverage, the NHS remains relevant as a prime example of the progress—and pitfalls—afforded by the largest single-payer and socialized health care system in the world.*

HISTORY

In 1911, nearly a century after the creation of the United Kingdom of Great Britain and Ireland, Chancellor David Lloyd George introduced the first national insurance scheme with health benefits as part of a campaign for wider social reforms. Prior to this legislation health care was considered a luxury, available only to the wealthy unless one was able to access free care through charity, a teaching hospital, or the socially stigmatized Poor Law, which provided local welfare services to the impoverished and almshouses to care for the sick. Lloyd George's legislation deducted a small amount of an employee's wage, combining it with contributions from employers and the state, in order to provide health insurance to wage-earning male workers. These workers could then choose a primary care physician from a select panel of local providers. As in Germany, this system did not initially cover workers' families or other non-workers.

Because only the employed were entitled to health care under the National Insurance Act, the system remained a hodgepodge of private, federal, and charity insurance plans until World War II. In 1939, UK hospitals banded together in expectation of a flood of civilian casualties from World War II. An Emergency Hospital Service was introduced in order to provide free treatment to any victims, including war evacuees. Additionally, the government expanded its infant, child, and maternity services during the war. A political consensus emerged that, in order to coordinate the hospitals and this increasing volume of health services, a kind of national health service was needed.

By 1940, the Labour and Conservative Parties had entered into a coalition and, in 1941, announced a new committee that would survey the UK's social insurance and health care services. In 1942, the results of this survey along with subsequent recommendations were published in the Beveridge Report. The report addressed the "five giants on the road of reconstruction . . . Want, Disease, Ignorance, Squalor, and Idleness." Among other recommendations, the Report proposed a flat-rate universal contribution in exchange for a standardized set of universal health benefits and social services. Upon its publication, the British Institute of Public Opinion found that 95% of the public had heard of the Report and that "there was overwhelming agreement that the plan should be put into effect."

In the postwar 1945 election, Labour won a landslide victory by running on a platform that included promises to enact Beveridge's 5 "giants." The Labour Party's newly appointed minister of health, Aneurin Bevan, proposed creating a nationalized health care system. At the time Bevan's proposal faced immense criticism. He was opposed by the Conservative Party, the British Medical Association (BMA), and even Labour members of Parliament. Nevertheless, Bevan did have the support of the Royal Colleges and ultimately won over the support of BMA physicians by cutting several deals with the association, which he described as "stuffing their mouths with gold." Two elements from Bevan's deal survive to this day: hospital-based doctors continue to do private work on top of their salaried employment, and general practitioners (GPs) are independent contractors rather than salaried providers.

Through Bevan's tenacity, the National Health Services Act was granted royal assent in November 1946 and came into effect on July 5, 1948. The Act established the National Health Service (NHS) as a national system in England and Wales, accountable to the minister of health. A separate NHS was created for Scotland, accountable to the secretary of state for Scotland, under the National Health Service (Scotland) Act of 1947. A similar service was established in Northern Ireland in 1948.

The NHS aimed to offer comprehensive health services that are free at the point of care and provided by public hospitals and primary care physicians (general practitioners, or GPs). However, the Act did retain power to charge for expensive medical appliances, home-based care, dental care, eye care, and services to privately paying patients. A representative Central Health Services Council advised the minister of health on any health-related matters. County councils and boroughs were designated as local health authorities, responsible for ambulance services, local health centers, and public health functions. Most hospital services were coordinated locally by hospital management committees, though overall hospital services were under the control of the minister of health. Responsibility for mental health care, previously under the supervision of the Board of Control for Lunacy and Mental Deficiency, was also transferred to the minister of health.

The 1950s and 1960s were focused primarily on the modernization of facilities and realignment of care to fit the NHS model. In 1952, small patient co-pays were introduced for prescriptions and dental care, a decision Bevan so opposed that he quit the cabinet in protest. In 1954, a Royal Commission was tasked with investigating the state of care for people with mental health conditions. It called for the integration of mental health more fully into the NHS and the expansion of local authorities' responsibilities to offer mental health services. In 1962, then minister for health Enoch Powell launched *The Hospital Plan for England and Wales*, which pledged £500 million over 10 years to develop a program of hospital building and improvements. In 1968, the Ministry of Health merged with the Ministry of Social Security to form the Department of Health and Social Security.

In 1973, the National Health Services Reorganization Act was passed. The Act sought to unify health and local authority services and resulted in the reorganization of the NHS into 14 regional health authorities and 90 area health authorities. The Act required area health authorities to set up family practitioner committees to provide general medical services and community health councils to act on behalf of the public and patients. In 1982, the NHS was again restructured. The area level health authorities were abolished, leaving 192 district health authorities that reported to regional health authorities.

In 1990, the Conservative government passed the National Health Service and Community Care Act, which introduced an internal market for the supply of health care, separating the public-payer functions from care provision. The idea was for the government to become a payer for health care, thereby encouraging public hospitals and community health care organizations to compete. The Act also created GP fundholding, which essentially offered the option for GP practices with at least 11,000 patients to become capitated payers themselves. These practices could then apply for an NHS budget to cover their staff and outpatient and inpatient services costs.

In 1997, Tony Blair and the Labour Party regained power partially on a pledge to reform the NHS. The Labour Party subsequently passed the Health Act of 1999, which established the Commission for Healthcare Improvement, an independent inspection body for the NHS, responsible for monitoring and reviewing the quality of health care services. That same year the National Institute for Care Excellence (NICE)—later renamed the National Institute for Health and Care Excellence—was established and entrusted with reducing the variation in the quality of NHS services through evidence-based guidelines and quality standards for health treatments and services as well as with ensuring that the most clinically and cost-effective treatments and drugs were made readily available. In 2000, the NHS Plan aimed to improve access to care, decrease wait times, recruit more physicians and nurses, and build more hospitals. In 2002, a white paper entitled "Shifting the Balance of Power" set out the devolution of responsibilities to the front line. The government abolished both regional and district health authorities, replacing them with strategic health authorities (SHAs) and 303 primary care trusts (PCTs) that assume responsibility for 80% of the NHS budget.

In 2003, the NHS was once again reorganized, with the establishment of NHS foundation trusts and 2 new bodies to regulate health care—the Commission for Healthcare Audit and Inspection (CHAI), replacing the Commission for Healthcare Improvement, and the Commission for Social Care Inspection. The CHAI was responsible for monitoring and inspecting all NHS health care providers as well as measuring and publishing NHS performance data. The Commission for Social Care Inspection assumed responsibility for the review of social care organizations.

In late 2008, during the global financial crisis, the first austerity measures were introduced to address the budget deficit and to lower the national debt. Although the NHS was largely protected, spending on mental health was curtailed. In 2009, the NHS Constitution was published, outlining the rights and responsibilities of patients and providers and enshrining the right of patient choice. Also in 2009, the Care Quality Commission (CQC) was established as an independent regulator of all health and social services in England, assuming the functions of CHAI, the Commission for Social Care Inspection, and the Mental Health Act Commission.

In 2011, a bill was introduced proposing to abolish SHAs and PCTs, create a new national NHS Commissioning Board and local clinical commissioning groups (CCGs), and establish a new patient-rights group, Healthwatch England. Despite fierce Labour Party opposition, it was ultimately passed.

The Health and Social Care Act of 2012 defines the current structure of the NHS. The NHS Commissioning Board—now referred to as NHS England—was responsible for authorizing 211 clinical commissioning groups (CCGs) across England and allocating funds to them. These CCGs are composed of local primary care practices and are led by an elected governing body made up of primary care physicians; other clinical providers, including a nurse and a specialist consultant; and members of the public. They "commission," or pay for, health care services for their local populations. NHS England oversees CCGs and is responsible for commissioning primary care and specialized services for patients across England.

In 2014, NHS England published the "Five Year Forward View," setting out a direction for the NHS to improve health, care, quality, and efficiency. NHS Chief Executive Simon Stevens described this as a road map for "triple integration of primary and specialist care, of health and social care, and of physical and mental health care."

In October 2016, local councils and NHS organizations set out to meet the long-term health and social needs of the population. They created Sustainability and Transformation Partnerships (STPs) in 44 local areas covering all of England. Partially informed by the 2014 new models of care program, the STPs represent what Sir Malcom Grant, former chairman of NHS England, called "the biggest shift toward integration of care of any health economy in the world, breaking down the division between physical and mental health provision."

In 2018, 70 years after the NHS was founded, UK Prime Minister Theresa May announced that NHS England's revenue funding would grow by an average of 3.4% in real terms over the following 5 years, constituting a $26.6 billion USD (£20.5 billion) increase over inflation by 2023–2024. This represented a departure from recent years of funding increases, which averaged 2.2%, against the long-term average of 3.7% per year since 1948. In response, in January 2019 NHS England published the "NHS Long Term Plan," which delineated service improvements over the next decade. The Plan had 3 aims: to create a new service model for patients, focusing on increasing investments in primary, community, and mental health services; to establish integrated care systems that would bring together local health and social care organizations; and to encourage a shift toward digital care. Each integrated care system operates similarly to an HMO in the United States and must decide how to plan and deliver care for their local populations. Simultaneously, a new contract was agreed upon between the BMA and NHS England regarding how GPs deliver care.

Ultimately the NHS has endured because it is immensely popular because, as one provider we interviewed explained, "Health is too important an issue to pass reform on without public support. In England this has meant enormous protection for the NHS."

The NHS is made up of 4 devolved health systems: England, Scotland, Wales, and Northern Ireland. The NHS model still broadly applies to all 4 countries. Given that the UK is a country of 66 million people, nearly 56 million (85%) of whom reside in England, England's health care system is the primary focus of this chapter.

COVERAGE

Mandatory Insurance

The NHS covers all citizens and residents of the United Kingdom; it is a single-payer socialized system. Patients can choose their primary care physician or GP, who acts as a gatekeeper and first point of contact. A patient may then be referred to specialists and hospital care if needed. A UK resident can receive health care anywhere in the UK, not just within their county or country of residence.

The NHS legislation ensures the delivery of necessary health services, though no explicit, positive list of covered services exists except for the drugs and new technologies appraised and ultimately approved by the NICE. The ministers of health in each country along with their respective health boards decide what services will be funded. As of 2019, each of the 191 English CCGs decide the actual services delivered in England. In general, the covered services are relatively comprehensive, including inpatient and outpatient hospital care, care in physician offices,

Figure 1. Health Care Coverage (United Kingdom)

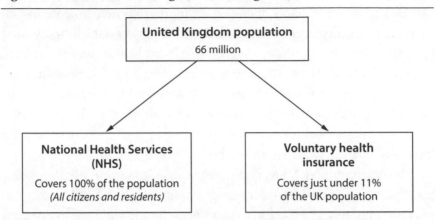

prescription drugs, mental health care, palliative care, some long-term care, rehabilitation care, and dental and vision care. However, because CCGs must make coverage decisions based on local budgetary needs, some areas end up covering services that others do not. Some patients have complained of such "postcode lotteries." NHS England oversees CCGs and remains responsible for commissioning—that is, paying for—primary care and highly specialized services, but CCGs have either joint or full responsibility for these. NHS England is also responsible for commissioning a range of public health services, such as immunizations and screenings, in conjunction with the Department of Health and Social Care (DHSC) as well as Public Health England.

Because the purpose of the NHS is to provide health care free at the point of care, any resident can use NHS services without having to pay. Nonresidents can receive emergency care and primary care for free, but they must pay for any subsequent care.

GPs provide a variety of primary care services under the NHS, including routine diagnostic tests, chronic care management, minor surgeries, referrals to specialists, outpatient prescription drugs, preventive and public health services, and family planning. In order for a patient to receive specialty care, they must first either be referred by their GP or admitted to a hospital due to an emergency. Emergency care services, whether provided in urgent care centers, hospital ERs, or emergency visits to GPs, are also provided free of charge.

Voluntary Private Insurance

Just under 11% of the UK population, about 7 million people, has some form of voluntary, private health care insurance; over 50% of privately insured beneficiaries reside in England. These plans can cover condition-specific care, such as chemotherapy for cancer, or elective therapies and diagnostic tests. About 82% receive their voluntary, private insurance from their employer, while 18% purchase their plans individually. Unlike other countries, the UK has seen a plateau in the percentage of people choosing private insurance, largely because of a boost in NHS funding. There are currently 9 main private health care insurers—BUPA, AXA PPP Healthcare, Aviva, Simply Health, Benenden, Allianz, PruHealth, Saga, and CS Healthcare. BUPA has the largest share of the market, covering just over 1 million people.

In these private plans the insurers charge premiums based on what services are covered, the risk of the patient, and the desired profit margins. The Prudential Regulation Authority regulates private insurers, and the Financial Conduct Authority acts as a consumer protector, making sure consumers in the private market are treated fairly.

FINANCING

In 2017, the UK spent about $260 billion USD (£197.4 billion), or 9.6% of the GDP, on health care. This translates to just under $4,000 USD (£2,989) per capita. Of the G7 countries, the UK has the 2nd-lowest percentage of GDP spent on health care, significantly less than the nearly 18% spent by the United States and the 12.2% spent by Switzerland. Only Italy spends a smaller percent of GDP on health care.

The whole NHS had a budget of $160 billion USD (£121 billion), or 61% of total spending, while NHS England had a budget of $140 billion USD (£107 billion), which accounted for 54% of total national spending ($148 billion USD, £114 billion) in 2018–2019. The largest nongovernmental expense in 2017 was out-of-pocket costs, including household spending on health care goods and services, such as residential and home-based long-term care provided by the private sector, totaling 16% of total spending, or $40 billion USD (£31 billion). The next-largest

Figure 2. Financing Health Care (United Kingdom)

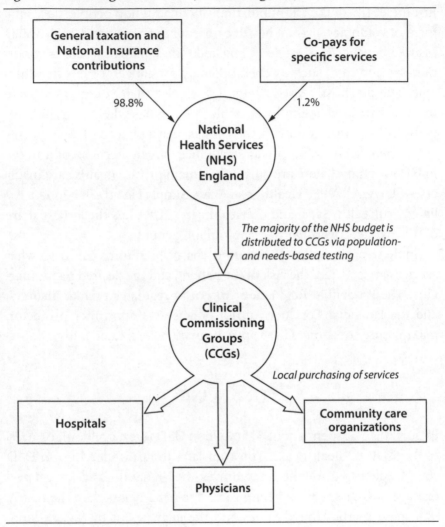

contributor was private health insurance, at 3% of health care spending, or $7.8 billion USD (£6.0 billion).

Mandatory Health Insurance

The UK Treasury sets the total budget for the DHSC in England, subject to parliamentary ratification. The NHS England budget exists within the total DHSC budget, and the NHS chief executive is then responsible for executing the budget of NHS England. The NHS allocates funds to the 191 CCGs in England based on population and health needs. In their respective geographic areas, the CCGs plan and pay for elective hospital care, primary care, community care, emergency care, and mental health care. In 2019, CCGs in England managed $104 billion USD (£80 billion). Separate allocations purchase specialized health care services, primary health care, and military health care services.

Almost 99% of NHS funding comes from general taxation and National Insurance (NI) contributions, with the remaining covered by co-payments on specific services such as dental care. NI contributions are income-linked payroll deductions. Those making less than a certain amount—$666 USD (£512) per month in 2019–2020—do not have to pay for NI but still receive the benefits. In 2019–2020, persons making between $930 and $5,400 USD (between £719 and £4,167) per month had 12% of their earnings deducted, and those who earned above $5,400 USD (£4,167) a month had a lower contribution rate, with just 2% of their earnings deducted. The remainder of funding comes from patient co-pays; charging overseas visitors for the cost of NHS care; and providing care to privately insured patients.

Voluntary, Private Supplemental Insurance

Most private health care insurance plans are offered by employers as part of employees' overall benefits packages. The contributions may be based on individual risk, community risk, or group risk, depending on the insurer. The average annual premium for a private health insurance plan is $1,865 USD (£1,435). Little public data exists on the variances in contributions by employers or employees for private plans.

Cost Sharing

Under the NHS there are no health care premiums, and almost all medical care is free at the point of service. However, there are small co-pays for certain services. In England, dental care incurs a co-pay ranging from $27 to $317 USD (£20.60 to £244.30), depending on the complexity of the service. Patients may also pay for private dental care through voluntary, private health insurance plans. In addition, approximately 10% of prescription drugs in England have a flat charge of $11.55 USD (£9). Children under the age of 16, adults over the age of 60, and those who have a specified medical condition, are pregnant, or recently had a baby are exempt from paying the charge for prescriptions.

Overall, nearly 90% of prescription drugs distributed in 2012 were free for patients. There are no prescription drug co-pays in Scotland, Wales, or Northern Ireland.

In 2016, out-of-pocket spending totaled $40 billion USD (£31.0 billion). It represented the largest area of spending outside of government-financed insurance. However, less than 1.5% of households have faced a threat of impoverishment due to out-of-pocket health care costs.

Long-Term Care

In 2017, the UK spent $63 billion USD (£48.2 billion) on long-term care. In the UK, the financing of long-term care is divided into 2 categories— financing for health care services, including assistance with activities of daily living such as eating and walking, and financing for social services, such as managing finances. For health care services 66% of total spending on long-term care was financed by the government, with another 31% financed by out-of-pocket payments, and the remaining 4% financed by nonprofit institutions. For social services 48% was financed by the government, 40% by nonprofit institutions, and 12% by out-of-pocket expenditures.

Long-term care spending is jointly financed by the NHS and the private sector. Local governments' funding of the majority of long-term care has dropped significantly. If a patient requires long-term medical care, the NHS provides that care for free. However, local governments fund personal assistance or custodial care. In England, a patient is not eligible for financial assistance for personal assistance or custodial care unless they have $30,000 USD (£23,250) or less in savings. For care in a nursing home, the value of the patient's home is counted toward the $30,000 USD (£23,250) threshold. Even then, the patient may still need to pay a share of the costs, depending on the area of England in which they reside. A patient has the option to delay paying their share of costs until after their death, at which time the government collects the payment from either the patient's estate or the sale of their home. For patients making above the threshold, the charge may range up to the full cost of care. Plans to cap out-of-pocket spending on long-term care at $94,000 USD (£72,000) were delayed until 2020, as the government could not decide how to fund the cap.

In 2017, long-term care was a major campaign issue. Prior to the election, Theresa May proposed changing the income cutoff from $30,000 to $100,000 USD (£23,250 to £130,000), including the value of patients' homes regardless of area of residence. Her proposal was expected to reduce out-of-pocket costs for most patients but would increase costs for homeowners. Dubbed the "dementia tax," the proposal was very unpopular. Taking note of May's disastrous proposal, Boris Johnson pledged to "protect you or your grandparents from the fear of having to sell your house to pay for the costs of care." For now the financing and affordability of long-term care remains highly controversial, with no clear solution in sight.

Public Health

In 2016–2017, the UK spent $13 billion USD (£10.3 billion) on preventive and public health care. Government expenditures accounted for 76% of total spending ($10.1 billion USD, or £7.8 billion), and out-of-pocket expenditures totaled 13% of spending ($1.7 billion USD, or £1.3 billion), with other sources, including private insurance, making up the rest.

Mental Health

In 2018–2019, NHS England spent $16 billion USD (£12.5 billion) on mental health care in England. The recipient of the largest portion of mental health funding was CCGs, with the remainder going toward more specialized mental health services. In 2015, the Mental Health Investment Standard (MHIS) was introduced to require CCGs to increase their investment in local mental health services to a level at least in line with the overall increase in money available to them. By 2018, all CCGs in England had met the MHIS, such that 13.9% of local health care spending went toward mental health care services. According to the NHS Long Term Plan, mental health investment will be at least $2.95 billion USD (£2.3 billion) higher per year by 2023–2024.

PAYMENT

In 2017, the UK spent $260 billion USD (£197.4 billion) on health care. The largest spending category was for curative and rehabilitative care

(65% of total expenditures), followed by long-term care (16%); medical goods, such as drugs, glasses, and wheelchairs (10%); and preventive care (5%).

Hospitals

In 2017, 49% of all government spending on health care was for care in hospitals, including care provided by hospital-based specialists. Beginning in 2003 hospitals in England began to be paid using a model similar to the US DRG system. Known as Payment by Results (PBR), the system links individual case groups, called Healthcare Resource Groups (HRGs), to specific reimbursement rates set by NHS England and NHS Improvement. If there are various episodes of care within one stay, the dominant episode is coded for. National average episode costs (self-reported by physicians) are adjusted for any technological innovations and for the market forces factor (MFF), which considers variations in cost by location in order to determine payments.

CCGs purchase care from trusts, reimbursing them for the care based on the PBR rates. The PBR system began by paying for elective inpatient procedures and now has expanded to cover 60% of all hospital activities. The remainder of hospital income comes from other activities, such as mental health services, health education, and research and training funds.

PBR has increasingly been criticized for its fee-for-service model, which incentivizes volume over quality and value. In response, commissioning of health care services in the UK is moving toward greater use of capitation and other alternative payment arrangements.

Payment for public hospital capital costs, such as buildings, equipment, and technology, is covered under the DHSC's capital budget and by providers' depreciation reserves.

In addition to public hospitals, there are also approximately 550 private hospitals and nearly 600 private clinics in the UK. Private institutions offer services either unavailable in the NHS or NHS services, such as bariatric or hip replacement surgeries, in which demand outstrips the public service's ability to provide and, consequently, have long waiting times. In England a patient may choose to receive an NHS-covered service at a private hospital so long as the private hospital can perform the procedure at NHS prices. Private institutions must register with both

Figure 3. Payment to Public Hospitals (United Kingdom)

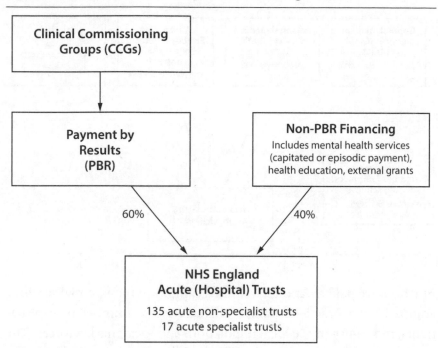

the CQC and NHS Improvement, but their charges to private patients are not regulated. A quarter of private hospitals' revenues come from NHS referrals; the remainder of care they provide is paid for either by private health insurance or by patients out of pocket.

Physician Payment

In 2017, 25% of all government spending on health care was for care delivered in ambulatory settings. Of this, $17.5 billion USD (£13.5 billion) was spent on services provided by GPs in their offices—or surgeries, as they are known in the UK. In addition, $3.8 billion USD (£2.9 billion) of government spending went to dental care, and $29 billion USD (£22.3 billion) was spent on care provided by other ambulatory providers. Under the NHS, specialists and hospital-based physicians are employees of the NHS, while GPs remain private practitioners who are paid by the NHS for their services.

GPs can be paid one of 3 ways. The predominant mechanism is through the General Medical Services (GMS) contract, under which GP

Figure 4. Payment to Ambulatory Physicians (United Kingdom)

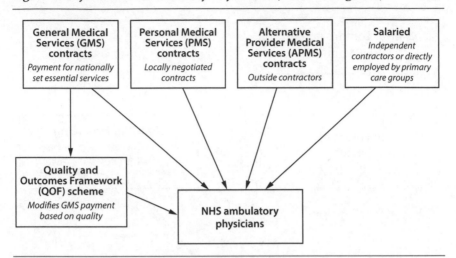

practices are paid a national weighted capitation for essential services, adjusted for a practice's patient characteristics, number of new patients, morbidity of the local population, and local market forces. The GMS is negotiated between the NHS and the British Medical Association. Practices can also agree to provide "enhanced services" in order to receive supplementary payments. To be paid extra for these "enhanced services," practices may need to enter and report data manually. In 2015, 62.5% of primary care practices operated under GMS contracts.

One alternative to being paid through GMS contracts is Personal Medical Services (PMS) contracts. PMS contracts are negotiated locally between NHS England and a practice. They offer more flexibility than national GMS contracts, as a practice can negotiate what services they will offer and the financial reimbursement for those services. Under a PMS contract a practice is paid a baseline sum for essential services, which is adjusted based on local population risk, and this may be supplemented with payments for enhanced services. In 2019, 26.3% of GP practices operated under PMS contracts.

There also exists a 3rd payment mechanism, Alternative Provider Medical Services (APMS) contracts, which are for primary care services provided by outside contractors, like international health companies. In 2018–2019, 2.3% of GP practices operated under APMS contracts.

GPs may choose to be salaried. These GPs are either employees of independent contractor practices or are directly employed by primary care organizations.

The NHS operates several different payment programs to incentivize quality improvement. Primary care physician practices may choose to participate in the Quality and Outcomes Framework (QOF), a voluntary payment structure that modifies GMS payments based on quality of care, primarily for chronic conditions. Practices are scored using a "quality scorecard," which can award a maximum of 1,000 points for performance on indicators such as patient education, medication management, and appropriate screenings. Data on quality is automatically extracted from a practice's electronic records. In its first year, the program was approximately $200 million USD (£155 million) more expensive than anticipated, as many practices achieved maximum performance that year. As such, the maximum percentage of practice income tied to QOF was subsequently decreased from 25% to 15%. Critics of the QOF suggest that it has eroded the relationship between physicians and the government. Dr. Donald Berwick reflected that "it was a dreadful period; doctors became convinced that they should do whatever the QOF says to be paid."

The standard contract the NHS uses for the majority of its commissioned services includes another pay-for-performance scheme, the Commissioning for Quality and Innovation (CQUIN). The CQUIN ties a certain percentage of provider income to quality improvement performance. The CQUIN pays 2.5% of a provider's income; at least 0.5% of this is tied to the provider accomplishing national quality improvement goals, with the remainder dependent on the provider accomplishing locally determined goals. Yet another pay-for-performance scheme is Best Practice Tariffs (BPTs), which were introduced in 2010 to incentivize optimal care according to guidelines. BPTs now cover over 20 areas of health care, ranging from managing acute stroke to diabetic ketoacidosis. This model includes a base payment for hospital admissions, plus additional payments for executing the best practices. For example, providers treating a hip fracture are paid a base rate of $5,620 USD (£4,326), with a potential total payment of $7,360 USD (£5,662) if the providers achieved all best-practice goals.

Most recently the NHS established Primary Care Networks (PCNs), which are organized around GPs that serve "natural communities of around 30,000 to 50,000" patients. In addition to GPs, PCNs will have funds to hire physician assistants, pharmacists, physical therapists and other health providers who can offer integrated, pro-active care to avoid exacerbations and other medical problems, not just respond to patients' illnesses. Payment to PCNs will be based on contract as well as shared savings if they reduce emergency room use, hospitalizations, and unnecessary office visits.

Mental Health

The NHS, local authorities, and private organizations all provide mental health services. Under the NHS mental health services are primarily purchased by CCGs. The NHS accounts for more than 80% of secondary mental health care, most provided by mental health trusts. These trusts provide health and social services to persons with mental health conditions. A patient may access a mental health trust through a GP referral or an admission to a hospital. There are currently 60 mental health trusts in the UK. Local authorities primarily fund housing and social services for people with mental health conditions.

In November 2016 the NHS published new guidelines for paying for mental care. Providers and commissioners can now choose between a capitated payment or an episodic payment.

Long-Term Care

In the UK, services are split depending on whether they cover long-term health needs, like support with activities of daily living (ADLs), which include bathing or eating, or social services, such as shopping or managing finances. NHS covers health needs, while local authorities generally cover social service needs. For patients qualifying for nursing care, their local CCG pays a direct contribution to the institution to reimburse them for the services provided. In England the standard reimbursement rate was $205 USD (£158.16) per week in 2019.

Local authorities are required to assess patients' needs for long-term care according to a national framework. With the exception of some home care and short-term rehabilitation services, long-term care is both needs and means tested. Full state support for home care is only available to patients with less than $18,500 USD (£14,250) in assets who also have high levels of need, with a sliding scale of support provided up to $30,000 USD (£23,250) in assets.

Government payments for institutional care have decreased in recent years, leaving much of the burden of long-term care to the private sector and even to patients themselves. Today some 95,000 people in residential and nursing homes must pay for their own care. Local government funding for long-term care continues to drop, even as the UK's population ages. Government projections estimate that within the next 50 years there will be an additional 8.6 million people ages 65 years and above, a population roughly the size of London.

Public Health

In England the DHSC, NHS England, and Public Health England coordinate public health services. The DHSC develops overall government policies on public health. NHS England is responsible for immunization programs and national screening programs. Public Health England is an agency within the DHSC that runs the national health protection service and advises local authorities on how to improve their local public health.

In 2012, the Health and Social Care Act established Health and Wellbeing Boards to determine how to best meet the public health needs of their communities.

DELIVERY OF HEALTH CARE SERVICES

Hospital Care

As of 2017 there were 1,920 hospitals in the UK, of which 1,370 were public and about 550 were private. The NHS has a relatively low number of hospital beds and high occupancy rates. In 2015, there were only 2.6 beds per 1,000 persons, well below the EU average of 5.1 beds per 1,000 persons. While the average length of stay has been decreasing, reaching a low of 7 days in 2015, occupancy rates remain at nearly 85%, the 2nd highest in the EU. High occupancy rates suggest that the NHS has little flexibility in dealing with increases in demands from, for example, a bad influenza season.

Publicly owned hospitals are organized within either an NHS trust or a foundation trust. There are currently 72 NHS trusts and 150 foundation trusts, many of which encompass multiple hospitals. NHS Improvement—made up of Monitor and the NHS Trust Development Authority and now combined with NHS England—regulates and oversees trusts and foundation trusts.

Patients in the UK have the right to choose both their hospital and their specialist so long as they obtain a referral from their GP.

Ambulatory Care

In the UK, primary care physicians—GPs—dentists, and pharmacists provide ambulatory care. Patients have free choice of the GP they must register with. Primary care visits serve both as the first point of contact and as gatekeeping for specialist care. Treatment for most common conditions and injuries can be obtained via primary care. GPs provide diagnostic tests, physical examinations, management of chronic conditions, vaccinations, drug prescriptions, basic life support when necessary, and referrals for urgent, specialist, and mental health services.

There are over 300 million GP practice appointments each year in England. A GP office will generally be run by a multidisciplinary team, which can include nurses, midwives, and pharmacists.

Hospital emergency departments provide emergency care. In some areas, urgent care centers or minor-injury units, which can be led by either nurses or GPs, handle less serious cases. Telephone advice for patients with urgent but not life-threatening conditions is available 24 hours a day through the hotline NHS 111.

Electronic Health Records

NHS England has been promoting the digitalization of health care, though the results are inconsistent. Innovations in the primary care sector are generally viewed as a success story. In the 1990s, practices began digitalizing, using software written specifically for them. Today 100% of GP practices are computerized. Since 2015, all GP practices are required to offer patients the option to schedule appointments and order prescriptions online. As of 2016 patients have a right to access their detailed electronic health record, which includes diagnoses, treatments, test results, medications, and immunizations, but not clinician notes.

Transitioning the hospital sector to electronic health records has been more challenging. In 2003, the government launched a massive program designed to computerize all NHS trusts (the National Programme for IT, NPfIT). A decade later, the program was disbanded, viewed as an example of the flaws of an overly centralized approach to a massively complex IT implementation. In recent years, the NHS has enacted several programs designed to achieve full computerization of the system, investing in training digitally facile clinicians and promoting digital interoperability across the hospital and primary care sectors. The complete digitalization of the NHS will not be possible until at least 2023. According to Richard Murray, chief executive of the English health charity The King's Fund, the resistance to transitioning to EHRs "is more of a cultural issue—there's a lot of concerns about data security. We're making progress locally, but not nationally."

Mental Health

GPs provide the first line of contact for mental health care, as they are expected to assess a patient's mental health status. When services exceed the clinical abilities of the GP, the patient can be referred for counseling for psychological therapy and/or drug and alcohol abuse to a local health center or a mental health specialist. Community mental health is often provided in teams, with GPs and community staff working together to provide services. With a primary care referral, a patient may access NHS mental health services for free. Community-based organizations may also provide mental health services, while mental health hospitals provide inpatient mental health services. The private sector provides about a quarter of NHS-funded inpatient mental health care.

A patient who needs mental health services has the legal right to choose any provider or care team able to offer such care. In England the CQC, an independent regulator of health providers, also has a specific responsibility to protect patients' basic human rights while they are being treated under the Mental Health Act.

While mental health remains a priority for the NHS, there are provider shortages that seem to be getting worse. In 2018, 2,000 mental health staff left their positions each month. Consequently, one in 10 mental health posts are unfilled. "It's fantastic what we've done in mental health," Mr. Murray explained, "but now we need to make good on our promise. We need to get more mental health providers."

Long-Term Care

In 2016, the Sustainability and Transformation Partnerships (STPs) were created to promote coordination between NHS and local authorities in order to improve health and care for patients. In 2018, 14 STPs evolved into integrated care systems (ICS), where NHS and local authorities are jointly responsible for budgeting and delivering health care and social services. The goal is to have ICSs covering all of England by April 2021 in the hopes of stronger care coordination.

Local authorities are required to assess the needs of patients who may need social services and provide such services if the patient is deemed eligible. However, there are no national standards for eligibility; it is up to the discretion of local authorities and often depends on year-to-year budget demands. Unsurprisingly, there exists wide variation in availability and quality of long-term care. Once a patient is eligible for long-term care, a social worker makes the necessary in-home or facility-based care arrangements. In England all long-term care providers are regulated by the CQC based on DHSC standards.

Preventive Care

The NHS covers, free of charge, a wide range of preventive screening and immunization services, including screenings during pregnancy and for newborn babies, cancer screenings, and diabetic eye screenings. Primary care physicians cover most of these NHS authorized preventive services. The majority of the decisions regarding what preventive services are covered are made at the local level by CCGs or Health and Wellbeing Boards.

Quality Controls

The quality of care provided in NHS England is measured primarily by 3 bodies. First, the CQC regulates all health and adult social services in England, undertaking regular inspections. All providers must register with the CQC, which sets national quality standards and may investigate any providers who do not adhere to these guidelines. The CQC also rates hospital inspection results and has the power to close down poorly performing hospitals.

Second, NICE provides quality and effectiveness guidelines for the most common conditions in primary, secondary, and social services. NICE has also established standardized recommendations regarding wait times for cancer, elective, and emergency treatment. Finally, NICE is responsible for analyzing the clinical and cost effectiveness of pharmaceuticals and other health technologies.

Third, information regarding the quality, location, and organization of services is published on www.nhs.uk, a website run by NHS Digital.

The proportions of NHS hospitals independently rated as "good" or "outstanding" doubled in the 5 years prior to 2019.

Patient Satisfaction

In 2018, The King's Fund asked NHS patients: "How satisfied are you with the way the NHS runs nowadays?" Of the sample surveyed, 53% were "very" or "quite" satisfied. This represents a 3% satisfaction drop from the previous year and the lowest satisfaction level since 2007, though this rate is still almost double that of 15 years before. Those over 65 years of age were happier with the NHS (61% satisfied) than younger persons (51% satisfied for ages 18 to 64). Patients were overall satisfied with their quality of care, the fact that care is free at the point of service, the variety of services available, and the behavior of NHS staff. Patients were overall dissatisfied because of long wait times, staff shortages, a lack of funding, and a perception that NHS funding is being wasted. Recent austerity budgeting under the Conservatives may be to blame for the lackluster support. "When you ask people what they think about the NHS," Mr. Murray explains, "they like the system but blame the government."

With respect to wait times, a recent NHS England survey found that 20% of patients seeking a primary care appointment must wait at least one week, a significant increase over the past 5 years. Additionally, 11% of patients are unable to secure an appointment when they first try.

In June 2019, the Public Accounts Committee published a report stating that 50% of NHS and foundation trusts did not meet the NHS maximum wait times of 18 weeks for elective treatment, and under 40%

met the 62-day standard wait time for cancer treatment. However, the median wait for planned surgery is under 10 weeks and has fallen dramatically since 2000. Wait times at emergency departments are also lagging; 84.4% of patients are seen, admitted, and treated or sent home within 4 hours of arrival, significantly below the NHS target of 95%.

PHARMACEUTICAL COVERAGE AND PRICE CONTROLS

The NHS currently spends around $24 billion USD (£18 billion) on drugs annually. This amounts to about $360 USD (£275) per capita—one of the lowest levels among all developed countries.

Market Access, Coverage Determination, and Price Setting

In the UK, the regulation of manufacturing, marketing, and pricing of pharmaceuticals is all decided at the national level. All drugs are licensed for marketing by the Medicines and Healthcare products Regulatory Agency (MHRA), an agency within the Department of Health, like the US Food and Drug Administration. In determining whether to permit the marketing of a drug, the MHRA authorizes clinical trials of drugs, assesses the results of those trials, and monitors the safety and quality of available drugs. It can also remove drugs from circulation if it deems them unsafe or ineffective.

There are 3 types of pharmaceuticals available in the UK, as delineated by the Medicines Act of 1968: (1) drugs sold on the General Sale List, which can be sold over the counter; (2) drugs dispensed only by pharmacists; and (3) drugs available only with a prescription.

The first step in establishing a price in the UK is approval by the National Institute for Health and Care Excellence (NICE). NICE is an official body that is operationally independent from but accountable to the Department of Health and Social Care. Using available research from pharmaceutical companies, peer-reviewed publications, professional organizations, patient advocacy groups, and others, NICE assesses the clinical benefits and cost effectiveness of the drug for a specific indication. It determines the incremental cost effectiveness ratio for a drug expressed as dollars per quality-adjusted life year (QALY). After this

Figure 5. Regulation of Pharmaceutical Prices (United Kingdom)

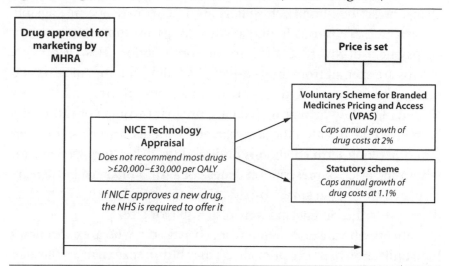

assessment, the Technology Appraisal Committee (TAC) evaluates the evidence. The TAC is composed of NHS employees, academic researchers, pharmaceutical industry representatives, and members of the public. While there is no firm QALY threshold, the TAC approves drugs that tend to fall at or below $26,000 to $39,000 (£20,000 to £30,000 per QALY). However, there are higher thresholds for drugs treating rare and life-threatening diseases, up to $390,000 (£300,000) per QALY.

To hold down total drug spending, the Association of the British Pharmaceutical Industry (ABPI) and the UK government announced in 2018 that they had reached a deal to update the voluntary scheme, which has existed for 50 years, with a new scheme for pricing branded drugs: the Voluntary Scheme for Branded Medicines Pricing and Access (VPAS). Begun in 2019, VPAS imposes a 2% cap on growth in the total NHS annual budget for brand-name drugs in exchange for a promise of faster drug approval. Companies who chose not to be in the VPAS fall under a statutory pricing scheme that limits annual sales growth for drugs at 1.1%.

Generic drugs prices are set via the NHS Drug Tariff, which dictates the amount that NHS repays pharmacies for generic drugs. The Drug Tariff usually uses market prices as its main reference. The pricing for over-the-counter drugs is not regulated.

Prices Paid by Patients

Drugs prescribed in NHS hospitals are free to patients. In England, prescription drugs used in outpatient settings are subject to a patient co-payment of $11.55 USD (£9.00) per prescription. However, many groups are exempt from drug co-pays, including children 16 years and under, children ages 16 to 18 who are in school full time, adults ages 60 and older, low-income individuals, pregnant women or those who have given birth within the last year, and patients with cancer or certain other long-term conditions or disabilities. Therefore, patients for whom the price of prescription drugs could be a financial burden are insulated from even small co-pays. Consequently, in 2015, 90% of all drugs prescribed in England were dispensed for free.

Patients who are not exempt from co-pays but who are expecting a high utilization of prescription drugs may buy prepayment certificates. A 3-month certificate costs $38 USD (£29.10), and a 12-month certificate costs $135 USD (£104.00). After purchasing a certificate, the beneficiary can incur no further charges during the 3- or 12-month period, regardless of how many prescriptions they need.

HUMAN RESOURCES

With approximately 1.5 million employees, the NHS is the largest employer in the United Kingdom and in Europe and is one of the world's largest employers, just behind Walmart and McDonald's.

Physicians

As of 2016, there were just under 9,000 GP practices in the UK, approximately 7,000 of whom were in England. There are a total of about 150,000 employed physicians in the UK, constituting about 2.9 physicians per 1,000 population, which is slightly higher than the United States but significantly lower than the average in the European Union of 3.6 per 1,000 population. But there are only about 35,000 GPs. There are also 35,000 dental practitioners and 66,000 pharmacists.

Until the last few years, the number of physicians in the UK has increased. This increase has not kept up with population growth. Even worse, over recent years the actual number of GPs has actually been declining, and the NHS in England currently does not have enough staff to meet demand. Between July and September 2018 alone, there were nearly 94,000 vacancies for full-time hospital and community service positions. Most of these vacancies are not of medical staff. Indeed, nearly half are of nurses and midwives. The precise shortfall of physicians is not quantified, although it is felt to be compromising access to care. These shortages are unequally distributed, with the largest vacancies in the southeast portion of the country: the Thames Valley and Kent, Surrey, and Sussex.

In 2016, the total average annual income of a full-time UK physician was $149,000 USD (£114,600). The average annual income for a full-time GP was $135,000 USD (£104,300), while the average annual income of a full-time specialist or consultant was $151,000 USD (£116,100). This is comparable to physician salaries in France and the Netherlands; higher than those in Norway, Taiwan, and China; and lower than those in the United States, Canada, Germany, and Switzerland. Consultants may also work in private practices to supplement their income or apply for Clinical Excellence Awards, which range in value from about $4,000 to about $100,000 USD (£3,016 to £77,320).

To become a physician, students after high school (completing British A level examinations) must complete a 5-year undergraduate degree at one of 34 UK medical schools. The 5 years are generally divided into 2 years of preclinical coursework, followed by 3 years of clinical experience. The educational programs are under the supervision of the United Kingdom General Medical Council (GMC), which approves the curriculum and assessments of each school. After graduation, students must then enter a 2-year foundation program analogous to internship and residency in the United States. Following this, graduates must decide to train as either primary care or specialist physicians. GPs train for at least 3 additional years, the first 2 years in a hospital and the last year in a GP practice. Specialists train in hospitals for 5 to 8 years. During these training years, they are referred to as junior doctors. After completing training, GPs can work as fully licensed physicians.

Junior doctors generally earn a base salary of about $35,500 USD (£27,689) in year one, which can increase to about $41,000 USD (£32,050) in the 2nd year of training. A junior doctor is expected to work no more than 48 hours per week. A physician beginning specialty training earns a base salary of $48,600 USD (£37,935), which can increase with training to $61,700 USD (£48,075). About 17% of physicians employed by the NHS are junior doctors.

The NHS and BMA negotiate the contract for all junior doctors. The negotiation of this contract, which began in 2012, was hotly contested. After several attempts, the negotiations failed, and junior doctors in England began a general strike across the NHS. Eventually a new contract with protected overtime rates was signed in October 2016.

Nurses
In 2018, there were about 307,000 nurses and midwives and an additional 16,000 practice nurses working in GP offices. There are 7.9 nurses per 1,000 persons in the UK, significantly lower than in the United States (11.6) and Norway (17.7).

As with other countries, there is also a nursing shortage in the UK. After the 2008 financial crisis, the number of nurses fell, and this was compounded by the introduction of English-language testing to qualify for nursing registration. In addition, about 33,000 nurses leave the NHS each year. In 2018 alone there were nearly 40,000 vacancies for nursing and midwifery positions in the UK.

To become a nurse, students must complete a 3- or 4-year degree. Generally, the first year teaches a common curriculum; students can specialize in subsequent years. After completing the degree, nurses register with the United Kingdom Nursing and Midwifery Council (NMC) and can begin to practice. Nurses must renew their registration annually and are evaluated by the NMC every 3 years to ensure they have met local standards for safe practice.

Annual salaries for a nurse in the UK range from $31,500 to $94,000 USD (£24,214 to £72,597), depending on the level of experience. By comparison, the average annual salary of nurses in Norway is $52,000 USD and in Switzerland is $57,234 USD.

CHALLENGES

The UK system is well known for its universality, both in coverage and access to care. All residents in the UK have reliable access to primary care services and free choice of provider. Primary and hospital services are free at the point of care. The strength of local authorities in determining how care is delivered is a major advantage of the UK system, as it gives authorities the flexibility to test new payment and performance pilot projects. When it comes to drug prices, the UK has what many people consider to be a model system, as it melds rigorous and objective cost-effectiveness analysis with public input. This has kept prices low and closely linked with drugs' purported health benefits. While this process has not been without controversy, especially with respect to cancer drugs, the system has remained in place to this day and has garnered significant respect.

Perhaps the biggest strength of the NHS is the public's trust and devotion to it. The public does not want to replace the system with an alternative. All the public wants is a fully operational NHS. To ensure the continued success of the NHS, there are at least 6 major challenges facing the system going forward.

Probably the biggest challenge facing the NHS is staffing shortages. While the number of physicians has increased over time, it has not increased in proportion to the population. Additionally, about 33,000 nurses leave the NHS each year, exacerbating this problem. Today there are nearly 100,000 job vacancies in the NHS; this is expected to increase to over 250,000 vacancies within the next decade if no efforts are made to combat the workforce shortage. The general perception is that these staffing shortages are compromising access and quality of care. Indeed, the 2019 NHS Long Term Plan identifies the workforce shortage as one of its most pressing problems. Though there are many causes of this problem, a central one is that while salaries for physicians, especially GPs, are competitive with those in many European countries, nurses' salaries are significantly lower than those in most other countries.

The NHS's staffing shortage relates to a 2nd major challenge: hospitals. Compared to the United States, the UK has fewer hospital beds and much longer lengths of stay. This has led to a high bed occupancy rate, about 85% across the system, leaving little room for any shocks to the system, such as those that arise from a bad flu season or other increases in utilization. Obviously, as hospitalization rates are decreasing over time across all countries, building new hospitals is not the answer. However, the system should shift the care of many patients with chronic conditions or those with simple operative needs, such as hip and knee replacements, out of the hospital. In addition, there needs to be an effort to reduce the length of stay for many admissions. These changes will require investing in new infrastructure, such as increasing home care services, thereby enabling the system to deliver more care at home, or increasing the number of beds in skilled nursing facilities and nursing homes in order to more smoothly discharge elderly patients.

The 3rd challenge facing the NHS is wait times. While wait times fell dramatically in the 2000s, the post-recession 2010 austerity measures have since increased them again. Attempts to address this issue have had minimal success. In 2013, NHS England rolled out legislation to standardize wait times for elective procedures. The guidelines called for most patients to receive elective surgery within 18 weeks of their primary care referral. Although performance initially improved, overall wait times have actually increased since the legislation's implementation. Similarly, wait times for GP appointments have increased, and wait times for cancer care are a persistent problem. Indeed, long wait times are an often-cited stereotype of the NHS and one of the problems that most drives the public's dissatisfaction with the system. To this day, wait times remain an ongoing sore point for physicians and the public alike.

These challenges—staffing, hospital occupancy, and wait times—can be at least in part traced to the overall funding of the NHS. While there is a governmental commitment to invest more in the NHS, only about 9.6% of the UK GDP is devoted to health care. This places the UK near the bottom of the rankings of health care spending by advanced OECD countries such as Canada, France, Germany, Netherlands, Norway, Switzerland, and the like, which all spend above 10% of GDP on health care. Undoubtedly, spending more money on health care, even if 0.5 to 1.0% of GDP more, would put the UK in league with peer nations. If spent prudently, this spending increase would make a significant dent in addressing the staffing and wait time problems currently troubling the NHS.

A 5th challenge is improving quality of care. In 2004, the NHS introduced the Quality and Outcomes Framework (QOF), the largest primary care pay-for-performance health scheme of its time. QOF was expected to provide quality targets and financially reward primary care physicians for proper management of patients with chronic conditions. Although QOF did modestly improve care for patients with diabetes and asthma and also helped low-socioeconomic areas catch up to national standards of care, several issues have jeopardized its future. A technical problem in the original payment formula unintentionally led to higher payments for larger practices than for smaller ones with equivalent levels of quality. Certain QOF indicators, such as those for diabetes, were poorly defined, leading to patients with less specific codes essentially vanishing from QOF registers. Finally, many providers felt that QOF targets, although evidence-based, achieved only marginal gains despite much higher workloads.

A 6th challenge is the deployment of electronic health records in hospitals across the UK. While the EHRs for GPs seem to work well, the roll-out in hospitals has not gone smoothly. Part of this is cultural, as many doctors and institutions still share suspicions regarding privacy. Part of this may be related to the general challenges of any large-scale deployment of a technology in a complex organization. However, going forward, having EHRs throughout the NHS is necessary and must be achieved to ensure the system's future.

Finally, long-term care has been a flash point in the UK system, especially in the 2017 election. As in most countries, there is no dedicated long-term care financing mechanism in the UK. Instead, funding comes from a hodgepodge of sources. Further stressing the system is the fact that funding from local governments has declined in recent years. Efforts attempting to change the funding formula to increase funding responsibilities for patients and their families have been highly unpopular. There remains no clear solution, yet the UK population continues to age. This issue will need to be addressed, especially as the number of elderly in the UK will increase substantially in the coming years.

Despite many criticisms, the NHS works relatively well. Medical care is of comparable quality to many peer countries, with no cost sharing at the point of care. Most of the problems and sources of dissatisfaction are not structural but rather can be traced back to persistent underfunding of the system. While this is an issue that will have to be addressed, it is very politically charged, as proven by the recent controversy over long-term care funding. Nevertheless, because of the British public's deep commitment to and trust in the NHS, there exists strong public support for change and perhaps even for change as sweeping as new funding legislation.

CHAPTER FOUR

NORWAY

While living in Norway, Vanessa developed new onset ulcerative colitis. She never selected a general practitioner, so when she got sick she had to call the urgent care center:

> While the healthcare professional on the other end of the line was super nice and understanding, [the doctor on duty] did not share my sense of urgency. [Instead he] arranged an appointment at a local GP office for me—who, in turn, sent me to the emergency room straight away.

During this first emergency room visit she was misdiagnosed and sent home, but her symptoms later worsened. The same GP referred her to the ER a 2nd time, where she was "finally admitted to the hospital and got a diagnosis one day later. [For all] this I mainly have to thank the GP who took me on even though I wasn't on his patient list . . . and who took me seriously right from the beginning and made sure to call the hospital."

In Vanessa's view the Norwegian system functions well. Although she could not get admitted to the hospital or see a specialist without either a life-threatening condition or a referral from a GP, she describes all the health care professionals who cared for her as very nice, and they never appeared rushed or stressed. And her medical treatment was low cost. A visit to a GP's office cost her $16 USD (150 kroner), an X-ray $27 USD (250 kroner), and a visit to the emergency room had a $38 USD (350 kroner) co-pay.

All this sounds very appealing, yet a major problem with the Norwegian health care system that seems to trouble everyone is waiting times. If *you do not have an urgent problem, there are waiting times for specialist care. In March 2018 the average wait time in Norway to receive a specialist appointment was 57 days.*

HISTORY

Norway is a small country with a population of 5.3 million. Beginning in the early 1970s North Sea oil production made it one of the world's richest countries per capita. As is typical in Scandinavia, it has an extensive, well-financed social safety net.

But these developments are relatively new. In the 19th century, Norway had few natural resources, relied on farming and fishing, and was ruled by Sweden. In 1838, elected municipal councils were established. Following the workers protests that swept Europe in 1848, trade unions were created and demanded legal equality regardless of social class.

In the late 19th and early 20th centuries Norwegian municipalities, the Lutheran church, and voluntary organizations established hospitals. Beginning in 1905, with full independence from Sweden, the Norwegian government enacted a series of social reforms, such as the 10-hour work day, unemployment insurance, and other worker protections. Modeled on Germany's Bismarckian system, the Compulsory Sickness Insurance Act of 1909 created a subsidized health insurance scheme but covered only workers.

After World War II Norway began consolidating its social democratic welfare state. In 1967, Norway enacted legislation to combine the many social insurance schemes for pensions, disability, sick leave, and other areas into a unified National Insurance Scheme (Folketrygden [NIS]) that was compulsory for all Norwegian residents, including noncitizens. The NIS became fully functional in 1971, and the Ministry of Labor administered it.

Beginning in the late 1960s the health system was repeatedly reorganized to improve equality of access to treatment, efficiency, and health outcomes. In 1969, counties were entrusted with responsibility for building and managing hospitals. The Municipalities Health Services Act of 1982 gave municipalities responsibility for primary care services.

The Patients' Rights Act of 1999 gave Norwegians the right to choose a personal primary care physician and required local municipal councils to guarantee fulfillment of this right and to finance physician care. It also gave individuals a right to specialized health care services. Then, in 2001, the Health Authorities and Health Trusts Act was passed, shifting hospitals' financing and operations from counties to the national government through newly created Regional Health Authorities (RHAs). In 2009, the Ministry of Health and Care Services, through the Norwegian Health Economics Administration (Helseøkonomiforvaltningen [HELFO]), assumed responsibility for the health care portion of the NIS budget.

Today 3 values govern the Norwegian health system: (1) universality, ensuring every Norwegian resident is covered for medical services; (2) full equality, ensuring access to health care regardless of geography and socioeconomic status; and (3) prioritizing children, ensuring that they get all care for free. Norway's health system is predominantly—but not totally—socialized. The government owns most hospitals and employs the physicians, nurses, and other hospital-based workers. The government pays for all hospital care. The municipalities pay for primary care. But primary care physicians are self-employed, not government employees. In a somewhat complex system (detailed below), the physicians collectively negotiate fees with and are paid by the government. Dentists are also self-employed. The government pays about 85% of all medical care and 75% of the cost of prescription drugs.

Almost everything in the Norwegian health system is divided into 2. Yet, as one health policy report notes, the traditional distinction of "'outpatient' and 'inpatient' are not relevant for describing the health system in Norway. Instead, the 2 sectors are defined as primary care and specialist care." Primary care is predominantly financed and overseen by the 356 municipalities. Conversely, 4 RHAs finance and oversee hospital and specialist care. The national Ministry of Health and Care Services, in turn, oversees the RHAs. This bifurcation extends to the payment for prescription drugs used in primary and specialized care. Counties are responsible for children's and adolescents' dental care. By providing payments to RHAs and block grants to municipalities, the Ministry of Health and Care Services essentially defines the national health care budget and priorities.

Figure 1. Health Care Coverage (Norway)

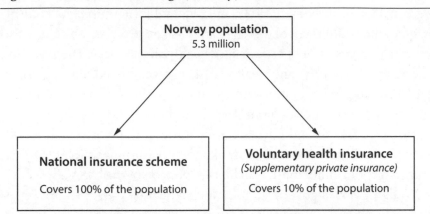

COVERAGE

The Norwegian system is a public health insurance scheme with supplementary private insurance for a small minority.

The National Insurance Scheme (NIS) is comprehensive: it covers pensions, disability, unemployment, parental leave, and health care. All tax-paying residents contribute to the NIS and, thus, are automatically enrolled in NIS without needing to make a positive selection of an insurer or sickness fund—and without paying a premium.

There is also private health insurance, called voluntary health insurance (VHI). It does not cover any acute or emergency services, such as treatment for heart attacks, and is mainly used to avoid the wait times for specialist consultations and elective surgery.

FINANCING

Norway is the 4th-most expensive health care system on a per capita basis, but the cost is relatively low on the basis of percentage of GDP. Overall Norway spends $7,400 USD (64,400 kr.) per capita on health care. But because of a high GDP per capita ($75,500 USD PPP 2017), it spends only 10.4% of GDP on health care, about $39.1 billion USD (340

Figure 2. Financing Health Care: Statutory Health Insurance (Norway)

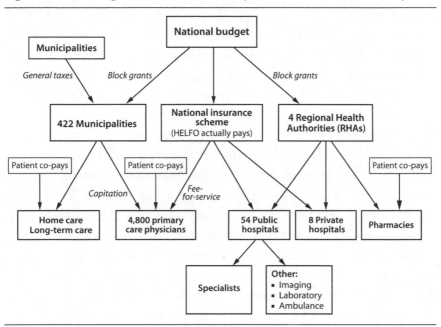

billion kr.) for 5.3 million people. Of this, approximately 85% is publicly financed, 15% is from out-of-pocket spending, and under 1% is from VHI.

Public Health Insurance

There are 4 sources of financing for health care: (1) general taxes, including national, municipality, and county taxes; (2) NIS funds; (3) individual out-of-pocket payments; and (4) employer and individual payments for VHI.

There are no earmarked health-specific taxes, such as the payroll taxes used in Germany and for Medicare in the United States.

Municipalities finance primary care, preventive services, long-term care, public health, and palliative care. Primary care and preventive services are financed by a combination of (1) block grants from the national government to the municipalities, (2) municipal funds, (3) fee-for-service payments from the NIS, and (4) individual out-of-pocket expenditures. The national government's block grant to municipalities is a single grant—without earmarks or allocations for specific services—that covers health care and many other municipal services, such as education. Municipalities determine how the funds will be divided among the various services they must pay for. They pay general practitioners' capitation, about $46 USD (400 kr.) per person on the GPs' panel list. The NIS also contributes to the financing of primary care by directly paying GPs fees for services rendered. NIS payments occur by transferring funds to the Ministry of Health and Care Service, which then gives the money to HELFO for actual payments.

From general tax revenues, the national government finances the 4 RHAs. The NIS also contributes funds to cover specialist consultations.

Counties pay 100% of dental care for children up to age 18 and 75% of dental care for young adults aged 19 and 20. Dental care for adults is totally private, paid 100% out of pocket by individuals. Similarly, children get free vision care, but adults pay 100% for vision care.

The Ministry of Health and Care Services sets an informal national budget for health care. It funds municipalities and RHAs for services. Beginning in 2013, the National System for the Introduction of New Health Technologies helps with setting priorities and ensuring high-value care by conducting Health Technology Assessments (HTAs) and cost-effectiveness studies of new drugs and other interventions.

Private Supplemental Insurance
About 10% of the population has VHI, but it constitutes only about 1% of health care spending. Employers provide about 90% of VHI through 8 for-profit insurers. Employers and employees receive no tax break for utilizing private insurance.

Long-Term Care
Currently 16.6% of the Norwegian population is over 65, with 10% over 70, and population growth is just under 2%. Long-term care, whether at home or in nursing homes, is financed by municipalities and out-of-pocket payments by the elderly.

Public Health
Municipalities pay for public health services. They fund GPs, who provide personal public health measures such as immunizations and cancer screenings. Municipalities are also responsible for school clinics and youth clinics that provide preventive services as well as the usual

health education around nutrition, physical fitness, contraception, vaccinations, and other public health measures.

PAYMENT

Payment to Hospitals

Overall, inpatient hospital services account for about 29% of all Norwegian health care expenditures. The dominant source of payments to hospitals is from the 4 RHAs, which, in turn, receive their money from the Ministry of Health and Care Services. The Ministry pays the RHAs in 4 ways:

1. About 70% of the revenue is paid as a block grant based on variables such as the types of services the hospital provides such as whether psychiatric services are provided, population size of the hospital catchment area, socioeconomic demographics, and health and mortality data.
2. About 27% of the payment to RHAs is based on services provided, also known as activity-based funding. The activity-based funding uses a Nordic version of the DRG system, with the weights based on average national costs.
3. Laboratory and radiology services are paid on a fee-for-service system, accounting for 2.3% of payments.
4. A quality-based financing payment is based on about 39 quality indicators; however, this method is less than 1% of hospital payments.

Each RHA determines for itself how to pay hospitals. As one official in the Directorate of Health noted, "There is no nationally determined system for the distribution of funds from RHAs to hospitals. [The RHAs] enjoy relatively large degrees of freedom to organize their activities and [in] how they use their funding." In general, the 4 RHAs pay hospitals in the same way they are paid: a combination of block grants, activity-based financing, and quality incentives.

These funds cover hospital operations, including salaries, pharmaceuticals, and other hospital-based goods and services. However, radiology and laboratory services are funded on a fee-for-service basis. These payments also include ambulance, same-day surgery, and hospital-based specialists, such as oncologists.

Importantly, the RHAs are responsible for planning and financing hospital capital expenditures. In 2017, capital investment in the hospital sector was less than 4% of total hospital expenditures. RHAs have wide latitude to determine budgets for capital expenditures as well as to determine how they will be paid. The 4 RHAs established an Agency for Hospital Construction to help rationalize and improve hospital planning and construction. Hospitals also have some control over capital investments, such as for imaging equipment, and finance them from their regular RHA payments. There are some Ministry of Health and Care Services funds for special capital initiatives.

RHAs also contract with private hospitals to perform elective procedures that relieve waiting times. About 10% of RHA budgets have gone to purchase services from private hospitals and physicians.

Municipalities are required to pay a fee to the hospitals when a patient is ready for discharge but stays in the hospital awaiting a nursing home bed or another municipally controlled service. The Parliament sets the fee in the national budget—about $550 USD (4,780 kr.) per day. Patients have no financial responsibility—that is, no co-pays—for hospitalizations.

Payments to Specialists

There are 2 types of specialists—those based at hospitals and a few who are in private practice. Hospital-based specialists are salaried employees. After hours, however, they are permitted to do private consulting outside the hospital to supplement their incomes. In addition, there are a few totally private specialists. The number of private specialists is limited by the number of licenses, which are determined regionally. Individual patients and VHI pay for these private services, but RHAs may pay to supplement public care to reduce waiting times.

Negotiations between the Norwegian Medical Association and hospitals determine pay, hours, schedules, coverage, and other work details of hospital-based physicians. In 2016, there was a strike over working and on-call hours because hospital-based physicians wanted to retain schedule predictability and family time, while hospitals wanted more

Figure 3. Payment to Hospitals and Specialists (Norway)

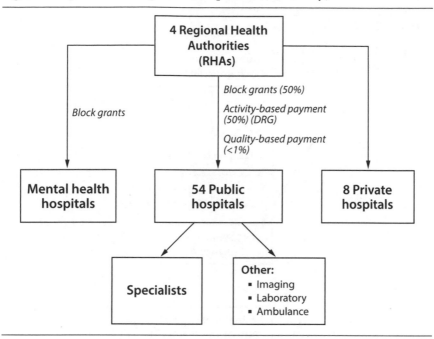

flexibility to modify on-call time. The Norwegian Medical Association won the court battle.

Payments to Primary Care General Practitioners

About 95% of GPs who provide primary care are private, self-employed workers, with the remaining 5% of GPs being full-time, salaried municipal employees. Primary care GPs are paid from 3 sources: (1) municipalities, (2) the NIS, and (3) patient co-pays.

GPs are required to take emergency calls for the municipality and could be required to work in the health and school clinics or municipal nursing homes. This municipal work is limited to one day per week, and they are paid a salary for these public health services.

Municipalities pay a capitated rate to GPs. This rate, about $46 USD (400 kr.) per patient, is not risk adjusted and accounts for about a third of GP income. Through HELFO, NIS pays on a fee-for-service basis to GPs for another third of their income. This amount has a small adjustment based on a patient's health complexity. Finally, individual patient co-pays account for the remaining third of GP income. Patients have

Figure 4. Payment to Physicians (Norway)

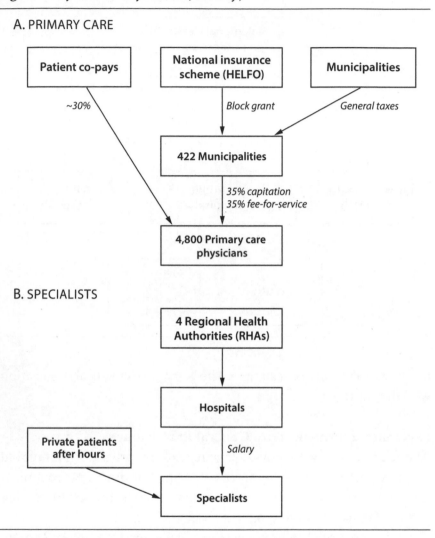

A. PRIMARY CARE

B. SPECIALISTS

a required flat co-pay for seeing the GP, amounting to about $23 USD (200 kr.) per visit. There are various limits on this payment. Cumulative annual patient co-pays are limited to about $250 USD (2,170 kr.) per year. After that amount patients have no more co-pays for any services, and HELFO covers the co-pays for the GPs. Certain groups of patients are exempt and have no co-pays for GP visits, including children under 16, pregnant women getting pre- and post-natal care, and HIV/AIDS patients.

The capitation rate, fee-for-service, and co-pay rates are all uniform throughout Norway and are negotiated nationally between the Norwegian Medical Association, which represents all physicians, and the Ministry of Health and Care Services.

Payments for Mental Health Services
As with everything else in the Norwegian health system, payment for mental health services is bifurcated, although the bulk comes from RHAs. Part of their payment from municipalities and NIS comes when GPs provide mental health care for patients with mild to moderate conditions such as depression and anxiety. However, specialists at district psychiatric centers, general hospitals, or specialized mental health hospitals provide services for patients with moderate to significant mental health issues. Unlike other specialties, the block grant largely covers these institution-based mental health services and specialized drug addiction treatments. The activity-based payments, or DRGs, cover about 15% of the outpatient mental health services that hospitals provide. It is projected that in 2021 mental health services in hospitals and outpatient hospital facilities will be paid in the same way as all other medical services.

Payments for Long-Term Care
Municipalities are responsible for paying for home-based and institutional (nursing home) long-term care. Municipalities own nursing homes and employ their workers. Special grants from the national government finance the construction of additional assisted-living facilities and nursing home beds.

There are substantial income-linked patient co-payments for home-based and nursing home custodial care. Importantly, there is no exemption or co-pay maximum for these services as there is for visits to GPs.

Payments for Complementary and Alternative Medicines
In Norway public resources pay for some minimal complementary and alternative medical care, particularly acupuncture. But practitioners outside the public health care system offer the vast majority of these

services, including homeopathy and naturopathy. These services are paid for by individual out-of-pocket payments without any reimbursement.

Payments for Preventive Services

Municipalities finance public health, school-based, and youth clinics that provide immunizations for children as well as health education on nutrition, exercise, contraception, and other matters. Municipalities set priorities for capital investments for these clinics and pay for them. GPs are also reimbursed for other preventive services, such as cancer screenings.

Out-of-Pocket Payments

Two "exemption card schemes" limit patients' out-of-pocket payments. Patients who exceed the maximum out-of-pocket payments automatically receive an exemption card (*frikort*) for public health services. They are then not required to pay any additional out-of-pocket costs for the calendar year. Group 1 exemptions include co-pays for GP visits, outpatient hospital clinic visits, X-ray and laboratory services, patient travel, and blue list—outpatient retail pharmacy—drugs. Legislation establishes the maximum co-pay per year before no additional payment is required. In 2019, the maximum out-of-pocket payment was $280 USD (2,460 kr.) for Group 1. Group 2 exemptions include co-pays for physiotherapy, certain types of dental treatment, and admission to rehabilitation facilities. In 2019, the Group 2 limit was $242 USD (2,085 kr.).

DELIVERY OF HEALTH CARE SERVICES

The Norwegian system is consumer friendly in its simplicity, choice, and limited financial barriers. Since 2002 residents have had the right to choose a GP *and* switch GPs up to 2 times a year. Patients can go to any hospital in the country and receive fully subsidized care. There are low caps on out-of-pocket costs for physicians and drugs. But, unlike in Germany, GPs are effective gatekeepers for more specialized care. There are significant waiting lists for services, and specialized services often require extensive travel to more urban centers. Also, long-term care is costly.

Hospital Care

There are approximately 60 hospitals in Norway, with just over 13,000 beds, about 2.4 beds per 1,000 residents. The number of hospital beds has declined by 23% since 1990. This is a much lower number than in Germany (8.2 per 1,000 population) and about the same as in the United States (2.4 per 1,000 population). There are about 540,000 hospital discharges, or just over one discharge per 10 people, about a quarter of the number in Germany and the same as in the United States. Consequently, length of stay is comparatively short—about 4.1 days per admission—and bed occupancy rates are at about 90%.

Almost all the hospitals in Norway are public hospitals. Aside from public hospitals, there are 6 university hospitals, which have over 45% of all beds, and 8 private hospitals.

How do patients get hospital care? For serious acute problems, such as crushing chest pain or loss of consciousness, the local on-call service calls an ambulance to take the patient to the hospital. Once admitted to a hospital, the hospital-based physicians—not the patient's personal GP—care for them. If the on-call services feel the problem is not that acute, they might send patients to a local urgent care or casualty center that operates 24/7. Physicians and nurses on staff then make an assessment.

In a nonemergency situation the patient sees their GP. If the GP believes the problem requires specialist care, the patient is referred to the hospital, where a specialist will administer care and, if necessary, admit the patient for medical or surgical care. Norwegian GPs thus act as gatekeepers to hospital services and hospital-based specialist care.

The hospital delivery system has several problems. One is that there are serious waiting times for elective procedures. Patients can see waiting times for a particular procedure at all hospitals in Norway and select hospitals based on wait times. For-profit hospitals do not provide acute care but rather are often contracted by RHAs to provide specialized elective procedures, such as cataract surgeries, to relieve these waiting times.

Another problem is the need for patients to travel for care. Norway is large but sparsely populated. It is only slightly smaller than California but has just 12% of California's population. This creates challenges in providing hospital care to the rural population. Over the ast few years several new programs have been established to improve quality and efficiency. There has been a push to close or consolidate some rural hospitals, although local public resistance has often stymied efforts to close them. In addition, specialized care has been centralized into "centers of excellence." For instance, percutaneous cardiac interventions are available at only 7 hospitals, 2 of which are in Oslo. Although this has increased standardization of care and quality, it has also required many Norwegians to travel great distances for specialized care and increased the need for air ambulances.

Specialist Care

Almost all specialist care is provided in hospital-based outpatient facilities. Specialist care thus falls under the RHAs' authority. There are about 15,000 specialist physicians. Hospital-based specialists provide free advice to GPs on managing patients with particular medical problems. These physician-to-physician consultations can help GPs provide follow-up care after a specialist consultation. In practice, however, these specialist consultations tend to be haphazard and not standardized.

Norway also has "mobile" specialists who visit patients in their homes. They most frequently provide geriatric and palliative care for home-bound elderly patients.

Some specialist physicians, such as obstetricians, dermatologists, oncologists, and others, are self-employed and practice privately.

Primary Care

The GPs provide primary care services and serve as gatekeepers to specialist care. As part of their payment from the municipalities, GPs are also required to work for municipalities, including by providing after-hours on-call services and covering nursing homes. Their municipal services may include work in local health clinics or stations overseeing nurses that provide primary care services, such as postnatal newborn and maternal care, services for children up to school age, adult preventive services, and some mental health services.

Norway has about 4,800 GPs who provide office-based primary care. Most GPs in Norway work in small groups of 3 to 8 physicians, which include nurses, lab technicians, and a secretary. On average each GP has a patient panel—or patient "list," as they are called in Norway—of just over 1,100 people, which is a comparatively low number of patients per physician. For instance, at Kaiser in the United States, physicians have an average patient panel of about 1,900 to 2,100 people.

The GPs' offices offer limited office hours (8:00 a.m. to 4:00 p.m.). Municipalities organize after-hours calls as well as nonhospital urgent care facilities. The municipalities require GPs to take after-hours call shifts on a rotating basis. In urban areas with relatively high numbers of GPs, the GP will do one on-call night about every 3 weeks.

Norwegians are not heavy users of physician services. On average Norwegians see GPs 2.7 times per year and visit the emergency departments only 0.25 times per year, a much lower rate than in Germany, France, and the United States.

Mental Health Care

As in most countries over the last 50 years, mental health care in Norway has undergone a shift from inpatient psychiatric hospitals to outpatient treatment. In 1998, the Parliament adopted the National Program for Mental Health, which made mental health a priority by requiring the municipalities to invest more financial resources and hire more trained personnel. Although there has been a decline in institutionalization, Norway still has a comparatively high number of psychiatric beds, about 4,000, 82 per 100,000 population.

As with all health care in Norway, mental health care is bifurcated. The first line of mental health care is the GP, who cares for patients with mild or moderate mental health conditions such as comorbid depression or anxiety. GPs can receive specialized training in cognitive behavioral therapy. In addition, there are psychologists and psychiatric nurses at the municipal level to supplement GP mental health care. There are private-practice psychiatrists and psychologists. GPs can refer patients to private practitioners, and the public system often pays for these services.

Patients with moderate to severe mental health conditions get specialized care from District Psychiatric Outpatient Services (DPOS).

DPOS provides outpatient services for chronic conditions such as eating disorders or bipolar disorders. DPOS care is hospital based and, thus, falls under RHA auspices. Finally, for the severely mentally ill there are 7 psychiatric hospitals and psychiatric wards within the larger hospitals. There are also private mental health hospitals that tend to care for patients with eating disorders as well as for geriatric psychiatric patients. Such private hospitals often provide services for patients— paid for by the RHAs—to relieve waiting lists.

All mental health care services have the same co-pays as GPs.

In 2004, substance abuse and alcohol treatment were deemed specialized mental health services and transferred to RHAs. Norway has a substance abuse problem, with over 17,000 patients currently being treated for substance abuse, and a high drug overdose death rate. Most such substance abuse patients get their care at specialized outpatient treatment units affiliated with hospitals. These specialized units can involve GPs in managing substance abuse.

Long-Term Care

About 15% of the Norwegian population is over 65. Municipalities are responsible for providing all long-term care services for the elderly and disabled, encompassing at-home care, adult day care centers, and nursing homes. Municipalities own the long-term care facilities, determine eligibility for services, and decide what combination of services to provide. The priority in municipalities is to keep people at home as long as possible, as this is far cheaper than moving them into nursing homes. Consequently over 100,000 Norwegian seniors receive personal or custodial care at home, about 45,000 receive care in nursing homes, and another 45,000 receive care in assisted-living facilities, also called sheltered housing.

These services require high co-pays. For instance, for nursing home care the first $760 USD (6,600 kr.) of income is excluded, but then patients pay 75% of income above that up to nearly $11,500 USD (100,000 kr.) and then 85% on all income above that level.

Preventive Care

Norwegians get preventive care services either from their GPs or the local, school-based, or youth health clinics.

Figure 5. Regulation of Pharmaceutical Prices (Norway)

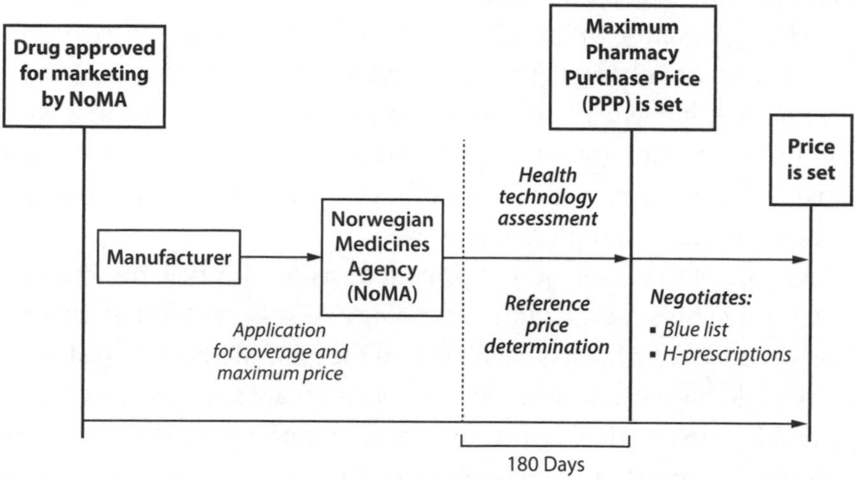

PHARMACEUTICAL COVERAGE AND PRICE CONTROLS

Pharmaceutical Market

The Norwegian market for pharmaceuticals is tiny, about $2.2 billion USD ($20 billion kr.). Overall less than 10% of national health care spending is devoted to drugs, amounting to just over $400 USD per capita. Norway has some of the lowest drug prices in Europe, and Norwegians consume a relatively low number of drugs per person, compared to other European countries. But, as in other countries, expensive drugs for cancer and rare diseases have pushed up total drug costs significantly. Public insurance bears about 75% of all pharmaceutical costs, while consumers pay about 25% out of pocket.

Coverage Determination

A branch of the national Ministry of Health and Care Services, the Norwegian Medicines Agency (Statens legemiddelverk [NoMA]), authorizes the marketing of drugs, monitors adverse events, and sets maximum prices. Its procedures for marketing approval are harmonized with European Union regulations. Marketing authorization is valid for 5 years. Although there is no cost-effectiveness requirement for marketing approval of a new drug, cost effectiveness is considered as part of the coverage decision.

After marketing approval, manufacturers must apply to NoMA for a maximum pharmacy purchase price, which constitutes a coverage and reimbursement decision. Because a drug cannot be marketed without a set price, the coverage and maximum pricing decisions are separate from the marketing decisions, even though the same agency is responsible for these different approvals.

As part of the coverage and pricing decisions for new prescription drugs, there must be a Health Technology Assessment (HTA). In 2013, Norway adopted what has been dubbed the New Methods to systematically evaluate new interventions in specialist care to ensure an orderly, equitable introduction of the approved technologies, including new prescription drugs. A major component of the New Methods system is the requirement for covered technologies to undergo an HTA, which informs decision making and price negotiations. In 2016, Parliament endorsed a report requiring new technologies—including prescription drugs, genetic tests, devices, surgical procedures, and other interventions—to be prioritized using 3 criteria: (1) overall benefit, (2) resource use, and (3) the severity of the condition. Since the publication of this report, the use of HTA has been extended to all new medicines, with the exception of Schedule 4 drugs for serious infections such as HIV/AIDS and tuberculosis (described below).

The most common form of HTA for prescription drugs in Norway—including all outpatient drugs—is single technology assessments. NoMA conducts all the single technology assessments for prescription drugs. Single technology assessments compare a drug to the best standard of care. The Norwegian Institute of Public Health conducts the full HTAs of other prescription drugs—finding the best therapy among multiple interventions for a condition—and all HTAs of other medical technologies.

Whether NoMA should use a cost-effectiveness threshold is controversial. An informal threshold of about $31,500 USD (275,000 kr.) per QALY, which is similar to the threshold used by NICE in Britain and the Pharmaceutical Benefits Scheme (PBS) in Australia, seems to inform decisions. However, the suggested threshold is higher for more severe illnesses, up to $94,500 USD per QALY (825,000 kr.) for life-threatening conditions.

The use of HTAs in approving drugs (as well as other technologies) constitutes a systematic and transparent way of evaluating new medical services' value.

LIKE EVERYTHING ELSE in the Norwegian health care system, the divide between primary and specialist care affects prescription drugs. The Directorate of Health within the Ministry of Health and Care Services makes a critical decision about whether the prescription drug is for primary or specialist care. This decision is triply important because it controls (1) how a drug's price is determined, (2) what patient co-pays are, and (3) which government agency pays for the drug.

Norway has a list of covered drugs for primary care, called Schedule 2 drugs, or *blue list* drugs. Blue list drugs are out-of-hospital drugs for chronic conditions—requiring 3 or more months of treatment per year—that the NIS reimburses through HELFO. Patients have a co-pay of 39% for these drugs, with a maximum of $58 USD (520 kr.) per drug and which is part of the annual out-of-pocket maximum of $275 USD (2,369 kr.).

In some cases, drugs will be prescribed for indications that have not been approved on the blue list or for rare diseases—Schedule 3a and 3b drugs. Physicians must apply for reimbursement for each individual patient, and the NIS decides on each individual reimbursement. There are also Schedule 4 drugs, used for infections such as HIV, tuberculosis, and hepatitis. These drugs are fully paid for, and patients have no co-pays.

There are *white list* prescription drugs that are not covered, and thus patients must pay 100% of the cost. These white list drugs include short-term and/or discretionary medications such as short-term antibiotics, sleeping pills, and painkillers.

Then there are *H-prescription* drugs, which are specialty drugs that are used out of the hospital, such as drugs for cancer, rheumatoid arthritis, multiple sclerosis, asthma, and hepatitis B. The Directorate of Health decides which drugs are on the H-prescription list. Less than 1% of prescriptions are H-prescriptions, but they account for nearly 20%

of drug costs. The number of H-prescriptions and their relative proportion of pharmaceutical costs have been increasing as more drugs are shifted from the blue list, such as drugs for hepatitis C. The 4 RHAs pay for the H-prescription drugs, and patients have no co-pays.

RHAs consider HTAs when determining coverage for both in-hospital and H-list drugs. The Commissioner Forum of New Methods, composed of members from the 4 RHAs and the Norwegian Directorate of Health, prioritizes the candidate topics and decides which assessments should be commissioned. The HTAs are eventually submitted to the Decision Forum of New Methods. Here the RHAs' CEOs have the authority to decide about introducing the new medicines and other technologies in specialist care. Because the 4 RHAs decide together, the assessed interventions are introduced across the country simultaneously.

There is no national coverage determination or price regulation for over-the-counter drugs. Prices are set by pharmacies and patients pay for them out of pocket.

Price Regulation
For blue list drugs, NoMA defines maximum prices and reimbursement levels. NoMA also sets the maximum pharmacy purchase price for nonhospital drugs. After marketing approval, manufacturers must submit pharmacoeconomic data such as price, clinical benefits, therapeutic comparator(s), number of patients, and budgetary implications to NoMA. The new prescription drug then undergoes an HTA. Using this HTA, NoMA then makes a coverage decision. It then determines the maximum pharmacy purchase costs based on a reference price that is established by averaging the lowest 3 prices for the drug in 9 European countries—Austria, Belgium, Great Britain, Denmark, Finland, Germany, Ireland, the Netherlands, and Sweden. If the drug is not sold in at least 3 of these countries, then NoMA uses the average price of the countries where it is sold.

Drugs cannot be sold at costs exceeding the maximum price, but they can be sold at any price below the maximum. Manufacturers may ask NoMA to reevaluate the maximum price if there are new data on European prices or clinical benefits.

For drugs covered by the NIS, there is also a total budget impact or affordability assessment. If the estimated annual incremental cost of the drug based on price and use exceeds $11.5 million USD (100 million kr.) for the whole country, the Ministry of Health and Care Services must review the drug. If it endorses the drug, the Parliament then needs to include its approval in a budget bill. Conversely, if the estimated cost is less than $11.5 million USD, then the Norwegian Medicines Agency (NoMA) decides on coverage of the drug.

There is a centralized procurement system for hospitals funded by the 4 RHAs, called the Hospital Purchases HF (Sykehusinnkjop HF). Through this system, price negotiations with drug wholesalers and manufacturers may be conducted to lower costs for hospitals.

In 2001, Norway began requiring generic substitution whenever possible. In 2005, Norway introduced *stepped pricing* to lower generic drug prices, thereby encouraging their use. In this model, after a patent expires, NoMA determines whether there is a suitable generic. If so, the price for the generic is lowered every 6 months. By 18 months after the generic is introduced, then, the price is lower than the brand-name maximum price by at least 90%. Pharmacies must inform patients if a cheaper generic alternative exists. If the patient refuses to switch to the generic, they will need to pay the difference in price between the 2 alternatives. Because profit margins on the generics are higher, pharmacies have a financial incentive to dispense generics. These policies have been successful, and generic drugs now constitute 70% of prescriptions.

Regulation of Physician Prescriptions
Reimbursement for drugs only occurs for approved indications, and physicians cannot prescribe drugs for unapproved indications. If they want to prescribe off label, they must apply for the drug to be given to a specific patient as a Schedule 3a.

Prices Paid by Patients
Patients have co-pays for out-of-hospital drugs. For blue list (Schedule 2) and Schedule 3 drugs, patients pay 39% of the cost, up to about $60 USD (520 kr.) per prescription. Payment for blue list drugs is included in the out-of-pocket maximum, which is about $275 USD (2,369 kr.) per year for a combination of services, including GP visits and X-rays. After they reach this out-of-pocket maximum, all prescription drugs are free. For children under 16, there is no co-pay for blue list drugs.

There are no patient co-pays for drugs prescribed during a hospital admission, H-prescriptions, and Schedule 4 drugs. For white list drugs, patients pay the full amount, up to $200 USD (1775 kr.) per year.

Norwegian pharmacy markups are strictly regulated. Pharmacies get 2 markups on blue list medications. One is a percentage added to the pharmacies' purchase price (2.25%), and the other is a fixed amount ($3.30 USD [29 kr.]) per package. In addition, all pharmacy prescriptions are subject to the 25% Norwegian value-added tax.

The Pharmacy Act of 2001 deregulated ownership to increase the number of pharmacies, resulting in an increase of about 25% since 2011, and to generate more competition. By law there is no direct-to-consumer advertising for prescription drugs, but companies may advertise over-the-counter drugs on TV and online.

Other

Recently Norway began pilot programs that pay pharmacies to train patients to use inhalers for asthma and to educate them when starting blood pressure and cholesterol-lowering medications. The goal of these programs is to improve medication compliance for patients with chronic conditions.

HUMAN RESOURCES

Physicians

Norway has over 26,000 physicians, or just over 5 per 1,000 population—the highest rate in all Nordic countries. Compared to all other Nordic countries, Norway has had the greatest growth—more than triple—in the number of physicians since 1980.

Of all physicians, approximately 4,800 (20%) are GPs, with about 60% of GPs practicing as specialists, which requires 5 years of training beyond an internship. Overall about 40% of GPs are women. Between 15% and 20% of Norwegian GPs are foreign born or have foreign citizenship. More importantly, nearly 40% of GPs were trained outside Norway, with the largest group trained in Poland. Over 90% of GPs are in group practice; they have relatively small panel sizes—just over 1,100 patients per GP.

There are over 15,000 specialists in Norway—over 3 times the number of GPs. Almost all are employed by hospitals, and there are 46 different recognized specialties.

Norway has a geographic maldistribution of physicians. About 20% of the population lives in rural areas, and this percentage has been slowly declining. According to the OECD, there are nearly twice as many physicians in urban areas as there are in rural ones—7 per 1,000 population versus 3.8 per 1,000 population. Like other countries with substantial rural populations, Norway has tried a number of programs to attract physicians to rural areas. In 1973, Norway opened a medical school in the far north's major city, Tromsø. Although the medical school induced more physicians to practice in northern Norway, they mainly stayed in more urban areas, like Tromsø, and are affiliated with the university hospitals.

Compared to those in many other European countries, Norwegian physicians' salaries are low. However, compared to other Nordic countries, Norwegian salaries tend to be high. According to Statistics Norway, the government statistical agency, GPs make an average of $92,000 USD (800,000 kr.) per year. Specialists, including surgical specialists, make an average of $110,000 USD (957,000 kr.) per year. The average Norwegian makes around $42,000 USD (365,000 kr.) per year.

Norway has 4 medical schools that together enroll a total of 600 students per year. Medical education is free, paid for by the national government. Norway even pays for students to study medicine in foreign universities. In Norway medical school takes 6 years, followed by 1.5 years of an internship and 5 to 6.5 years of specialization training. About two-thirds of all medical students are female, indicating that the profession will soon become predominantly female.

Nurses

Norway has about 103,000 nurses. This is the 2nd-highest number of nurses per population: over 17 per 1,000 population and about 3.5 nurses per practicing physician. Despite these high numbers, Statistics Norway predicts a shortage of 28,000 nurses by 2035. Many nurses in Norway are recruited from other European countries.

Nurses' salaries are comparatively high. According to Statistics Norway, full-time nurses earn on average about $67,000 USD annually (over 576,000 kr.). There is relatively high nurse job satisfaction, with few wanting to leave the profession or not recommending it.

Although there are some specialties, such as nurse anesthetists and geriatric nurses, the nurse practitioner position is at the earliest stages. To date, Norwegian nurses are not permitted to write prescriptions or order tests.

CHALLENGES

The Norwegian system has many strengths.

It is absolutely universal based on paying taxes. There is no access barrier, such as enrollment in an insurance plan or paying a premium. Patient choice is real and extensive. Patients can choose any GP, may change their GP twice a year, and have minimal co-pays. They can go to any hospital in the country for care and have no co-pays. And all medical, dental, and vision care services for children are free. Physicians have low panel sizes and manageable work hours. Although there is some controversy about whether the latest drugs are somewhat delayed in their introduction to the Norwegian market, the country has the latest technology and all drugs. Norway has taken high costs and resource allocation issues seriously, establishing the New Methods to create a systematic process for conducting health technology assessments and integrating them into coverage decisions for drugs and other technologies. Finally, of all the systems I surveyed, Norway's seems the least complicated and easiest to navigate.

Nonetheless, there are 6 serious challenges, with each tracing back to some dimension of the system's structure. The first 2 challenges relate to different aspects of care coordination. First, the rigid distinction between GPs and hospital-based specialist care—as well as the different ways they are paid, incentivized, and held accountable—fosters poor coordination between primary care and specialized, hospital-based care. Municipalities largely finance and oversee GPs and home care, but specialty care is organized by separate RHAs that are operated regionally, not locally. This makes it hard to get patients optimal care. As one academic health policy expert stated, "There is no dialogue between GPs and specialists. GPs refer patients. Specialists accept the referral, and the patients return to their GP. Information back from the specialists to the GPs is haphazard at best."

The multiple sites of care for patients with complex illnesses exacerbates this poor coordination. For instance, a patient with cancer might get surgery, radiation therapy, and chemotherapy at 3 different facilities in 3 different locations as well as have a GP in a 4th community. This dispersion of care *can* ensure high-quality services at each step, but there are transition challenges and barriers to coordinated care. Much of this coordination can be facilitated because Norway is small and people know each other. Even the biggest cities are small—Oslo has only 630,000 people and Bergen has just over 250,000. But care coordination that relies on informal networks will be haphazard and frequently fail—often for the patients who need it most. Indeed, as one health policy expert put it, "A Norwegian needs to be quite healthy to become sick, because there are a lot of things to organize and it is hard to line everything up. GPs are supposed to coordinate care, but they don't." Efforts to incentivize more coordination—such as requiring municipalities to pay for patients ready to discharge from hospitals without available outpatient services—have failed to solve the problem. Adequately addressing the problem requires clinical, financial, and administrative alignment of GPs, specialists, and hospitals. The rigid divide between the primary and specialist care systems, however, complicates such alignment.

Second, and relatedly, the care coordination infrastructure necessary for optimal management of patients with chronic disease is lacking. Like all other health systems in developed countries, Norway's evolved in the 20th century to address acute medical conditions. But the predominant medical issues of the 21st century are multiple chronic conditions that cannot be solved by episodic visits to the GP or hospital. Optimal chronic care requires a lot, including:

- extended office hours;
- after-hours care by someone who knows the patient or at least has access to their medical record;
- open-access scheduling so physicians can see patients in their offices instead of sending them to urgent care or emergency rooms; and

- chronic care coordinators who work in GP offices and proactively engage with and educate patients daily or weekly to ensure compliance with medications and other medical interventions.

The problem, as one expert stated, is that "geriatric care for patients with chronic conditions is not well coordinated. It is not prioritized by the health care system. And there is little integration of social services and medical services." Although Norway has excellent community health clinics, even as they are good at delivering immunizations, preventive services, and postnatal care for mothers and children, they are not optimal for coordinated chronic care for elderly patients. A well-developed system of home-based nursing care may partially compensate for this.

In addition, GPs have little incentive to redesign how they provide care. GPs are paid by capitation and on a fee-for-service basis, neither of which provide any financial incentive to reduce hospital admissions. GPs get a fee for medication reconciliation and coordinating care, although that fee is low, does not incentivize comprehensive care, and is too low to incentivize care redesign. And GPs have no responsibility, accountability, or incentive to limit the total costs to the system of patients' care. GPs also receive no feedback on the quality of their care or pay adjustment based on quality or excessive hospital admissions. Paying pharmacists to educate patients who are initiating chronic medications, such as for high blood pressure or cholesterol, is good, but it hardly ensures medication adherence and does not constitute coordinated care. Providing more chronic care coordination would require municipalities to make significant changes in terms of how they pay and incentivize GPs, quality reporting and feedback, and after-hours care. It is unclear whether municipalities have the human and financial resources to do this.

A 3rd challenge is waiting times. The caricature of socialized medical systems is that patients must wait and wait for care services. Although this is exaggerated in many ways—including the fact that waiting times are also long in nonsocialized medical systems—Norway has a serious waiting time problem. This is indicated by the recent growth in supplemental private insurance, the main purpose of which is to circumvent waiting times.

Part of the problem may be an attitude among health care experts that a waiting time can be useful. For instance, some Norwegian experts thought that patients with back pain on a waiting list for surgery may find that their pain stops on its own, eliminating the need for surgery. And some hospital administrators may manipulate waiting lists to increase their leverage in budget negotiations. There have been multiple efforts to address the problem, including publicly listing hospital waiting times for various procedures at different hospitals and allowing patients to select hospitals based on waiting times. Another partial solution has been for the RHAs to pay private hospitals and practitioners to perform elective procedures. The problem persists, though, and Norwegians feel annoyed and are losing confidence in the system.

The previous problems relate to a 4th challenge: the system is not patient centered, although some elements are focused on how patients will use the services. For instance, the location and operation of community, school, and, especially, youth clinics seem attuned to particular patient populations' needs. But in general, the system is still physician centric. Physician office hours are limited, and few use open-access scheduling. Pharmacy times have also been limited. After-hours care is performed by rotating physicians who often have no detailed information about the patient. Home care is limited, and to see a specialist or get imaging or laboratory tests, patients must travel to one of the major hospitals because there are few community-based specialists. This can work for acute, one-off problems but not for chronic conditions.

Some efforts are being made to solicit patients' experiences and make the system more responsive. For instance, the RHAs have patient ombudsmen, all hospitals are required to have patient boards, and there are patient experience surveys. But these efforts are only the first steps in creating a patient-centered system.

A 5th challenge is quality. In general, Norway provides high-quality care, but the quality data that the system collects is not integral to operations and payment. The Directorate of Health in the Ministry of Health and Care Services collects quality data on hospital infections, survival rates for various conditions, waiting times, and related data. Unfortunately, as one official in the Directorate of Health said, "Not even results from the best registries are used to follow up patients or to routinely monitor and improve quality."

Relatedly, many Norwegian health policy experts worry that there is a great deal of wasted, unnecessary, and inefficiently delivered care. Quality payments affect less than 1% of hospital payments. Although waiting times are publicly available, other quality data, such as about physician performance, are not. For instance, data on ensuring that people with diabetes have their blood glucose, blood pressure, and lipids under control is not collected or disseminated to physicians or the public. Similarly, quality and waste data related to the frequency of ER visits and hospital admissions for patients undergoing chemotherapy or with diabetes or other chronic conditions are not routinely assessed or given back to physicians with comparisons to other practitioners. The Minister of Health and Care Services has urged the RHAs and hospitals to reduce unnecessary care. Quality data to inform patients which GPs are high performers are not available, nor are data used for bonuses or to modify capitation or fee-for-service payments to GPs.

Finally, some key services are not well integrated into the system. That dental and vision care for adults are paid 100% out of pocket seems outdated. More importantly, Norway does not seem well positioned regarding long-term care. There is no national long-term care insurance; municipalities are responsible for funding both home-based and institutional long-term care. One consequence of this is that elderly Norwegians pay for a substantial portion of long-term care services, which consumes most of their pensions and other resources. This may be a wise policy choice when combined with free care for children, but it means that long-term care is more unequally distributed. Over the last few years there was significant investment in building thousands of nursing home beds. But as the senior population grows—thus increasing the needs for more custodial and nursing services—the system will need to expand in-home and nursing home care. Municipalities might not be able to afford and organize such care. Inadvertently this may lead to increased use of hospital services if outpatient services are unavailable. Although policymakers are aware of this problem, solving it is another issue.

All of these challenges, though, are at the margins of a system that is easy to use and generally works well: it is universal, provides extensive choice, has no co-pays for children and limited co-pays for adults, and may be the least complicated system in any developed country.

CHAPTER FIVE

FRANCE

"Every country's health care system is driven by a core national value. For the United Kingdom, it's utility. For Germany, responsibility. For the United States, liberty. [And for France,] equality," says Dr. Laurent Degos, vice president of the Pasteur Institute.

As Dr. Isabelle Durand-Zaleski has said, the French system truly is a "chimera." It combines a wide but shallow compulsory public health insurance with practically essential supplemental private insurance to cover high out-of-pocket costs. Simultaneously, it merges largely centralized financing and strong national regulation with privatization in its delivery systems.

The French love their freedom to choose any private physician and among many private hospitals, and they can go to any specialist without primary care gatekeeping or a referral. But this cherished freedom of choice creates what is probably the biggest challenge of the French system: extreme fragmentation of care. As one patient reported, whenever he goes to his physician he makes sure to bring his own X-rays and other test results; otherwise the consulting physician will not be able to access them. At a time when most of health care is focused on chronic conditions, this fragmentation of care raises the question of whether the French system lives up to its esteemed reputation for equal, accessible, and high-quality care for all.

HISTORY

France adopted a national health care system relatively late. Whereas Germany enacted its employer-based Bismarckian system during the 1880s, France did not pass its first form of national health insurance until 1928. Prior to this, medical care was largely accessible only through sporadic employer benefits, fraternal associations, and direct fee-for-service purchases.

This original national health insurance was narrow in scope. It only covered low-wage salaried workers in industry or commerce. It excluded their families, moderate- and high-wage workers, farmers, the self-employed, students, and the unemployed. It reimbursed physicians exclusively fee-for-service and offered limited benefits. It did expand over time, however, so that by the end of the 1930s it covered roughly two-thirds of the French population.

World War II decimated French society and displaced many entrenched institutions and interests. Many medical leaders were killed during the Nazi occupation, while others were delegitimized by their collaboration. In particular, mutual funds—the equivalent of German sickness funds—were maligned for their collaboration with the Vichy state. French physicians, however, kept their respected place in society. They famously defied the Nazis and continued to treat all wounded persons—both French and German—in accordance with their oaths.

In the postwar period, the French looked to rebuild and, under Pierre LaRoque's guidance, crafted their first modern system of social security. As part of this, they sought to improve national strength by expanding health insurance to all workers and their families, irrespective of their income. Mutual funds had been providing these services but were shunted aside as the primary vehicle for coverage and were forced to reposition themselves by offering supplemental insurance on a voluntary basis for services *not* covered by the mandatory national plan.

Despite significant pressure to move toward socialized medicine, physician groups kept their financial independence. Under the new, postwar system, French physicians were granted much of the professional autonomy they desired. They preserved private practice with fee-for-service reimbursement as the cornerstone of French health care. France eventually adopted a uniform fee schedule, but it took years of debate, culminating with Charles de Gaulle himself quipping "I saved France on a colonel's pay" after physicians kept arguing for higher wages.

Figure 1. Health Care Coverage (France)

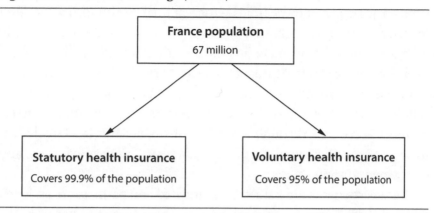

Over the next 50 years, this national health care program under-went piecemeal expansion. In 1961, agricultural workers were included, and in 1966 the self-employed were brought in as well. But it was only in 2000, with the passage of the Universal Health Coverage Act (CMU), that universal coverage was officially achieved. The Universal Disease Protection Act's (PUMA) passage in 2016 finally granted automatic and continuous eligibility to the national health insurance for all legal residents.

COVERAGE

The French health care system has 2 layers of coverage: mandatory basic health insurance provided by the national government and voluntary, albeit nearly universal, supplemental health insurance provided by private insurers.

Public, Statutory Health Insurance

The entire French population is covered by national statutory health insurance (SHI). Like the German sickness funds, the French statutory health insurance is not a single-payer system; instead, patients are covered through one of a handful of health care funds. However, unlike the German sickness funds, the French are *assigned* to their health care fund based on employment status. The French cannot "shop" between funds. The largest of these funds—the National Health Insurance Fund for Salaried Workers (CNAMTS), or the General Fund—covers nearly 90% of the population, including most salaried workers and their families. Two other funds, Mutualité Sociale Agricole (MSA) covering agricultural workers and Regime Social des Indépendants (RSI) for the self-employed, cover about 8% of the remaining population. The remainder is covered through a handful of smaller funds—largely historic—for specific populations such as miners, railway workers, and clergymen, among others.

Because benefits are nationally mandated and patients are assigned to funds based strictly on employment, the differences between the funds is minimal. They all cover the same basic package, and they all reimburse at the same rate.

In general the SHI benefits are quite broad and include inpatient care, outpatient services, prescription medications, medical goods, long-term care, and health-related transportation costs. Coverage is more limited for preventive services. And like many other countries, dental and vision coverage are, in the words of one physician, "nominal."

Though broad, coverage under SHI is not deep, placing substantial out-of-pocket costs on patients. Coinsurance rates tend to be quite high with SHI alone. Inpatient care is generally covered at 80%, leaving 20% of hospital bills to patients. Similarly, in the outpatient setting 60% of laboratory tests are paid for by SHI while 70% of physician services are. Although patients are free to choose any physician, SHI will only cover 30% of specialist fees without a referral. Pharmaceutical reimbursement averages around 65%, but it varies from 15% for low-therapeutic products to 100% for nonsubstitutable and/or expensive medications. Thus, patients have substantial costs if they are only insured by the SHI.

SHI has also introduced small co-payments to raise revenues and reduce consumption. In 2005, a $1.08 USD (€1) deductible (*participation forfaitaire*) was introduced for every physician visit, laboratory test, and imaging procedure. In 2008, a 54 cent USD (€0.5) deductible was added for each prescription medication. These deductibles are capped: the maximum is $54 USD (€50) per year for medications and $54 USD (€50) for consultations. Importantly, there is no overall spending cap for out-of-pocket payments.

Most specialists and some general practitioners are also legally permitted to charge extra, beyond the official SHI payment. Such "balance billing" is not covered under SHI. As of 2018, these rates ranged from slightly higher than the nominal reimbursement rate to over 10 times the official SHI rate for certain specialists and specialties. While the 2015 Health Reform Law attempted to curb these excesses by containing an agreement for "responsible contracts," balance billing remains a hotly debated issue in France.

Private Supplemental Insurance

Because of this high degree of cost sharing and out-of-pocket costs with the statutory health insurance alone, 95% of the French population has purchased private, supplemental voluntary health insurance (VHI). While only a handful of mandated health care funds deliver SHI, the voluntary health insurance is different. Myriad private insurance companies compete in an open market. Most of these plans are offered as part of an employment package, although individual plans are available. For the poorest parts of the population VHI is provided free of charge.

These plans largely serve 2 purposes. First, they reduce the degree of cost sharing for standard benefits covered under the national plan by covering coinsurance and certain amounts of balance billing. These plans thus function similarly to older Medigap plans in the United States. Second, they cover select benefits that the SHI does not cover. Almost all these voluntary plans cover dental and vision care, and many cover a wide range of additional services, such as complementary and alternative medicine. Unlike in other countries, French VHI is not used to increase access to desired providers or to avoid waiting times.

As VHI has historically been available only to the wealthy, recent legislation has aimed to increase access for all French citizens. In 2004, a new voucher system gave a "health check" (*cheque santé*) to everyone with income between 100% and 135% of the poverty line. These annual vouchers range from $108 to $615 USD (€100 to €550), depending on age, and they must be used to purchase private health insurance. Tax rebates encourage employers to provide VHI benefits to their employees. Since 2016, the government has required many employers to offer VHI. For individuals who cannot afford VHI by themselves or do not receive it through their work, the government offers its own state-sponsored VHI to around 10% of the population.

In this way, the French value of equality has caused the private voluntary coverage to become nearly universal. It remains an ongoing debate whether it would be better if the SHI simply expanded what it covers. Proponents argue that it could reduce the significant administrative costs associated with the VHI, while opponents are concerned this would disrupt the current system.

Special Coverage for Chronic Illnesses
The French approach seniors and the chronically ill by assuming complete financial responsibility for their medical care through the Chronic Disease (Affection de Longue Durée, or ALD) program. Each year the Ministry of Health defines 30 such categories of illness—including diabetes, asthma/COPD, heart failure, stroke, cancer, and long-term psychiatric disease. Patients who suffer from any of these afflictions are exempt from all costs related to the treatment of their illnesses, except for balance billing (if applicable) and the $1.08 USD (€1) *participation forfaitaire*. However, they are still responsible for paying for treatment for concurrent, nonchronic illnesses, such as an injury unrelated to their chronic condition. For patients with low incomes, most co-payments and coinsurance are waived.

FINANCING

Overall, France spends 11.5% of its GDP on health care, or $4,600 USD per capita. But it represents the 3rd-highest share of GDP in Europe, 2nd only to Switzerland and Germany. Around 80% of total healthcare spending is covered by statutory health insurance, 15% by voluntary health insurance, and 5% by out of pocket costs.

Statutory Health Insurance (SHI)
SHI has 4 funding sources: (1) a highly progressive system of payroll taxes (50%), (2) national income taxes (35%), (3) excise taxes on tobacco, alcohol, pharmaceuticals, and automobiles (13%), and (4) subsidies from the state (2%).

Figure 2. Financing Health Care: Statutory Health Insurance (France)

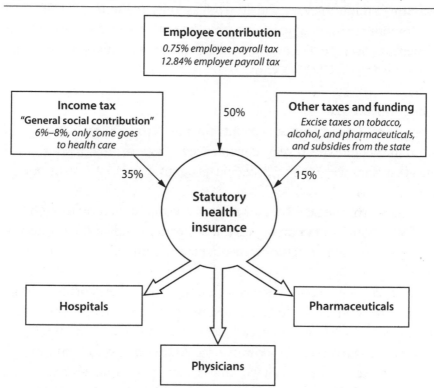

These funds are based on which industry each person works in, not by geographic location. In 2016, the payroll tax rate was 0.75% for employees and 12.84% for employers. The national income tax is known as the General Social Contribution (CSG). Its rate is based on the source of income. For instance, the CSG rate is 6.6% of pension income, 7.5% of earned income, 8.2% of capital gains, and 8.2% for gambling winnings. Only a fraction of the CSG goes to health insurance.

Voluntary Health Insurance (VHI)
A diverse market of largely private organizations funded through premiums provides VHI. Cumulatively, VHI accounts for about 13% of total health care spending. Most private insurance plans are obtained through an employer. Most private insurance funds use income-linked premiums and limited-risk rating. These organizations *can* consider age, health status, and region. Although age and region are commonly

used, health status is rarely used in practice to establish premiums. Monthly premiums vary widely, from as low as around $16 USD (€15) per month for scant coverage to over $108 USD (€100) per month for generous coverage. For a 55-year-old couple, the annual premium can be about $2,700 USD (€2,500).

Long-Term Care

Long-term care in France accounts for over $50 billion USD (€45 billion) in spending each year. It is financed through 3 major sources: (1) health insurance, (2) social benefit programs, and (3) out-of-pocket costs.

Long-term medical care for seniors is covered directly though SHI and VHI. SHI covers nursing care and inpatient end-of-life services at the standard rates of coinsurance, unless exempted as an ALD program.

A meshwork of national and local programs covers custodial long-term care services, including housing payments for residential care facilities and certain home care services. The largest of these programs, the Personalized Allowance for Autonomy, is funded through a solidarity contribution all working citizens pay (equal to one unpaid working day). To increase revenues, an additional 0.3% excise tax was introduced on all retirement and disability plans. Smaller benefits are covered through a variety of other directed national and local taxes.

Finally, patients and their families bear a large—and increasing—proportion of long-term care. Despite the generous social and medical benefits offered through France's system of social security, rising costs for long-term housing and insufficient levels of funding have left patients and their families to fill in the gaps. One study estimated that around 18% of supportive services, 81% of room and board, and 5% of health care services related to long-term care are paid for by families out of pocket.

Public Health

Historically, with the exception of maternity care, the French have lagged behind other nations in their embrace of public health measures and preventive medicine. On the individual level preventive services such as cancer screenings and vaccinations are largely covered by SHI, although co-payments exist for some preventive measures. To combat low rates of vaccinations, vaccination for 11 diseases is now free—and obligatory—for all children. Since 2017, a special incentive has been offered to general practitioners to advise adolescents and young adults on the prevention of sexually transmitted diseases.

On the systems level, general taxation pays for funding for public health offices responsible for tasks such as disease surveillance and national campaigns.

PAYMENT

Since 2004, payments for inpatient hospital stays have been based on DRGs. For the past century payments for physician services have remained largely fee-for-service. Recently, however, there has been a push toward pay-for-performance and capitated payments for French generalists, and these now account for approximately 10% of their reimbursement.

Payments to Hospitals

As of 2016, 73% of total hospital financing comes from DRG payments, while 27% comes from other sources, including annual payments and directed funding.

The Ministry of Health sets the DRGs and reimburses acute inpatient stays. These are referred to as the Homogeneous Group of the Sick (Groupe Homogène des Malades, or GHM). They were first introduced in 1986, and by 2004 there were 600 groups. As of 2009, there were over 2,300, each with 4 levels of severity.

Each year the Ministry of Health sets the rate of reimbursement for each GHM. Annually the Ministry of Health conducts a comprehensive bottom-up cost study that compares the most recent official French reimbursement with the real-world unit cost from about 16% of French hospitals. This is called the National Cost Studies with Common Methodology (Études Nationales de Coûts à Méthodologie Commune, or ENCC). The Ministry of Health then uses these data in the context of the overall budget established by Parliament and public health priorities to set the official French reimbursement levels, or tariffs, for the

Figure 3. Payment to Hospitals (France)

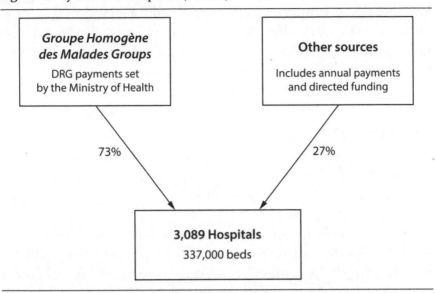

next year. Although this database is well done, the process has been criticized for a lack of transparency and public debate. It has also been criticized for its significant pricing inertia, in which prices for overvalued procedures are slow to come down.

Interestingly, payments are different in both amount and what is covered between public and private hospitals. To start, DRG reimbursement levels (tariffs) for private, for-profit hospitals do not include physician fees, while tariffs for nonprofit hospitals do. Moreover, certain imaging procedures are included in the DRG for public hospitals but not for private hospitals. Imaging performed by private hospitals outside DRGs is paid at a negotiated fee-for-services.

Emergency room visits are also handled differently. This stems from private hospitals being tasked with negotiating their own contracts with the government. They have engaged in favorable patient selection and also tend to assume fewer research and teaching responsibilities.

In addition to DRG-based payments, hospitals also receive direct activity-based payments for emergency room visits and experimental or novel procedures as well as block grants to promote activities of national importance, such as public health measures, clinical research, and cost-effectiveness research.

Figure 4. Payment to Ambulatory Physicians (France)

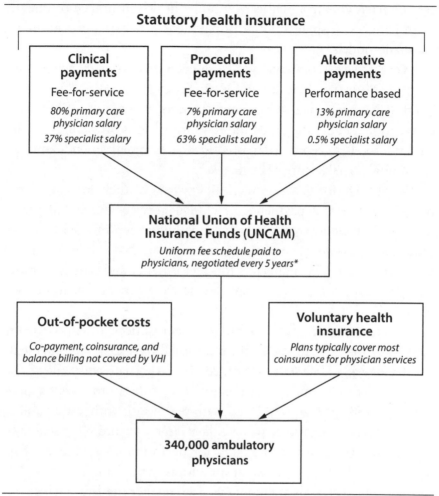

Statutory health insurance

Clinical payments	**Procedural payments**	**Alternative payments**
Fee-for-service	Fee-for-service	Performance based
80% primary care physician salary	*7% primary care physician salary*	*13% primary care physician salary*
37% specialist salary	*63% specialist salary*	*0.5% specialist salary*

National Union of Health Insurance Funds (UNCAM)
Uniform fee schedule paid to physicians, negotiated every 5 years*

Out-of-pocket costs	**Voluntary health insurance**
Co-payment, coinsurance, and balance billing not covered by VHI	*Plans typically cover most coinsurance for physician services*

340,000 ambulatory physicians

*Convention 1 accepts fee schedule without balance billing; Convention 2 accepts fee schedule and balance bills; Convention 3 only accepts VHI and out-of-pocket expenses

There are limited efforts to penalize hospitals for poor quality or for high readmissions.

Payments to Ambulatory or Office-Based Physicians

About 85% to 90% of payments to French physicians are based on a fee-for-service model. This includes psychiatric physicians, who receive fee-for-service payments from statutory health insurance, as well as nonphysician providers such as psychologists, who receive fee-for-service payments from either voluntary health insurance or directly from patients. A small amount of payments are based on alternative payment models.

Every 5 years representatives from each professional society meet with the Ministry of Health and National Union of Health Insurance Funds (UNCAM) to negotiate a contract, known as a convention. These conventions set the standards and rates for various procedures and interventions. Between conventions there are annual amendments via the annual Social Security Finance Act.

On average for general practitioners 87% of their income comes from fee-for-service payments for clinical services (80%) and procedures (7%). Patient payment for balance billing represented less than 3% of their income. The remaining 13% came in the form of alternative payments models, including pay-for-performance and capitation models. Since 2007 this percentage of alternative payments has more than doubled.

Generalists have several reimbursement options to choose from. First, they may opt to stick with traditional fee-for-service payments and receive $27 USD (€25) per office visit. Alternatively, if they practice in a medically underserved region, they can opt to accept a guaranteed income of $7,700 USD (€6,900) per month. If they are publicly employed, they can also be paid a salary largely according to seniority. In addition, generalists can qualify for performance payments of up to $5,600 USD (€5,000) per year for adopting meaningful use of electronic medical records and doing well on quality metrics, such as immunizations and compliance with chronic disease guidelines. They can also receive an additional $45 USD (€40) per patient by participating in programs designed to help manage patients with chronic illnesses.

Almost all payments to specialists and surgeons are traditional fees-for-service payments. In contrast to generalists, 16% of specialist total compensation stemmed from balance billing and only 0.5% from alternative payment models. Since 2006, the share of procedural fees and the amounts of balance billing have risen.

The amount and type of balance billing depend on the sector in which specialist physicians choose to practice. Sector 1 physicians (conventionnés) have completely accepted the fee schedule from the every-5-year meeting. They must assume the standard reimbursement rate and are not allowed to charge any additional fees. In exchange, the national health insurance reimburses all fees, and the Sector 1 physicians receive a credit toward their social security contributions via a 2% reduction in their retirement contribution rate. Over 91% of generalists and 55% of specialists practice in Sector 1.

Sector 2 physicians are permitted to charge higher rates than those set by the meeting, but they must do so with "tact and measure." SHI will still reimburse the standard rate, but patients are required to pay the difference between what the physician charges and the SHI fee. In exchange, these physicians relinquish several of the social and financial advantages granted to Sector 1 physicians, notably the reduced social security contribution. Providers must apply to become a Sector 2 physician, as the area is tightly regulated and the majority of Sector 2 physicians are required to concurrently have a full-time public hospital position. In total, 45% of specialists practice in Sector 2, while only 8% of generalists do.

Finally, Sector 3 physicians have completely rejected the negotiated fees and can charge whatever price they want. As a consequence, they are not eligible for any reimbursement through SHI. Only 1.2% of generalists and 0.4% of specialists practice in Sector 3. In general these physicians run boutique practices limited to the most affluent regions in France, such as Paris.

Nonphysician practitioners, such as nurses, pharmacists, and therapists, negotiate similar contracts with the Ministry of Health every 5 years and continue to be reimbursed through fee-for-service or salaried models.

Payments for Mental Health Care

The DRG activity-based payment model has not been extended to acute psychiatric hospitals. In public and nonprofit hospitals payment for mental health is by an annual prospective global budget. This budget is paid by SHI and allocated by regional health agencies on the basis of historical costs adjusted by the expected annual growth rate of hospital spending. Payments to for-profit hospitals are based on predetermined daily rates fixed according to the type of care provided, such as full-time or part-time hospitalization.

Payments for Long-Term Care

All citizens are automatically covered for medical benefits for long-term care through SHI and VHI. For custodial and residential services citizens must generally apply and demonstrate need. The largest national program, the National Solidarity Fund for Autonomy (CNSA), provides a Personalized Allowance for Autonomy (APA) to all citizens aged 60 and above who cannot perform daily activities independently. The monthly payment is based on the severity of disability and can be up to $1,900 USD (€1750) per month. Although it is not means tested, this benefit is discounted so that people with higher incomes can only earn 20% of the maximum benefit. There are various other benefits and tax incentives aimed at reducing the financial burden of long-term care.

Payments for Complementary and Alternative Medicine

Unlike many other countries, complementary and alternative medicine in France enjoys widespread health insurance coverage. SHI covers acupuncture, reimbursing it at half the cost of a general practitioner visit. SHI covers homeopathic products at a rate of 30% unless the products make certain health claims or contain high concentrations of medically active ingredients. VHI plans commonly contain additional coverage. Other forms of alternative medicine, such as osteopathy, are generally only covered by VHI or out-of-pocket spending.

Preventive Medicine

Most immunizations and recommended screening tests are paid for via SHI without coinsurance. The majority of preventive care, however, is not incentivized directly, and standard coinsurance rates apply for preventive care. However, there have been some recent initiatives targeting general practitioners to provide more preventive services.

DELIVERY OF HEALTH CARE SERVICES

While French health care is largely financed publicly, provision of care remains overwhelmingly private. Most medical practitioners are self-employed, and nearly twice as many hospitals are private and for profit in France than in other developed countries. Given this high degree of autonomy, fragmentation of care constitutes a major issue.

Hospital Care

France has 3,089 hospitals, with a total of 377,000 beds for approximately 67 million people, equal to 6.3 hospital beds per 1,000 people. This is more than double the number of hospital beds per capita in the United States (2.9 per 1000 people), while Germany has more beds per capita but fewer hospitals. Hence, hospitals are typically much smaller in France than they are in Germany. Although the total number of hospital beds has decreased over the past decade, closing hospitals remains politically perilous. According to one policymaker: "We're unable to close hospitals that need to be closed because it would be politically unacceptable." This has led to many small, isolated hospitals.

Many more of the French hospitals are private than in other European countries. Fully 36% of all French acute care hospitals are private. Of those, nearly three-quarters of them are for profit. Taken together, these hospitals employ nearly 300,000 physicians. Similar to other countries, private, for-profit hospitals in France typically specialize in a limited number of highly profitable procedures, such as elective percutaneous coronary angiograms, upper and lower endoscopies, and joint replacement surgery.

FRANCE LAGS BEHIND other developed countries in introducing EHRs and other information technologies. In 2004, France launched its first attempt at a national health record, the Personal Medical Record (Dossier Médical Personnel, or DMP). Despite high hopes, adoption rates were poor and, even after a redesign and relaunch in 2010, uptake continued to languish. As of 2014 the overall adoption rate was only 67%. As one physician explained, "It's unclear to whom the EMR 'belongs'... interconnectedness is poor, and there's a low level of trust."

When combined with an already fragmented delivery system, the lack of a uniform electronic record has significantly impeded high-quality care. France also has less advanced imaging equipment per capita, although it has similar levels of use. Further, although all

French citizens have an electronic health insurance card (Carte Vitale), the card doesn't currently contain any health information.

Ambulatory or Outpatient Care

At a rate of 6.3 annual consultations per person per year, the French visit physicians slightly less often than people in other developed countries but much more frequently than Americans. French physicians see an average of 2,020 patients per year, similar to the rate of other developed countries but substantially lower than Canadian and Taiwanese physicians.

As with hospitals, fragmentation of care remains a central issue for France. Most practitioners remain in solo practice and are largely autonomous. As one physician observed,

> Physician practices are largely single-person practices. Groups and co-ordination are rare. . . . There's very little incentive, given the current fee-for-service structure. . . . And specialists don't talk to generalists—there's a sense that "they wouldn't understand."

Another physician I spoke with noted, "It's not rare for patients to have to repeat tests 2 to 3 times. . . . It's to the point where you have to carry around your own X-rays." However, this situation is changing, and most younger physicians are beginning to work in group (*maison de santé*) and multidisciplinary practices (*pluridisciplinaire*).

There are no preferred provider networks of physicians and hospitals. There is no selective contracting in France with physicians' groups and only limited ways for health funds to penalize underperforming physicians. Moreover, as Dr. Durand-Zaleski explained, enforcement of gatekeeping—preventing patients from seeing a specialist without a primary care physician referral—is quite limited: "You just have to tick a box saying that you have a gatekeeping physician" to bypass this hurdle.

Mental Health Care

Similar to other developed countries, since the 1960s France has undergone a slow trend of deinstitutionalization. Most mental health care is now provided on an outpatient basis under the responsibility of a local team attached to a psychiatric hospital. According to one's area of residence, patients are automatically attached to a psychiatric sector (*secteur*), a geographical area of roughly 70,000 inhabitants. In each sector a mental health team decides the most appropriate type of care. Mental health care in the sector is free of charge. In addition, patients can choose to be treated by a private mental health physician and/or a private mental health hospital with the same financing rules as any other disease. SHI provides funding for inpatient and ambulatory psychiatric care and covers it at the same rates as nonpsychiatric care. However, care by a psychologist is not included under the statutory health insurance, although some VHI plans do cover their care.

Long-Term Care

In France a relatively high proportion of inpatient beds (about 15%) are dedicated to rehabilitative care, while fewer are dedicated to long-term care. The majority of long-term care institutions are public (54%), although the number of private, not-for-profit and for-profit institutions is increasing.

Preventive Medicine

Ambulatory physicians typically administer cancer screening and immunization. Historically, the rates of screening for breast, colon, and cervical cancer in France have been significantly below the European average. The same goes for vaccination rates for hepatitis B (83%) and measles (91%). Dr. Fabian Calvo, chief scientific officer for Cancer Core Europe, notes that this is part financial and part cultural: "There is a lack of funding for preventive care, including cancer screening, and these fields are not considered as prestigious for providers."

Recently the national government has introduced nationwide screening campaigns. For instance, for colon cancer the government will mail eligible individuals reminders to undergo a colonoscopy twice and will then send them a fecal-occult blood test at home if they do not see a physician. Similarly the government has made childhood vaccination both free and obligatory and offered physicians incentives to council adolescents on sexually transmitted diseases. The definitive impact of these measures is yet to be fully assessed.

PHARMACEUTICAL COVERAGE AND
PRICE CONTROLS

Pharmaceutical Market

France is the world's 5th largest pharmaceutical market, with an approximate size of $37 USD billion. This translates to 12% of total health care spending, or $637 USD per person per year. This is about 45% of US spending and 67% of Swiss spending per person. In absolute dollars, this is 12% higher than the OECD average. High consumption of prescription medications drives this higher-than-average expenditure.

Coverage Determination

After the European Medicines Agency (EMA) evaluates a drug for safety, effectiveness, and quality, it is automatically approved for licensure in France.

The French High Authority on Health (HAS) then evaluates the medication's scientific validity and grades its absolute and relative benefits.

The HAS Transparency Committee first categorizes the degree of absolute health benefit—known as the medical service rendered (service médical rendu, SMR)—by examining the new drug's clinical attributes. It considers the drug's demonstrated efficacy, side-effect profile, and the severity of the condition being treated. It then grades the drug's health benefits on a 5-level scale ranging from irreplaceable to major, moderate, weak, or insufficient. This designation is important: patients taking medications designated as irreplaceable are reimbursed 100% of the cost, while patients taking drugs providing a major improvement are reimbursed at 65% by the statutory health insurance. Conversely, drugs designated insufficient are not paid for at all. Prescription drugs deemed moderate are covered at 30% of cost and weak prescription drugs at 15%.

The HAS then assesses the new drug's relative efficacy by comparing it to existing therapies already on the market. This is known as an improvement in additional benefit (IAB). It rates the new drug's relative performance in one of 5 tiers: (1) major therapeutic improvement, (2) significant improvement, (3) moderate improvement, (4) minor improvement, or (5) no improvement. Thus, a drug, such as a statin, could

Figure 5. Regulation of Pharmaceutical Prices (France)

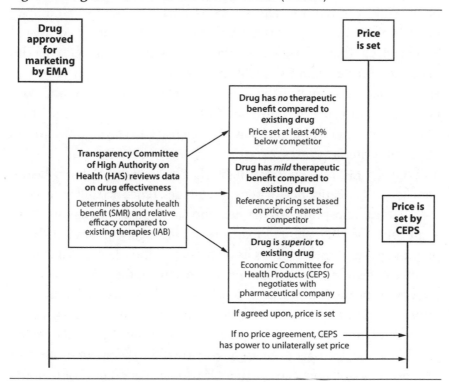

have major health benefits in an absolute sense but represent no improvement over drugs already on the market.

These absolute and relative health benefit designations last for 5 years by default but can be reassessed at any time if new data emerge. Recently HAS received criticism for being slow to review products. As one physician noted: "HAS decides when they decide to decide.... The entire process is getting slower and slower, with more and more committees."

Price Regulation

After approval and grading by HAS, the Economic Committee for Health Products' (CEPS) pharmaceutical section reviews the available clinical and economic data to negotiate a price with the pharmaceutical company.

First, CEPS collects an economic dossier that includes a proposed price and sales projections. Using an informal external reference pricing, the proposed price must be in line with neighboring countries or else CEPS can reject it. This serves as a price ceiling for reimbursement. In addition, drugs classified as having a relative benefit compared to other drugs that is designated as major or significant as well as a sales projection greater than $22.5 USD million (€20 million) per year have an additional economic analysis performed by the Economic and Public Health Assessment Committee (CEESP), a committee within HAS. This was the result of a 2012 law that increased HAS's power to use economic criteria to assess drugs.

Second, CEPS reviews the available data by assessing absolute health benefit (SMR), relative health benefit (IAB), reference pricing indexed to the 4 largest European nations neighboring France—Germany, Italy, Spain, and the UK—and comparisons with drugs with similar therapeutic benefits. It then submits its own price proposal. For medications deemed to be of minor therapeutic improvement, the price is set at the level of the nearest competitor. Generics and those deemed to have no improvement have discounted pricing, generally at least 40% below the brand-name drug's cost. Importantly, SHI is not legally allowed to reimburse medications deemed to have neither therapeutic nor cost benefit. For novel medications there is usually a good deal of negotiation between the company and CEPS. If negotiations fail, CEPS has the power to unilaterally set prices.

Ultimately, CEPS submits a final price proposal, which is then put to a vote. Once passed, it becomes national law. After this, National Union of Health Insurance Funds (UNCAM) sets the reimbursement rate based on the absolute and relative health benefits, and then the health minister then gives final approval before listing the new medication in the official register. Subsequently, prices are reevaluated at least once every 5 years.

To keep prescription drug costs low, France has adopted 2 additional practices. First, France has established a national limit on annual pharmaceutical spending growth. Above the growth cap, companies must pay the government 50% to 70% rebates on any additional revenue. The 2020 target growth rate for total pharmaceutical spending is 0.5%.

Second, CEPS has frequently used price-volume contracts to lower sales of high-cost drugs. Reimbursement for Gilead's hepatitis C drug Sofosbuvir (Sovaldi) is illustrative. In 2013, Sovaldi was approved in the

United States at a price of $84,000 USD (€75,000) for a 12-week course and made widely available. Citing its immense price, the UK initially refused to cover the treatment. France took an intermediate approach and negotiated a price-volume contract in which they paid $46,000 USD (€41,000) and capped volume at 15,000 doses. CEPS then gave strict prescription criteria so that only the medically sickest 15,000 of the 200,000 hepatitis C patients in France would be treated. Costs were limited because, as is law in France, if total sales went over the negotiated amount, Gilead would be legally obligated to pay back the difference.

CEPS's strong central negotiating power has achieved remarkable control over drug pricing. The pharmaceutical retail price index for France is 61, nearly half that of the United States (100), Germany (95), and Switzerland (88). And this translates into real savings: whereas Germany consumes 6% fewer pills per capita, it spends nearly 40% per capita more due to higher prices. For instance, in the case of the statin Crestor, when it was branded, a one-month supply cost $86.40 USD in the United States, $40.50 USD in Germany, $25.80 USD in the UK, but only $19.80 USD in France.

This system has kept prices under control despite France's high share of branded drugs. In fact, only 30% of the prescriptions are generic, significantly lower in other developed countries.

Regulation of Physician Prescriptions
The French have several mechanisms regulating how physicians prescribe medications. First, certain classes of medications are only covered in specific settings. Some medications, such as powerful antibiotics and antifungals, can only be prescribed in hospitals. Others, such as certain forms of anticoagulant medications, can only be started on an inpatient basis. Prescribing these medications in inappropriate settings is not covered under SHI, and providers could be held liable for adverse events.

Second, certain medications can only be prescribed by certain specialists (prescription réservée à des médecins spécialistes). For instance, ivabradine, a drug used in advanced heart failure, can only be prescribed by cardiologists, while riluzole, an expensive orphan drug used for amyotrophic lateral sclerosis (Lou Gehrig's disease), can only be prescribed by neurologists.

Third, certain exceptional medications (médicaments d'exception) can only be prescribed with preapproval. These exceptional medications are either expensive or innovative and have very specific indications delineated in the drug information sheet (fiche d'information thérapeutique).

France continues to have high levels of prescribed medications. There are no penalties for physicians who prescribe significantly more drugs than their peers. Whereas France has average prescriptions for antihypertensive drugs, cholesterol-lowering agents, antidiabetic drugs, and antidepressants, it has high levels of other types of medications, including benzodiazepines. As one physician explained, "In France, there is a perception that if I visit my primary care physician and he didn't prescribe me a drug, then what did he do? He must not be a physician!"

Prices Paid by Patients
In France the price of drugs for patients is quite low compared to other countries. All medications deemed to be irreplaceable are covered 100% of the pharmacy cost, while VHI typically handles the coverage gaps for prescription drugs with lower therapeutic ratings. Moreover, medications deemed to have lower health benefits that are used to treat chronic illnesses are covered 100% through the ALD program. This lack of cost sharing has affected the French public's relative insensitivity to pharmaceutical costs and perpetual high sales volumes.

HUMAN RESOURCES

Physicians
France has 226,000 physicians serving a population of 67 million, or roughly 3.3 physicians per 1,000 population. This is in line with the OECD average. Of all physicians, nearly 46% provide primary care. The preponderance of generalists is due to the Ministry of Health limiting the number of specialist training spots in an effort to curb spending. The majority of both generalists and specialists are either fully or partially self-employed.

Roughly half (44.3%) of French physicians are female, in line with other developed countries and significantly higher than the percent in the United States (34.6%). In addition, France has a relatively low share of foreign-trained doctors, just 10.4%, while the percentage in Norway is 38% and Switzerland is 27%. France also has among the oldest physician workforce in the world. In 2017, nearly half were aged 55 or older. This is significantly higher than the OECD average. This is largely driven by a lower-than-expected rate of retirement by older physicians. (Reforms in 2003 and 2009 enabled retirement-age physicians to continue to practice.) To compensate, the French Ministry of Health increased the number of training spots by about 15%.

France's physicians are some of the most geographically concentrated. For instance, there are 2.7 physicians per 1,000 people in rural areas, with 3.9 per 1,000 people in urban areas. However, for some specialties there are 8 specialists in urban areas for 1 in a rural geography. The maldistribution and "physician deserts" are a consequence of the freedom that France offers its practitioners. As Dr. Agnes Couffinhal described, in the French system the physician is "the king. He sets up shop anywhere he wants and can leave as he pleases." Moreover, incentive programs to encourage physicians to move to more rural and underserved areas have been largely unsuccessful, as many physicians who take advantage of them only stay for a year or 2. As policymakers say, they "take the money and go."

In general French physicians make more than their European counterparts but half of what their US counterparts earn. Privately employed primary care physicians earn about $127,000 USD (€113,000), while privately employed specialists and surgeons earn an average of $208,000 USD (€186,000). However, primary care physicians working in public facilities earn much less, about $95,000 USD (€85,000) per year. The divide between compensation for specialists and generalists has increased over the past several decades. Between 2005 and 2015, while specialists' take-home pay increased 1.6% per year, generalists saw their wages increase by only 0.8% per year.

While there is a comparatively low salary, especially compared to Germany and Switzerland, French physicians have other financial advantages. They do not pay for malpractice insurance. Moreover, depending on their sector placement, they have a variety of government financial benefits, including subsidized social security taxes.

Similar to other European nations, college and medical school are functionally merged in France. After completing high school, aspiring French doctors begin with 2 years of basic science education, referred to as "Cycle 1" (Premier Cycle d'Études Médicales), similar to US pre-medical coursework, and then take a competitive exam that determines eligibility to move forward, similar to the United States' MCAT. They then take 4 years of in-classroom and in-hospital medical education, referred to as "Cycle 2" (Deuxième Cycle des Etudes Médicales), similar to US medical school curricula. They then have 2- to 5-year residencies at hospitals to complete their clinical training, similar to US residencies but generally shorter in duration. When combined with 2 fewer years of tertiary education, French physicians can begin to practice independently 3 or more years sooner than their American counterparts.

There are 34 medical schools in France that train just over 8,000 physicians each year. The Ministry of Health sets the number of training spots available each year centrally (numerus clausus), although this strict quota will be eliminated in 2020. There has been considerable controversy surrounding the Ministry of Health's restriction of the number of physician trainees. Medical education in France is free.

Nurses

As of 2015 France had 9.9 nurses per 1,000 people, about the average of developed countries. Nurse practitioners have not yet been nationally recognized, and expanded scopes for nonphysician providers remain rudimentary.

Compared to nurses in neighboring countries, nurses make significantly less money. French nurses earn on average $42,500 USD (€38,000) per year, compared to $53,700 USD (€48,000) per year for nurses in Germany. In fact, French nurses are some of the only nurses in the world to earn less than the average workers.

To obtain a bachelor's degree in nursing in France, a student must first pass an entrance exam and then complete a 3-year training program at a university-affiliated program. Upon completion, nurses routinely pursue additional training to subspecialize in field such as pediatrics. Despite the president calling for the nation to embrace nurse practitioners in 2014, their roles are yet to be defined, and higher payment has yet to be realized.

CHALLENGES

There are 5 major challenges facing the French health care system. First, France must find a way to coordinate care better, especially for the elderly and individuals with chronic illnesses such as diabetes, heart failure, and COPD. The current system of care delivery is highly fragmented, and the vast majority of physicians practice independently and without a functional national electronic health record. Care coordination is in its infancy and has led to lackluster chronic disease management and increased spending over unnecessary testing. As Dr. Zaleski stated bluntly, "Care coordination is a disaster." This is exacerbated by difficulties modernizing the hospital system and closing smaller hospitals and limited abilities to regulate quality of care. With the growing burden of chronic illnesses, this is a major challenge for improving care.

Second, while France has controlled prices through strong central oversight, its continued dependence on a fee-for-service payment model for physician services and DRG payments for most hospital care creates systemic incentives for wasteful spending. Volume thus remains high and rising rapidly in terms of office visits, hospitalizations, and consumption of pharmaceutical products. This has led to high costs and increasing physician and nonphysician provider dissatisfaction and burnout. Although alternative payment models have been successfully implemented for some generalists, they remain a tiny fraction of total payments. Bundled payments and other alternative models must be expanded to include the majority of generalists and specialists.

Third, preventive health care services, both vaccinations and cancer screenings, are relatively poor and need improvement. Although many in France live long lives, a significant proportion of this can be tied to healthy diet and higher-than-average levels of physical activity. Rates of immunizations and cancer screenings are among the lowest in Europe. Preventive health care is underfunded and underutilized. Some efforts in this direction have been undertaken, such as making vaccinations for children both free and obligatory. However, further public health measures to reduce tobacco and alcohol consumption, especially among the young, are also warranted.

Fourth, inequalities in care must be addressed. Although France undeniably has excellent access to care, it continues to use an awkward 2-tiered payment system. With recent reforms continuing to expand access to VHI, the line between what is mandatory and what is voluntary is being blurred. Perhaps it is time to expand the range of covered services to include the "fringe" benefits of dental and eye care. Moreover, France continues to struggle with encouraging physicians to move to more underserved rural areas of the country.

Finally, the French health care workforce remains largely traditional and physician based. Expanded roles for nurse practitioners should be explored.

Good truly is the enemy of great—at least in France. French health care is, if not anything else, assuredly "good." Life expectancy is high, costs are not unbearable, and—although there remain significant areas in need of improvement—there is broad domestic approval of the current program. As one physician put it, "everyone agrees . . . health care is not a salient political issue in France." In this way the hybrid French system largely delivers what it promises: universal access to health care in an easily accessible and largely affordable way.

CHAPTER SIX

GERMANY

For people who cherish patient choice, Germany is pretty close to ideal. There is free choice of sickness fund (insurance company), hospital, and physician, all with pretty minimal co-pays. Physicians and hospitals are extremely convenient, and access is pretty convenient too. On average Germans have a primary care physician within 15 minutes of where they live. And Germany is one of the few countries to have solved the financing of long-term care with a dedicated tax.

Although Germany has a reputation for efficiency, the health care system—with over 100 sickness funds—is anything but efficient. As one health policy expert said, "It is hard to know what [the sickness funds] add to quality, cost, or care coordination." About 99% of benefits are the same between funds. In addition, all the funds collectively bargain with physicians, hospitals, and pharmaceutical companies regarding fees and prices. They have almost no selective contracting and networks of high-performing providers. "While sickness funds could be more active in checking quality of performance and ensuring appropriate utilization of services, they are lazy."

Every expert and government health official recognizes there are too many German hospitals, many of which lack essential services such as stroke units or cardiac catheterization facilities. But, as one government official noted, Germany is doing so well that no one wants to confront the hard choices and expend the political capital it would require to close unnecessary and underperforming hospitals: "A booming economy means it is easier to buy out people than change the health care system."

HISTORY

The Franco-Prussian War ended in 1871, resulting in the official political and administrative unification of the German state. Kaiser Wilhelm I became the head of state, and the conservative aristocrat Otto von Bismarck became the chancellor. In response to industrialization, which fostered worker unrest, the desire for unionization, and advocacy for socialism, Bismarck instituted a number of social welfare programs, from workman's compensation and disability insurance to retirement pensions. His aim was to undermine workers' support for socialism and the Social Democratic Party by acceding to some of their demands for better protections against risk during the tumultuous societal transformations caused by industrialization.

The Health Insurance Act of 1883 was a major component of Bismarck's social welfare program. It created the world's first statutory health insurance scheme. At first, health insurance was limited to urban industrial workers, skilled craftsman, and other blue-collar workers in commercial enterprises—just 10% of the population. "Sickness funds" administered the health insurance, and these were mainly attached to workers' place of employment and governed by boards elected from the workers and employers. Based on the preexisting guild system, there were initially almost 19,000 sickness funds associated with different companies across the country. Contributions from both workers and employers financed the system. Workers paid about two-thirds of the premiums and employers about one-third.

By the start of World War I, workers in the transportation, agriculture, and service sectors were covered by mandatory health insurance, and by the end of the war in 1918 the unemployed were integrated into the insurance scheme. By 1926, half the German population had health insurance coverage through the statutory health insurance (SHI) scheme. Farmers, however, did not receive coverage until 1972. Three groups have been excluded from the statutory health insurance scheme and are required to purchase private health insurance: civil servants, the self-employed, and high-income earners.

Initially the point of health insurance was not to pay for health services but to mitigate wage loss due to illness. But as the effectiveness of medical services improved and costs for these services increased, sickness fund payments shifted to covering diagnostic and therapeutic medical services. At the start, sick workers received up to 50% of their wages in cash for 13 weeks, with additional coverage of ambulatory care, drugs, and treatments. Over time additional services were covered: mandatory maternity pay in 1919, hospital care in 1936, and preventive care and annual check-ups in 1970.

Early in the 20th century, physicians became worried about encroachment on their professional autonomy by sickness funds and began demanding higher fees. In response, the government created the Imperial Committee of Physicians and Sickness Funds to define the health insurance benefit package and the delivery of ambulatory services. This committee made fundamental changes in governance and payment in 1931, when the Weimar Republic was collapsing and hyperinflation was ravaging the German economy. Ambulatory physicians were granted a legal monopoly over outpatient care. They were required to be members of their Regional Association of Statutory Health Insurance Physicians. Payment for services flowed from the sickness funds to these regional associations that, in turn, paid their physician members for their ambulatory care services. This abolished individual contracts between physicians and sickness funds, replacing them with a uniform contract covering all ambulatory care physicians and sickness funds. Another consequence of this was that it rigidly divided care between ambulatory care physicians, governed by and paid through these regional associations of physicians, and hospital-based physicians, paid by the hospitals. This division persists today.

When Germany reunified in 1990 after the fall of the Berlin Wall, the Communist East German health system was disassembled and integrated into the West German system. It is the West German system that exists today.

Since reunification there have been 14 major pieces of health reform legislation, 3 of which have ushered in fundamental changes. First, the Health Care Structure Act of 1993 replaced geographical, occupational, and employer-based assignment to sickness funds with free choice by the individual, with the option of changing sickness funds annually. To minimize risk selection, sickness funds were paid a risk-adjusted amount from the central health fund. Second, the Statutory Health Insurance Modernization Act of 2004 increased workers' financial contributions for insurance by 0.9% of wages, fully instituted DRG payments for hospitals, and created the Federal Joint Commission (Gemeinsamer Bundesausschuss [GBA]) to negotiate most of the reimbursement rates and other policies between sickness funds, physicians, hospitals, and other entities in the health system. The SHI Modernization Act also introduced co-pays of $11 USD (€10) per day for hospitalizations, $5.40 to $11 USD (€5 to €10) for ambulatory care services and products, and $11 USD (€10) per quarter for physician and dentist visits—this quarterly co-pay was eliminated by a unanimous parliament vote in 2012. Finally, the Act to Strengthen Competition in Statutory Health Insurance, enacted in 2007, made health insurance mandatory and universal for all Germans and created a central financing pool that collected payments and redistributed risk-adjusted premiums to the sickness funds.

Despite extensive reforms over nearly 150 years, the German health care system has 3 enduring and defining characteristics. First, it is committed to the fundamental principles of solidarity and universality. All Germans both contribute to fund the system based on income and receive the benefits based on health need, not geography or wealth. In addition, spouses who do not earn an income as well as children are covered without an additional contribution or co-payments, and those with serious chronic diseases are further subsidized through rather generous exemption regulations.

A 2nd characteristic of the system is self-government by the payers, hospitals, physicians, and patients. From the beginning, government involvement in the health system was minimized in favor of self-government by collective organizations that represented the various actors in the health care system. Bismarck wanted the federal government to collect premiums and pay out benefits, but his political opponents worried this would give his government excessive power. Instead, the administrative and financial power was assigned to the nongovernmental sickness funds based around employers. As a result, various nongovernmental commissions have been empowered with legally binding authority to negotiate details of the health insurance system, such as reimbursement rates and benefits. During Hitler's rule these self-government arrangements were preempted, and the government enforced some of the worst Nazi practices, such as prohibiting Jewish physicians in the statutory health system from treating non-Jews. Because of this abuse, the commitment to empowering nongovernmental, self-governing commissions with administrative and financial authority was reaffirmed and strengthened. Today it is fair to say that the most important body overseeing health care in Germany is not the federal government but the Federal Joint Commission.

Finally, the German statutory health system has shown impressive endurance over the past 135 years. Despite abuse by the Nazis, the fundamental values of the system have persisted. As health policy expert Reinhard Busse and colleagues note, Germany's health care system has had

> remarkable resilience: it survived, with key principles intact, different forms of government (an empire, republics, and the dictatorships), two world wars, hyperinflation, and the division and subsequent reunification of Germany.

COVERAGE

The German health care system has 2 major and one minor component, each of which covers different segments of the population.

First, the SHI scheme—the descendant of the original Bismarckian system—covers approximately 87% of the population, including privately employed workers and their dependents, students, the unemployed, and retired workers. The SHI is not a single-payer system. Instead, patients are covered through the approximate 105 sickness funds (as of January 2020). Traditionally, individuals were assigned to sickness funds based on geography or occupation, but the Health Care Structure Act of 1993 granted Germans the right to choose among sickness funds annually beginning in 1996. The 5 largest sickness funds have over 33 million members, representing 47% of the SHI market.

Individuals insured through the statutory health insurance system can purchase supplementary private insurance to cover amenities and benefits not covered in the SHI, such as private hospital rooms and

Figure 1. Health Care Coverage (Germany)

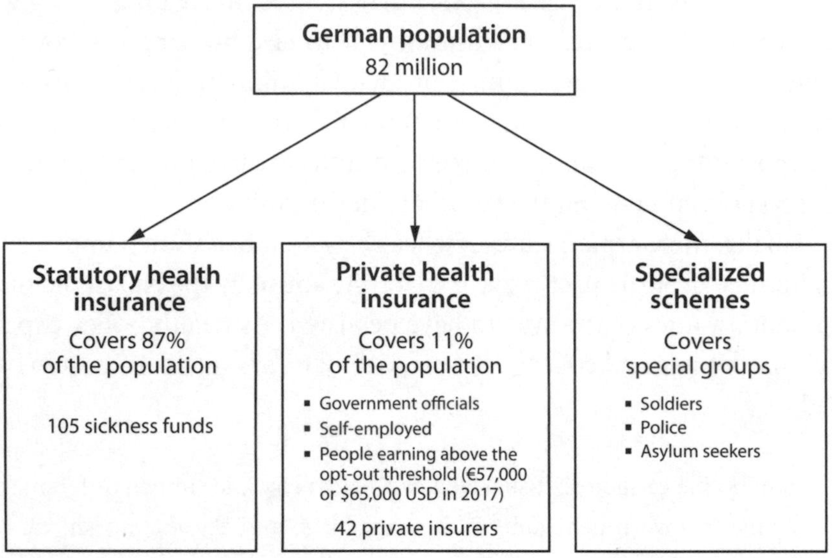

---

dental prostheses. A large number of Germans—just under 30% of the population—purchase this supplementary private insurance.

The 2nd main component is the private health insurance system. It covers 11% of the population. Three groups are eligible to purchase private health insurance: (1) government officials—ministers, members of Parliament, and civil servants, including current and retired government workers as well as teachers; (2) the self-employed; and (3) people earning over the "contributory income," or opt-out threshold, which was $62,200 USD (€57,600) in 2017, for 3 calendar years in a row. The self-employed and employees with high incomes can opt out of the statutory system and buy private health insurance. In order to prevent gaming—insuring with the private system when young and healthy and switching to the statutory system when older with more chronic conditions—opting into the private system is a onetime, lifetime, and (nearly) irrevocable decision. Once a person is in the private insurance sector, it is almost impossible for them to return to the SHI system. In 2018, there are 42 private health insurers in Germany.

Finally, a small minority of special groups, such as soldiers, police, and asylum seekers, receive their own special government health insurance.

FINANCING

Overall, Germany spends 11.5% of its GDP ($406 billion USD, or €376 billion) on health care, accounting for about $6,200 USD (€5,740) per capita in purchasing power parity. Of this, approximately 77% is publicly financed.

Statutory Health Insurance (SHI)

The SHI is funded from 5 distinct sources: (1) employee contributions, (2) employer contributions, (3) government subsidies, (4) sickness fund supplementary premiums, and (5) patient out-of-pocket payments.

Employees' and employers' contributions are progressive, based on a worker's income below the contributory income or opt-out threshold into a SHI funding pool. With both worker and employer contributions, the assessed amount totals to 14.6% of a worker's income. Between 2015 and 2018, the contributed amount was not evenly split. During this period workers paid more than employers, contributing about 53% of the total, or about 7.7% of their income. As of 2019 the share between employees and employers is equalized again. Retirees contribute based on their pensions, the unemployed contribute based on their unemployment benefits, and university students contribute a uniform amount based on the government stipend for students. There are no contributions for nonearning spouses or children. Since 2009 this money is collected by the sickness funds but deposited directly into the Central Reallocation Pool (Gesundheitsfonds) administered by the Federal Insurance Authority.

The 3rd source of funds comes from the federal government in 2 forms. Because the payroll payments are insufficient to fully finance sickness fund expenditures, the government provides a subsidy of about 7% of total expenditures directly to the Central Reallocation Pool. In addition, the government pays sickness funds a fixed amount for providing specific services, which are not directly linked to health insurance, such as contribution-free coinsurance and reproductive services such as maternity care, in vitro fertilization, and contraceptives. Fourth, when expenditures exceed revenues from the Central Reallocation Pool, sickness funds charge enrollees supplementary premiums, which, beginning in 2019, are shared equally between employers and

Figure 2. Financing Health Care: Statutory Health Insurance (Germany)

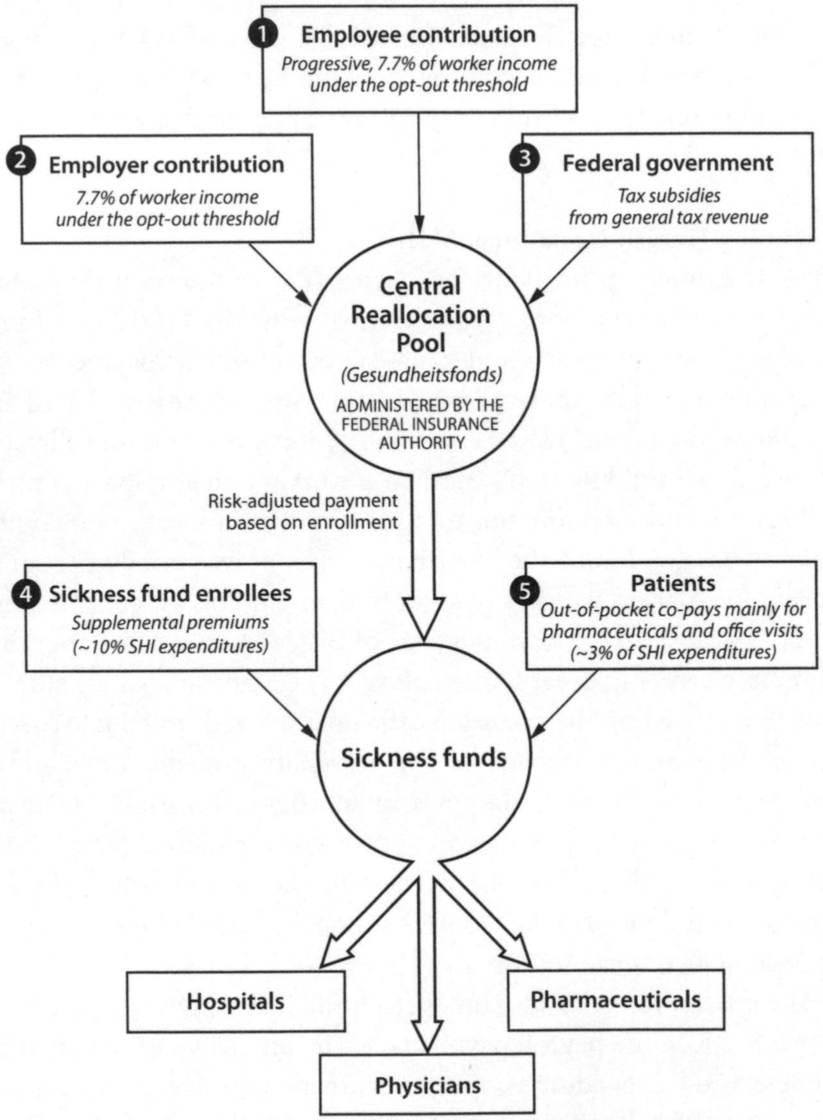

❶ Employee contribution
*Progressive, 7.7% of worker income
under the opt-out threshold*

❷ Employer contribution
*7.7% of worker income
under the opt-out threshold*

❸ Federal government
*Tax subsidies
from general tax revenue*

**Central
Reallocation
Pool**
(Gesundheitsfonds)
ADMINISTERED BY THE
FEDERAL INSURANCE
AUTHORITY

Risk-adjusted payment
based on enrollment

❹ Sickness fund enrollees
*Supplemental premiums
(~10% SHI expenditures)*

❺ Patients
*Out-of-pocket co-pays mainly for
pharmaceuticals and office visits
(~3% of SHI expenditures)*

Sickness funds

Hospitals

Pharmaceuticals

Physicians

employees. These premiums are in the range of 6% of sickness fund expenditures, or 1.1% of wages. But these premiums are highly variable between sickness funds based on their efficiency and are a main basis for competition among the funds.

The final piece of financing for health care services in the SHI is patient out-of-pocket expenditures. The 2 largest out-of-pocket expenditures are the purchase of pharmaceuticals and co-payments for physician office visits. Some groups are exempt from co-payments: low-income individuals, patients with high health needs, and children under 18. For instance, the average German is exempt from co-pays once they have spent more than 2% of their gross income, while a patient with a chronic illness is exempt once they exceed 1% of gross income in co-pays. Co-payments are a very small part of SHI expenditures, only about 3% of the total, but are very visible and politically charged.

After collecting all the money, the Central Reallocation Pool pays the sickness funds a risk-adjusted amount for each enrollee. The risk adjustment is based on age, sex, and the actual illnesses of patients. Sickness funds cannot run a deficit.

Because contributions to the sickness funds are linked to workers' income below the contributory threshold, the amount of money available depends on employment, wages, and population. A high unemployment rate, a high number of dependents, and a high number of pensioners all decrease the amount of money flowing into SHI. Conversely, a good economy with a high labor force participation rate increases the amount of money going into sickness funds.

Sickness funds are capitated and carry full financial risk for their enrollees. Although the SHI system covers 87% of the population, overall contributions to the SHI only account for 57.4% of the total German health care spending.

Private Health Insurance
Private insurers can offer a variety of insurance packages. The packages usually contain benefits that are better than those available in the SHI, such as choice of physician to treat a person in the hospital. But it is also possible to buy high-deductible plans and plans that exclude specific benefits. Premiums are risk rated and, consequently, vary by age, sex, and medical history at the time of enrollment. Unlike the SHI scheme, premiums must be paid for spouses and children. Thus, young, healthy individuals and childless couples with incomes above the contributory threshold have the most incentive to enroll in private health insurance.

To protect people who might not make substantial incomes, such as the self-employed or retired, there is a minimum-benefits package, or *basic tariff*. The basic tariff must cover benefits equivalent to those in

SHI at a premium that cannot exceed the worker assessment at the contributory limit to the SHI—that is, the highest contribution level to the SHI. This price is available only to those who are over 55 years of age, low income, or newly entering the private health insurance system.

Civil servants have 50% of their health bills covered by the government and must buy private health insurance to cover the remainder of the costs. Employed individuals with private insurance have 50% of their premium paid for by their employer, up to 50% of the average SHI contribution.

Because opting into private health insurance is nearly irreversible, private insurance companies are legally required to set aside a portion of the premium from working individuals to cover their health care costs when the workers retire and are no longer earning income. As of 2009 a substantial share of these reserves follow the insured individual even if they switch private insurers.

In general, private health insurance plans in Germany are indemnity plans; patients pay physicians and other providers and are then reimbursed by the insurer. This reimbursement is limited to fixed multiples (1.7 or 2.3, depending on the services) of the official price list set by the government in the official Catalogue of Tariffs for Physicians.

The private health system, distinct from supplementary insurance for SHI, covers 11% of the population and accounts for approximately 9% of expenditures.

Long-Term Care

Currently 21.4% of the German population is over 65, and general population growth is low. Historically, municipalities financed long-term care, but this became a drain on municipal budgets as the population aged. Thus, in 1994 the government enacted *mandatory* statutory long-term insurance. All Germans must contribute to long-term care insurance. Overall 87% of the population receives social long-term care, and about 12% have supplemental private long-term care insurance.

Long-term care insurance is financed like health insurance. Employed individuals pay 1.275% of monthly gross income, and employers match that payment. Pensioners pay the entire 2.55%. Childless individuals pay an extra 0.25% based on the understanding that they are less likely to get family care in the home as they age. Because payments do not cover the full cost of long-term care, people are encouraged to buy supplemental private long-term care insurance. The government subsidizes these purchases.

Public Health

Individual preventive services, such as cancer screenings, are part of SHI and funded through the health insurance system. States (*Länder*) establish and cover the cost of public health offices responsible for the nonindividual public health measures such as surveillance of communicable diseases, diagnosis of STDs, supervision of infections in hospitals and outpatient offices, and food and drug contamination. The Federal Ministry of Health is responsible for funding population-wide health education and promotion.

PAYMENT

Payments to Hospitals

Overall hospital payments account for approximately one-third of total German health care spending—about $108 billion USD (€100 billion) in 2017. Since 1972 hospital funding has been bifurcated.

Capital expenditures for building hospitals, expanding and renovating facilities, and purchasing big equipment come from the individual German states to the hospitals in their geographies and are financed at the state level through state taxes. Capital investment by the German states in hospital facilities and equipment is approximately $3 billion USD (€2.8 billion) per year and is widely considered too low. There have been recent efforts to increase this funding, especially for IT.

Hospital operations costs are paid by sickness funds, private insurance, and self-paying patients.

As of 2004 German hospitals are paid for operations based on DRGs. Each patient is assigned one of over 1,100 DRGs based on major diagnosis, secondary diagnoses, medical procedures, demographic characteristics, and length of stay. These DRGs are created and updated by the Institute for Reimbursement in the Hospital (Institute fur das Entgeltsystem im Krankenhaus [INEK]) at the federal level. Relying on actual cost and utilization data from German hospitals, the German

Figure 3. Payment to Hospitals (Germany)

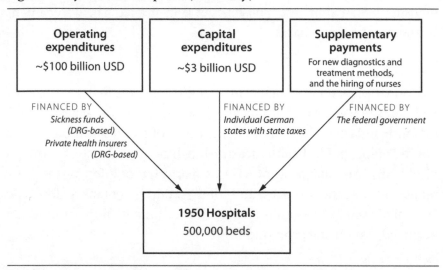

Hospital Federation and the associations of sickness funds and private health insurers negotiate each year on the cost weights for each DRG—how much each DRG is worth and will be paid. These cost weights are calculated at the state level; hence, DRG payments are the same within each state but vary among states by about 10%.

There are many exceptions to the DRG payment system. Supplementary payments are made to hospitals for highly specialized services, specialized centers, and very expensive drugs. Similarly, there are so-called new diagnostic and treatment methods (Neue Untersuchungs-und Behandlungsmethoden [NUB]) payments, which are payments to hospitals covering innovative diagnostic or treatment interventions such as experimental cancer therapies. These payments are determined on a case-by-case basis by the Federal Joint Commission and mainly benefit university-affiliated hospitals. There are also supplements to help hire more nurses. Altogether these supplements account for almost 20% of payments to hospitals.

The statutory health insurance and private insurance pay the same DRG with the same cost weights. But depending upon their plan, privately insured patients may have supplementary payments that cover amenities such as single rooms and ensuring that the chair of the department is their attending physician. These extra payments incentivize hospitals to admit more privately insured patients.

To ensure hospitals do not skimp on care because of DRGs, they must submit data on over 400 process, structure, and outcome indicators. They are subject to regular review for how they code patients in order to prevent upcoding and the use of low-value interventions. To further incentivize improvements in quality, 2016 legislation requires sickness funds to initiate pay-for-performance reimbursement.

Patients have little financial responsibility for hospital payments. Within the SHI they are assessed $11 USD (€10) per day for a maximum of 30 days. And, as with other co-pays, the poor and individuals with chronic illnesses are exempt.

Payments to Ambulatory or Office-Based Physicians

There are 5 different kinds of payments to ambulatory physicians, 3 of which come from the public SHI system. First—and by far the largest—is a morbidity-based payment for services delivered to patients. This payment is subject to an overall budget cap determined at the regional (state) level. Second is a potential supplementary payment based on unexpected medical emergencies, such as a bad flu season. Third are payments for specific services such as immunizations, ambulatory surgery, and cancer-screening tests. These are paid on a fixed fee schedule and are not subject to a budget cap. The 4th payment is fees for services rendered to patients with private insurance. The final payment is out-of-pocket patient payments for services not covered by the SHI, such as travel vaccines.

The actual payment to physicians is a bit more complex and reduces compensation because of an overall cap for SHI services. Annually, the overall payment to ambulatory physicians providing SHI care is negotiated at the regional (state) level between the association of sickness funds and the association of SHI physicians. The level of payment is supposed to reflect anticipated services and be based on the health needs of the state's population, derived from data on the use of services from 2 years prior to the actual negotiations, such as using 2014 data for 2016 payments. The sickness funds then transfer money to the physician association, which in turn pays the individual physicians based on their submitted billings.

The payments to physicians from the regional physician association are based on the Uniform Value Scale, negotiated by a committee

Figure 4. Payment to Ambulatory Physicians (Germany)

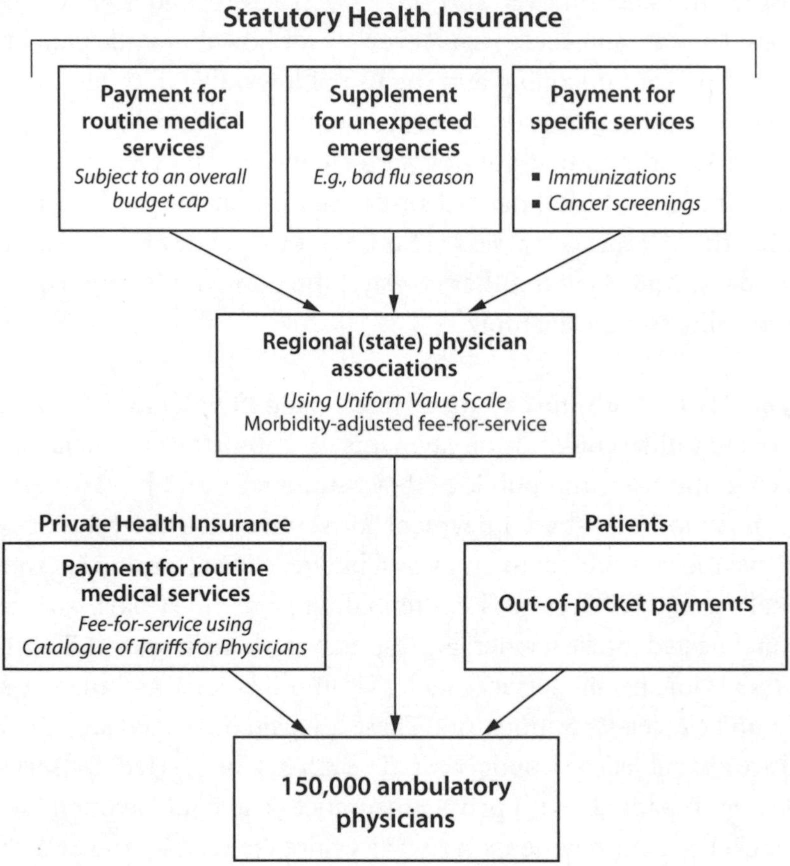

Statutory Health Insurance

Payment for routine medical services	Supplement for unexpected emergencies	Payment for specific services
Subject to an overall budget cap	*E.g., bad flu season*	▪ *Immunizations* ▪ *Cancer screenings*

Regional (state) physician associations

Using Uniform Value Scale
Morbidity-adjusted fee-for-service

Private Health Insurance

Payment for routine medical services
Fee-for-service using Catalogue of Tariffs for Physicians

Patients

Out-of-pocket payments

150,000 ambulatory physicians

of the Federal Joint Commission, which specifies the billing point value for every possible service covered by the SHI. Like the US RVU system, these points are based on 2 components: (1) the physician's time and (2) technical support needed to deliver the service. Thus, procedures requiring substantial technical supports have high points, whereas services such as home visits or office discussions that do not require technical support have few points. The points are converted to actual money values at the regional level and vary between regions.

Every quarter, physicians submit the number of billing points they actually provide to all patients. The regional physician association checks these points and then pays the physicians. In most states, the number of billing points submitted by physicians exceeds the total remuneration negotiated with the sickness funds, so physicians' actual payment is lower than the value of the billing points they submit and, thus, the services they rendered. How much lower is not known until all physicians in a region have submitted all their billing points and the regional physician association can determine how far over budget the points are for that year. Reductions are a fixed percentage across all physicians in the 2 pools.

There are 2 further complexities in the payment system for ambulatory physicians. The total budget to pay physicians is divided into 2 different pools, one for family and primary care physicians and one for specialists. Consequently, if specialists bill significantly more points, this does not lower payments to primary care physicians. Second, there are special services provided only by some physicians, such as bronchoscopies or ultrasounds. These are termed qualification-based services. Specifying a budget for these special services ensures that their volume does not increase, thereby siphoning significant payments to the few physicians that perform high volumes of these procedures.

Ambulatory physicians caring for patients under the SHI complain that they end up providing a significant amount of uncompensated care. They submit their quarterly points but do not know how much they will actually be paid until months later. And if the collective points of all physicians in the region exceeds the budget, they are penalized. Despite this penalty, they feel an obligation to provide care and not turn away patients even if they are not compensated for the services. A member of the Federal Association of SHI Physicians described physicians' frustrations with the payment system:

> After a quarter of the year, a physicians' office sends the number of visits and procedures to the state Gesetzliche Krankenversicherung [statutory health insurance system]. Those numbers undergo control mechanisms to check the times and ensure they comply with regulations. Eventually they are finalized, and about 6 months later the doctor gets paid by the state Gesetzliche Krankenversicherung. But it looks in its cash register and finds out "we don't have 100% of the money to pay you, we only have 90%." Then the physician only gets 90% of what was sent in, even though [the physician] rendered the services and they were approved as valid. And even worse, you never know in advance

how much you will be paid because you don't know personally how many patients have been seen by all the other doctors in the state. It is a blind flight, no instruments.

This perspective about the deficiencies of payment to physicians is not universally shared. The uncertainty in payment is not large. Moreover, the reason for the cuts in payments are because physicians tend to overtreat, and as a group, physicians have rejected other policy approaches to reducing overtreatment. Plus, German physicians find other ways to make income, such as charging patients for activities not typically covered by SHI, such as travel vaccinations.

Physicians treating patients with private insurance, however, receive fee-for-service payments. They are compensated based on the billing points in the Catalogue of Tariffs for Physicians, not the Uniform Value Scale used for SHI services. The points are multiplied by a factor to convert them to actual money values. Treating physicians can then multiply the money value by 3.5 to produce the maximum charge rate. Payments are typically lower than this maximum charge rate, usually around 1.7 to 2.3 times higher than the calculated money value. But only physicians who work in certain areas—urban areas with high incomes, such as Munich, and high numbers of civil servants, such as Berlin— are likely to have a sizable number of privately insured patients.

Payments for Long-Term Care
People must apply for long-term care payments. The Medical Review Board reviews applications, and approximately two-thirds are approved for one of 3 types of payments. First, there are monthly cash payments to reimburse for in-home care provided by family members. Second, there are fee-for-service payments for professional home care services. Finally, there are per diem payments for institutionalized nursing home care.

Payments for Complementary and Alternative Medicine
Sickness funds do not cover most complementary and alternative medicine services. Payments for these services come from private, supplementary insurance, or from out-of-pocket payments made by individuals.

Preventive Medicine

Sickness funds and private health insurance pay private, ambulatory physicians for most primary prevention services such as immunizations, cancer-screening tests, and health education. These payments are negotiated between the associations of sickness funds and SHI physicians. However, they are separate payments not subject to the budget caps.

DELIVERY OF HEALTH CARE SERVICES

The German health care system is a consumerist paradise. Patients with SHI have totally free choice of sickness funds, hospitals, and physicians, and co-pays are very low. Although there are wait times, especially for high-demand specialists, patients nonetheless have no gatekeepers and have access to any physician in the country. As a physician put it, "A patient can see any doctor, in any region, at any time. You can see 3 orthopedic surgeons and 3 GPs a day if you want. And you can see them all again the next day if you want. There is no limitation for the patient. The patient just walks into the doctor's office and gets service."

Hospital Care

There are approximately 1,950 hospitals, with nearly 500,000 beds for approximately 82.3 million people, with 8.2 beds per 1,000 population. This ratio is about 2.5 times that of the United States and is exceeded only by Japan. About 50% of hospital beds are in public hospitals owned and operated by municipalities. Of these public hospitals, 33 are university hospitals. The other hospitals include religiously affiliated, Red Cross, and private hospitals. There are about 19.5 million hospital admissions each year, about 55% of the admissions of the United States, a country with 4 times as many people as Germany. Trends show that the number of hospital beds has slowly declined, but hospital admissions have increased, though with shorter stays. Even with these changes, the average length of hospital stays is comparatively long, at 7.6 days. Experts and commentators suspect that there are many unnecessary hospitalizations, especially for ambulatory-sensitive conditions such as exacerbations of chronic conditions like COPD and uncontrolled diabetes.

Hospitals are mainly inpatient facilities providing surgery, treatment for exacerbations of chronic medical conditions, and other typical inpatient services. When a patient is admitted, a hospital-employed physician takes over managing the care from the patient's primary care or specialist physician.

Some hospitals—mainly university hospitals—have the right to operate outpatient facilities. These focus on specialized services such as for oncology, hemophilia, pulmonary hypertension, and other complex or rare diseases. There has also been an increase in ambulatory surgical procedures, some of which take place at hospital facilities. Hospitals have a very limited right to or responsibility for post-acute care, such as rehabilitation services or post-treatment home care.

Importantly, hospitals are regulated by the Ministry of Health in each region, not at the federal level. Although they can go to any hospital in the country for the same co-pay, Germans expect to have a hospital within 25 kilometers (about 15 miles) of their homes. As a result, closing hospitals is a highly charged political decision.

Ambulatory (Outpatient) Care

Germans are heavy users of physician services. There are over 150,000 ambulatory care physicians, 45% of whom are primary care physicians. Visits to ambulatory physicians have increased over time and now average about 10 per person per year.

There is very limited selective contracting and a limited but steadily increasing number of physician networks. Sickness funds must pay all physicians who are members of the regional association of SHI physicians, giving patients free choice of any SHI physician. Since the 1990s there have been various efforts to incentivize more integrated care, delivered by a network of physicians coordinated with hospitals. Patients who select these integrated care models can have lower co-pays for physician visits and pharmaceuticals. But both the tradition of free choice of physicians and the rigid divide between hospital-based and ambulatory care physicians mean that Germany is not conducive to integrated care delivery. Thus, in 2015 only 1.5% of all sickness fund payments went to selective contracts for integrated care.

One important change in care began in 2003 through the introduction of disease management programs (DMPs) for patients with chronic conditions. Unlike a formal provider network, which limits access, the DMPs are an attempt to efficiently coordinate care among outpatient providers—both primary care and specialist physicians—using an evidence-based protocol. All the regional sickness funds, in conjunction with the regional associations of SHI physicians, create these DMPs. They include standardized reporting requirements and quality measures as well as patient reminders and reports to physicians on their performance. Sickness funds are paid an administrative fee of about $162 USD (€150) for each patient enrolled in a DMP. Currently there are over 10,000 DMPs covering diseases ranging from type I diabetes and asthma to breast cancer, and they have enrolled over 7 million patients.

Mental Health Care

Beginning in the 1970s Germany underwent a process of deinstitutionalization for patients with mental illness. East Germany followed West Germany, with a lag of about 20 years, deinstitutionalizing after unification. Although the number of inpatient psychiatric beds steadily declined from 150,000 in 1976 to under 40,000 today, community-based care has been inadequate. About a quarter of acute care hospitals have inpatient psychiatric wards, and many have outpatient psychiatric departments. Private psychiatrists and psychotherapists assume the bulk of outpatient mental health care, but there are long wait times for appointments, which is exacerbated in rural communities where psychiatrists are often scarce. These providers oversee a sociotherapeutic benefit that covers housing and social services intended to help avoid unnecessary hospitalization for acute exacerbations of mental health conditions.

There are a growing number of for-profit, private hospitals focusing on substance abuse and psychiatric care.

Long-Term Care

Nearly 3 million (3.6%) Germans receive long-term care payments, and 55% of Germans over 80 years of age receive such payments. About 70% receive payments for in-home care, mostly cash benefits for family care, and about 30% for institutionalized nursing home care. Most ambulatory long-term care is provided by private, for-profit companies, while nonprofit organizations mainly provide institutionalized nursing home care.

Preventive Medicine

Ambulatory physicians provide most individually focused primary preventive activities, such as immunizations and cancer-screening services. Preventive care that is considered relevant to public health, such as the diagnosis of STDs, may also be provided through regional public health offices established by the states. In addition, recent reforms have strengthened prevention, with a focus on health promotion in schools, businesses, and long-term care facilities.

PHARMACEUTICAL COVERAGE AND PRICE CONTROLS

Pharmaceutical Market

Germany is the world's 4th-largest drug market by revenue, accounting for $58.6 billion USD (€54.3 billion) in revenue in 2014. Approximately 14% of health care spending—or $780 USD (€722) per capita—in Germany goes to pharmaceuticals. Out-of-pocket payments by consumers for drugs make up about 16% of the total drug spending, and Germans consume a relatively high proportion of prescriptions per person.

Coverage Determination

In Germany drugs are granted a license and marketing approval based on European Union regulations embodied in German law. The Pharmaceutical Act of 1976 made the licensing of drugs mandatory. The Paul Ehrlich Institute oversees the licensing of vaccines and blood products, while the Federal Institute for Pharmaceuticals and Medical Devices reviews applications for licensure of all other drugs. Drugs approved by the European Medicines Agency are automatically approved for licensure in EU member states, including Germany. Manufacturers must demonstrate that the drugs they submit are safe and effective, although marginal effectiveness is all that is necessary; there is no cost-effectiveness requirement necessary for the licensure of a new drug, nor is there mandatory postmarketing surveillance of drugs for their side effects and/or effectiveness. Licensing lasts for 5 years, but it can be renewed. The Federal Institute for Pharmaceuticals and Medical Devices does not review homeopathic drugs; they merely register with the Institute.

Figure 5. Regulation of Pharmaceutical Prices (Germany)

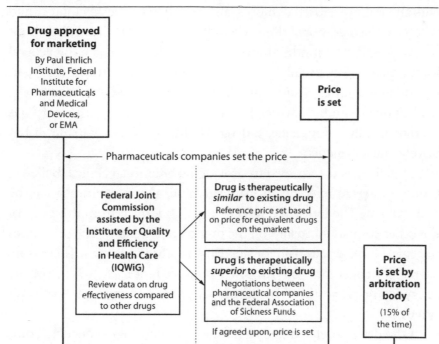

Germany does not have a list of covered drugs. However, the Federal Joint Commission does specify the indications for the appropriate use of a drug and, thus, what will be paid for. Therefore, a physician may not prescribe a drug not licensed for a specific indication; patients can only be reimbursed for off-label use of a drug if (1) there is no other treatment, (2) it is used to treat a life-threatening condition, and (3) there is some scientific evidence suggesting benefits.

The SHI also does not reimburse over-the-counter drugs except for children under 18 and for adults with select chronic conditions.

Price Regulation

Germany has a rigorous multistep process for determining the price of a new drug that occurs in the 12 months after a drug is allowed to be marketed (Figure 5). For the initial 12 months after market launch, pharmaceutical companies can sell a drug at any price. At market launch manufacturers must prepare and submit a dossier on the clinical benefits and risks of a drug, demonstrating its therapeutic advantages and whether it has additional clinical benefits compared to drugs already on the market. For 6 months after submission of that dossier, the Federal Joint Commission, usually with the assistance of the Institute for Quality and Efficiency in Health Care (Institut für Qualität und Wirtschaftlichkeit im Gesundheitswesen [IQWiG]), determines whether a drug is therapeutically comparable to drugs on the market or whether it has novel clinical benefits.

If the drug is determined to provide no additional clinical benefits, then an internal reference price determines the maximum price the SHI will pay. The internal reference price is derived from the price of the other comparable drugs on the market in Germany. The price does not refer to the prices paid for the drug in other countries. There is no co-pay for consumers on drugs whose price is at least 30% below the reference price, so there is substantial consumer pressure for lower prices.

If the drug is determined to have additional clinical benefits compared to existing drugs, the Federal Association of Sickness Funds and the pharmaceutical manufacturer negotiate to determine the price. The price premium is supposed to reflect the added therapeutic value of the drug, as determined by the Federal Joint Commission. These negotiations decide the price for both the SHI and private insurance systems. If after 6 months of negotiations no agreement is reached, the price is determined by an arbitration body, which has 3 months to render a decision. Price negotiations go to arbitration about 15% of the time.

Sickness funds get 3 types of rebates on the price they pay for drugs. The first rebate comes from pharmacies. The law requires pharmacies to give sickness funds a mandatory rebate, currently under $2.20 USD (€2) per prescription. Second, pharmaceutical manufacturers must provide sickness funds a legally specified mandatory rebate, currently set at 7% for patented drugs and 6% for generics. Finally, there is a rebate, mainly on generics, that is determined through negotiations between pharmaceutical manufacturers and individual sickness funds. In the typical agreement the manufacturer gives the sickness fund a discounted price and the sickness fund designates the manufacturer's drug the one generic in a specific class of drugs, such as statins, that it will cover for its insured members. This is one of the rare cases in which individual sickness funds do the negotiations instead of the Federal Association of Sickness Funds. Pharmacies are obligated to honor the negotiations by dispensing the specific drug to sickness fund members. This discount/rebate system has significantly reduced drug spending.

Pharmacies set prices for over-the-counter drugs without regulation.

Regulation of Physician Prescriptions

There are 3 mechanisms to shift German physicians' prescribing behavior to use fewer and lower-cost prescriptions. First, the Federal Joint Commission issues guidelines for the proper use of costly drugs, and physicians who do not comply can be fined. Second, each physician is given a prescription budget based on drug utilization data for a similar group of patients. If a physician exceeds the budget by 15%, they receive a warning; if they exceed it by 25%, they may need to reimburse the sickness funds. Finally, physicians are given maximum quotas for heavily prescribed drugs, set by negotiations between the associations of the sickness funds and SHI physicians. They are encouraged to use lower-cost drugs in these therapeutic areas. If physicians exceed these quotas, their reimbursements may be reduced.

Prices Paid by Patients

The price patients pay for a drug is the same throughout Germany. Pharmacies are only able to mark up drug prices by a legally predetermined fixed amount—$9 USD (€8.35), plus a 3% margin. Since 2004 German patients have been required to pay a co-pay for drugs, at a maximum of $11 USD (€10) per prescription. These co-pays can be waived if patients are in an integrated care network.

Importantly, unlike in many other countries, German drug prices include the 19% national value-added tax (VAT), making German drugs unusually expensive. If a pharmaceutical manufacturer sets the price above the maximum reference price, the patients pay the difference. Due to the resulting consumer pressure, few prices are above the reference price maximum. In addition, there is a mandatory generic substitution law; if a drug is prescribed, the pharmacist is required to dispense the generic unless the physician specifies not to.

HUMAN RESOURCES

Physicians

There are approximately 350,000 physicians in Germany for a population of 82 million, or 4.5 physicians per 1,000 population, which is well above the international average. Of these physicians, 151,000 are ambulatory physicians, and approximately 190,000 work in hospitals, including trainees. About 45% of the ambulatory care physicians are primary care physicians. Primary care physicians tend to be older, whereas younger physicians are increasingly entering specialties. Over 95% of ambulatory physicians take SHI patients; only about 4% of physicians exclusively see privately insured patients. As in most countries, German physicians are more heavily concentrated in the urban areas.

In general there is a rigid separation of ambulatory and hospital-based physicians, but a few hospital-based specialists (mainly chiefs of hospital departments) have ambulatory offices as well. A growing number of specialists are also performing surgical procedures in hospitals on a part-time basis. Although the number of multi-physician group practices and employed physicians has increased, the vast majority of German physicians are self-employed. They work in private, solo, or very small group practices that own their own equipment and employ staff. Self-employed physicians tend to work longer hours than those employed by other physicians or centers. The shift to fewer work hours and more externally employed physicians is associated with an increase in female physicians. If the causal link is accurate, this trend will continue, as 70% of current German medical students are female.

Physician salaries in Germany are lower than in the United States and Switzerland. For instance, an average general practitioner earns approximately $124,000 USD (€115,000). Radiologists are the highest earners, at about $432,000 USD (€400,000), with surgeons earning about $238,000 USD (€220,000). These salaries are from SHI payments. Private insurance contributes about 20% of the total physician salaries in the ambulatory care setting, although this is not evenly divided across the country because patients with private insurance are concentrated in larger urban areas.

There are 35 medical schools in the country, which produce about 11,000 medical graduates each year. Medical schools are funded and operated by regions. Because medical schools are expensive, regional governments do not want to expand their numbers, even though the health system demands more physicians.

Countries that can offer higher salaries, such as Switzerland, are increasingly recruiting German-trained physicians. In turn, Germany is recruiting physicians from Eastern European countries such as Romania.

Nurses

There are approximately 1.1 million nurses in Germany, or 13 per 1,000 population. Approximately 400,000 work in hospitals. There is no real pathway for nurses to become nurse practitioners, nor is there much use of medical assistants or other non-nursing personnel to take over tasks performed by nurses that do not require nurse training.

There is a widely held perception that there is a serious shortage of nurses in Germany. The reasons for the shortage are multidimensional but include stringent staffing rules, like the requirement in neonatal intensive care units that there be one nurse per neonatal patient, 24 hours per day. Recently, the government altered hospital payments to provide an incentive to hire more nurses. There is a proposal to separate the payment to hospitals for nurse salaries, which would dictate to hospitals how to allocate their budget for nursing. To satisfy demand, Germany has undertaken several policies, such as increasing the training of nurses, improving nurses' working conditions, and recruiting nurses from other countries.

In Germany, nursing is neither a profession nor a guild—that is, a specialized craft. Nursing schools are run by a relatively small number of hospitals and are not part of the university education system. Nursing training takes 3 years, and approximately 40,000 nurses are trained each year. Sickness funds pay for nursing education by deducting a small amount from the payment to hospitals without nursing schools and reallocating it to hospitals with these schools.

CHALLENGES

There are at least 7 major challenges facing the German health care system over the next decade. First, the biggest challenge may be the excessive number of hospital beds and hospital admissions. For a country with 25% of the US population, Germany has 40% the number of hospitals, 60% the number of hospital beds, and 55% the number of hospital admissions per year. However, closing hospitals and reducing the number of beds is very difficult. Because capital costs for hospitals are made at the state level and many hospitals are owned by municipalities, closing hospitals is a local political decision, and no politician who wants to be reelected will voluntarily close a local hospital. The only politically feasible reason to close hospitals is demonstrated poor quality or a lack of adequate nursing staff. Whether this will succeed in reducing the number of hospital beds is unclear.

Second, there is perceived to be a severe shortage of nurses. However, Germany has 13 nurses per 1000 people, one of the highest ratios in Europe, indicating that this shortage is more a result of the structure of the system and how nurses are deployed than a real shortage of personnel. This perception also seems to be due to the excessive number of hospital beds in Germany and the lack of clear roles for non-nurses, who could assume many functions currently performed by nurses that do not require nurse-level training. Until the hospital-bed issue is resolved, there may be no resolution to the perceived nursing shortage.

Third, there is a lack of care coordination for patients with chronic illness. The rigid divide between hospital-based and ambulatory physicians as well as the limited use of home health care services have made care coordination difficult. Attempts to improve coordination through DMPs and integrated care have met with some, but limited, success. There are thousands of DMPs, yet they guide care for fewer than 10% of the population. And, despite being available, integrated care is not widely utilized. Care coordination might be improved—although not completely fixed—by requiring hospitals to assume responsibility for posthospital discharge and readmissions, but this would probably be met with fierce opposition from ambulatory physicians. Two policies are needed: reducing the rigid divide between hospital-based and ambulatory physicians and providing greater incentives for integrated care through selective networks. These are major structural changes that will take a long time to occur.

Fourth, it is unclear whether the high number of sickness funds adds value. Patients can choose among different sickness funds, but structural constraints mean that there are not significant differences among them in terms of quality, cost, or service. Sickness funds do have different DMPs and could do more integrated care and quality monitoring, but these do not seem to justify the costs of having over 100 of them. More quality monitoring and the creation of high-quality networks could be valuable, but it is not clear whether this is part of any of the funds' strategic plan.

Fifth, there is a perceived unfairness of private insurance. There are advantages of having a private insurance system. It provides competition to the SHI. It has large reserves, over $270 billion USD (€250 billion), that will help pay for medical services as the population ages. Nevertheless, there is some sense that well-off individuals and civil servants receive private insurance that is experience rated, so many of them have greater benefits but lower premiums than SHI. But because the very people who have the power to reform private insurance are the ones who benefit from it—politicians and civil servants—reform seems unlikely.

Sixth, Germany is trailing in digitizing health care and adopting EHRs. There are several major digitization initiatives that need to be completed: ensuring medications and emergency data are available on each patient's health card and the full adoption of a platform that can be used by all stakeholders in the health care system with interoperable EHRs for patients. This may be politically difficult to accomplish. At least at the hospital level, improving the electronic health infrastructure would require capital funding by states that already underinvest in capital projects.

Finally, there is the challenge of long-term care. By 2030, 30% of the German population will be over 70 years of age. This will increase the need for both home and institutional long-term care services. Institutional care is very expensive, and as of 2018, public long-term care insurance covers only about 50% of the cost of institutional care. As the need for long-term care increases, the number of nursing home beds required and the overall cost will strain the system. This demographic and financial challenge will become a major issue in the next decade.

Currently Germany has one significant advantage that is simultaneously a liability. The economy is doing tremendously well with low unemployment, and because the financing of the sickness funds is linked to wages, the system is currently very well-funded. Hence, the system is not under financial threat, even though there are focal areas of financial strain, such as capital investment by states in hospitals and long-term care. But the good economy also creates 2 problems. First, because unemployment is low, there are not many people available for nursing and other lower level health jobs such as medical assistants. This makes it hard to address the need for more nurses and geriatric caregivers. Second, with a good economy and adequate funding, there is little sense of crisis to drive health care reform. There is no real financial pressure to reduce the number of hospitals and hospital beds and develop more integrated care. Few policymakers will face these hard choices if they can avoid them; the system's strong financial position allows politicians, officials at the sickness funds, physicians, hospitals, and other stakeholders to "kick the can down the road." But when there is an economic slowdown, these issues will intensify, requiring more comprehensive solutions.

CHAPTER SEVEN

NETHERLANDS

"*Dutch huisartsen [general practitioners] are notorious for sending you home with advice to rest and take a paracetamol [Tylenol]. Come back in 2 weeks if you're not feeling better.*"

This is a common complaint about Dutch health care, especially from expatriates. Dutch physicians have a strong tradition of conservative care, intervening hesitantly because, in their view, nature fixes most minor ailments.

This philosophy is embodied in the Dutch health care system. Patients may select any insurer and general practitioner. Primary care physicians have both extensive responsibility and authority. They act as true gatekeepers. General practitioners (GPs) are clinically and financially responsible for chronic and mental health care—often delivered by a nurse practitioner in the office—and a GP referral is required before seeing any specialist. GPs are fastidiously noninterventionist and manage most issues. But when needed, an advanced, innovative, comprehensive, and supportive health care system kicks in, as described by a mother of an infant with a cardiac abnormality that required a month's hospitalization and surgical repair:

> Support from the child developmental staff, pastoral workers, a nutritionist, a pre-speech therapist, a world class surgeon, pediatric home nurse when needed, and incredible nurses, consultants, and trainee consultants. . . . [W]e had stellar support and amazing care.

All this care was essentially free at the point of service. While adults have a $435 USD (€385) deductible, primary care visits are exempt, and all children under 18 have no deductible or cost sharing.

Special financing extends to the elderly as well. The Netherlands is one of only a few countries to have a dedicated, tax-financed long-term care arrangement for the disabled and elderly. Is it any wonder the Dutch system consistently comes out on top of the Euro Health Consumer Index?

HISTORY

Guilds, Sickness Funds, and Hospitals
Before the 20th Century

The Netherlands has a long history of providing health benefits through insurance funds. The German occupation during World War II influenced the modern system, but it has evolved into what is plausibly the world's purest form of managed competition.

In the middle of the 19th century there were a number of health insurance funds run by physicians, trade unions, and corporations. In 1908, the Netherlands Medical Association (NMG) established the Schreve Commission, which advocated for independent physician practices, free patient choice of doctors, and having nonwealthy patients purchase health insurance while wealthy patients pay out of pocket for services. The Commission also proposed physician representation on the governing boards of health insurance funds so as to ensure physician autonomy was protected. The Commission's proposals were not immediately enacted.

The 1913 Sickness Act (*Ziektewet*) was the first attempt at a government mandate for health coverage. It actually provided a kind of unemployment payment to workers who were out of the job due to illness. Further governmental attempts to institute compulsory health insurance schemes were stalled due to World War I, but after the war the NMG, unions, and commercial insurers sponsored a proliferation of competing health insurance funds. To some degree this was successful: by 1941 nearly 50% of Dutch citizens had some form of health insurance.

World War II changed everything. The Nazi occupation brought with it an imposition of the German Bismarckian model of compulsory state insurance provided through competing sickness (insurance) funds and financed by taxes assessed on both employees and employers. The covered benefits included hospital, specialist, and dental care.

As in the German system, the well off above a certain income threshold were exempt from the statutory health insurance and purchased private health insurance. The self-employed and elderly could choose between being in the statutory insurance system or purchasing private health insurance. The German rules reduced the number of sickness funds and nearly eliminated all physician-run funds.

The imposed German system remained largely intact until 1966. After World War II premiums in the private health insurance market rose rapidly, driven by the enrollment of larger numbers of elderly and disabled people. Several attempts at addressing the problem—such as transferring the lower-income elderly, disabled, and children into the statutory sickness fund system—failed to fully address the high premiums. In 1966, the Health Insurance Act, *Ziekenfondswet*, was implemented. In reality, it essentially copied and codified most of the German system wholesale. The only notable change was that the new Health Insurance Act allowed funds greater flexibility to determine their geographic region of operation and introduced an income-based premium. The main goal of the Health Insurance Act was a political one: the Dutch finally had their own system, not one directly tied to the Nazis.

In 1967, the Dutch Parliament passed the Exceptional Medical Expenses Act (AWBZ) to address the issue of long-term care, including care for the disabled. This effectively bifurcated the Dutch system, with one part focusing on curative care, which was further divided into statutory and private systems, and a 2nd part encompassing long-term insurance.

By the 1980s, premium costs had grown rapidly, prompting a growing consensus that the system needed reform. The Health Care Prices Act of 1981 empowered the national government to set global hospital budgets that covered total yearly operational expenses, excluding capital costs. In addition, the government also capped medical specialist expenditures, although these caps were frequently exceeded. In 1986, the Insurance Law on Access to Care abolished much of the private system and moved nearly a million people into the statutory sickness fund system. It also required private insurers to provide benefits nearly identical to those in the statutory system.

Rising costs continued to plague the health care system, and in 1987 the government appointed the Dekker Committee to propose systemic reform. The Committee recommended combining the statutory and private insurance systems into a single system of competing private insurers that all had to provide the same basic benefit package. Income-linked taxes collected by the government and nominal premiums set by insurers would finance the system. People would have the option to purchase supplemental insurance for services not in the basic benefit package, and the Dekker Committee also recommended direct negotiations of fees between insurers and providers. The government tried and failed to enact the Committee's recommendations multiple times. Finally, in 2006, the Dutch Parliament passed the Health Insurance Act (ZVW), which implemented many of the Dekker Committee's original recommendations. This is the legal framework for the current Dutch system.

The Dutch system has evolved into one that features competition between insurers for patients, negotiations between insurers and providers, and regular national collaboration across parties to deal with systemic problems as they crop up. On the one hand, the principles of local, managed competition between private, mostly nonprofit providers and private, nonprofit insurers underpins the system. On the other hand, competition is restricted: insurers must offer the same basic benefits package, and negotiations between insurers and providers are far from cut-throat. National agreements—led by the government—between insurers, providers, and politicians identify target levels of health care cost growth, setting a benchmark for reasonable price increases. The ultimate responsibility for the functioning of the health care system lies squarely on the government.

Thus, the Dutch health care system has gone through 3 phases of evolution. From the 19th century until World War II, there was the system of health benefits through an amalgam of insurance companies run by physicians, unions, and commercial entities. From World War II until the mid-2000s, the system was structured with a statutory public system funding private sickness funds and a parallel private insurance system. And, since the 2006 reforms, there has been a managed competition system, with the government allocating premiums to competing sickness funds and residents purchasing supplementary private insurance.

Figure 1. Health Care Coverage (Netherlands)

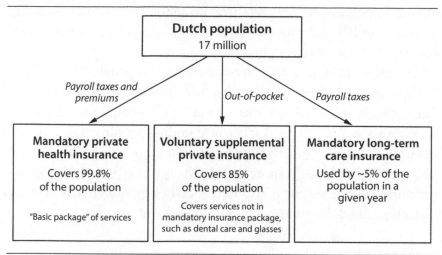

COVERAGE

The Netherlands is a country of 17 million citizens. Fully 99.8% have health insurance. Just over 24,000 people are uninsured, although 223,000 (1.7%) have not paid the entire premium. In addition, 85% of the Dutch population purchases private supplemental insurance.

Insurance coverage in the Dutch health care system is divided into 3 main components: universal statutory insurance provided by competing sickness funds, voluntary supplemental insurance provided by private insurance companies, and mandatory long-term care provided by the government.

Statutory Health Insurance
The entire population (99.8%) is covered under the compulsory statutory health insurance system set up by the Health Insurance Act of 2006. Competing, nonprofit insurance companies set premiums for the same mandated benefits package. Individuals choose which insurer they want for coverage. Payroll taxes cover most of the basic premium, and individuals need to pay a nominal premium for the remainder. The government provides income-linked subsidies to individuals to help

pay for these premiums, with about half of all Dutch households receiving some form of subsidy. There are approximately 24 competing insurers that fall under 9 umbrella organizations. The 4 largest groups cover 90% of the Dutch population.

Coverage is essentially universal because the penalty for not having insurance is stiff. As a government official noted, "The penalties are rather tough, and of course, this is a nation of accountants and bookkeepers. So they are also very efficient at finding people who are simply not insured." After 3 months without insurance, people are fined about $440 USD (€367). After 3 more months the fine is repeated. Finally, the tax office has the authority to automatically sign individuals up for a plan and deduct the premium (minus fines) from wages.

Voluntary, Private Supplemental Insurance

There also is the supplementary, private health insurance system that is voluntary. Voluntary supplementary insurance can only cover services not in the basic benefit packages, such as eyeglasses, adult dental care, and physical therapy. There are no tax breaks or subsidies specifically earmarked for voluntary supplemental insurance, and there is some evidence of adverse selection in the voluntary market. Nearly all enrollees purchase supplementary insurance from the same insurer that provides them with the basic package.

Long-Term Care Insurance

Finally, there is mandatory long-term care insurance funded by payroll taxes. Since 2015, all Dutch residents are enrolled in a government plan that provides up to 24-hour custodial and nursing care, either in institutions or at home. The Social Support Act encourages independent-living initiatives and is administered by municipalities. The Long-Term Care Act finances intensive home health care and institutional care in nursing homes.

FINANCING

In 2017, according to the Dutch government's statistical bureau (Statistics Netherlands, or CBS), the Netherlands spent $109.3 billion USD

Figure 2. Financing Health Care: Mandatory Private Health Insurance
(Netherlands)

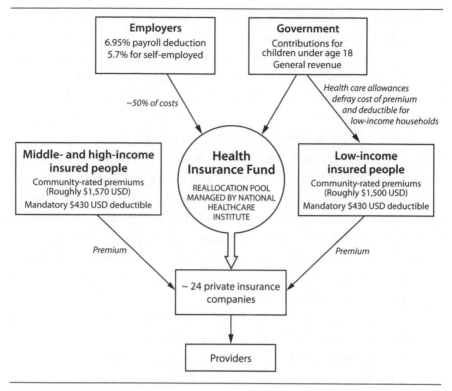

(€97.1 billion) on health-related activities, including social supports.
Just considering health care services, the Netherlands spent $83.7 billion USD (€74.5 billion), or 10.1% of GDP, equal to roughly $5,000 USD
(€4,400) per capita. Fully 80% of health-related spending is either publicly financed through taxes or compulsory health insurance premiums and income-linked subsidies.

Spending on all health care and health-related services breaks down
such that about 44.6%, or $48.8 billion USD (€43.5 billion), is spent
through the compulsory health insurance system; 4.6%, or $5 billion
USD (€4.5 billion), comes through supplemental insurance; and 19.1%,
or $21 billion USD (€18.7 billion), is spent on compulsory long-term
care insurance. Spending on long-term care is actually higher because
much of the funding for long-term care services comes through the
compulsory curative care insurance system, such as payment for home
nursing care. Individuals contributed about $12 billion USD (€10.7

billion) in out-of-pocket spending, accounting for about 11% of overall spending.

Each year the Minister of Health, Welfare, and Sport sets the national Health Care Budget (BKZ), which creates target growth rates for different categories of spending, such as hospital care and primary care. The minister of health has the authority to order claw-backs from providers and insurers when the Health Care Budget is exceeded.

Statutory Health Insurance for Curative Care

The statutory managed competition system is financed through 4 sources: (1) income-linked payroll deductions from employers, (2) community-rated nominal premiums, (3) state contributions from general revenue, and (4) individual out-of-pocket payments. All insurers cover the same services specified in the basic package by the minister of health. Insurers may only compete on price and quality of the basic package, and price and quality of voluntary supplementary insurance packages that they offer to members.

The government collects payroll deductions, which were 6.65% of income, with a limit of about $60,500 USD (€53,701) per worker in 2017. In 2019, the limit was increased to 6.95% for those with a maximum income of $63,000 USD (€55,927). For self-employed persons the contribution was 5.4% of wages in 2017 up to the same ceiling, which also increased to 5.7% up to a maximum of $63,000 USD (€55,927) in 2019. These taxes are collected in a central health insurance fund that the government then pays to each sickness fund on a risk-adjusted basis. The payments are based on expected health risks, and insurers bear the full risk for medical care, with the exception of long-term mental health services. These payroll taxes account for approximately half of the spending on statutory health insurance.

The National Health Care Institute (ZIN) manages the risk-adjustment process. Insurers must submit claims data. The risk adjustment formula used to pay individual insurance companies is managed by several universities and includes about 200 different variables, from age and sex to drug utilization and socioeconomic status. It does a very good job of reducing insurers' incentives to engage in risk selection. One professor involved described the process:

> A lot of people are coming to the Netherlands to understand how we
> risk adjust the insurance pool. It is quite comprehensive how we dis-
> tribute [the premiums], in fact. So there is no real incentive to do some
> risk selection. . . . We have more than 200 variables in the model at the
> moment . . . we are quite lucky that we have actually quite good data.
> What happens is that every insurer [reports quarterly what is] reim-
> bursed . . . to the information center. Here we have algorithms, and we
> use that increasingly. The quality [of the data] is excellent.

Additionally, regulation prevents insurers from certain types of cream
skimming. For example, it is illegal to advertise specifically to young
students or higher-income individuals.

Second, households pay a nominal premium to their selected insurer. These premiums are community rated. For an individual the
average annual premium was about $1,525 USD (€1,353) in 2017, increas-
ing to $1,550 USD (€1,378) in 2019. The government subsidizes these
premiums for joint-filing households with incomes under $42,200
USD (€37,500) and individuals earning under $33,300 USD (€29,500).
Importantly, the government pays the full premium for all children under 18.

Private Supplementary Insurance
In addition to compulsory insurance to cover most routine care, individuals decide whether they want to purchase voluntary supplementary health insurance (VHI). VHI plans use experience rating to set
premiums and can reject applicants. Individuals are responsible for the
full cost of payment. There are neither tax preferences nor other subsidies or incentives for purchasing supplementary insurance. About 85%
of Dutch residents have VHI.

Long-Term Care
The Dutch Healthcare Authority (NZA) establishes the national budget
for long-term care. Long-term care is financed through 3 sources: (1)
payroll taxes, (2) general tax revenue, and (3) out-of-pocket payments.

The Long-Term Care Act, enacted in 2015, assesses a 9.65% payroll
tax on employee wages up to $38,600 USD (€34,300) in 2019. This

covers about 73% of the cost of long-term care. The National Health Care Institute manages these funds. They are distributed to regional care offices (*Zorgkantoren*), run by private insurers, in order to pay long-term care providers, and to the Social Insurance Bank (SVB), which manages personal budgets for long-term care recipients.

General taxes are also used to fund custodial care provided by municipalities. These funds are not earmarked but rather are part of government payments to municipalities covering all governmental activities in addition to custodial care, such as roads and sewers. Almost all recipients of long-term care must also pay some portion of the cost out of pocket. The system for deciding how much a beneficiary should pay is complicated, but in general, out-of-pocket costs are means tested based on income and assets. Typically beneficiaries must pay about 10% to 12.5% of their income. Total out-of-pocket costs for long-term care were capped at roughly $2,471 USD (€2,200) per year in 2015. Municipalities may require co-payments for domestic help and social support provided under the Social Support Act.

Out-of-Pocket Costs

Out-of-pocket costs apply for both the basic insurance package and for long-term care. All compulsory insurance plans carry a mandatory $430 USD (€385) deductible, although many services are exempt from the deductible, including GP visits, home nursing care, and services for children. Every year enrollees can voluntarily increase their deductibles to up to $990 USD (€885) in exchange for a lower premium. About 12.6% of enrollees opt for voluntary higher deductibles, and 9.6% take the maximum deductible.

For long-term care, beneficiaries pay some portion of the cost directly to the Central Administration Office (CAK), and municipalities have considerable flexibility to set additional co-payments.

PAYMENT

Since the liberalizing reforms in 2006, payment rates for nearly 70% of all curative care services—including most hospital care and physician services—are negotiated between insurance companies and providers.

Figure 3. Payment to Hospitals (Netherlands)

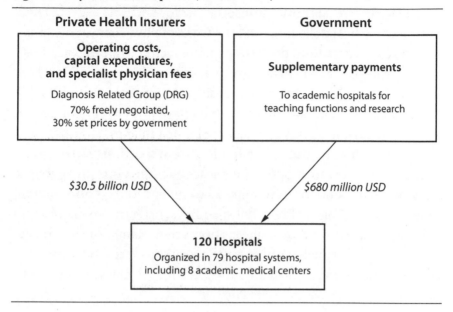

The prices for the remaining 30% of services, such as for long-term care, are set nationally by the Dutch Healthcare Authority. The specific mechanisms for negotiation and payment to hospitals and providers are exceptionally byzantine, having been described by experts as "governance by confusion."

According to the OECD, which only measures health care spending (excluding social supports), in 2017 the Netherlands spent a total of $83.6 billion USD (€74.4 billion) on health care. Of that figure, $28.9 billion USD (€25.7 billion), or 34.6%, of health care spending was for hospital services; $21.8 billion USD (€19.4 billion), or 26.0%, was for residential long-term care facilities; $15.3 billion USD (€13.6 billion), or 18.2%, went to physicians and other providers of ambulatory health care services; and $9.4 billion USD (€8.36 billion), or 11.3%, was spent on medical goods and pharmaceuticals.

Payment to Hospitals

Insurance companies negotiate directly with hospitals. Each insurer establishes its own hospital networks and uses selective contracting. Most negotiations occur on the basis of price and volume. Insurers and hospitals rely on a modified DRG system called Diagnosis Treatment

Combinations (DBCs). There are approximately 4,400 DBCs, and the Dutch Healthcare Authority is responsible for updating the list. DBCs cover fees for hospitalization and the work of physicians in hospitals. Insurers can negotiate on the basis of price, such as a rate for each DBC. Insurers can also reach an agreement about a volume of services they will pay for. Insured persons who visit noncontracted providers will typically pay a larger portion of the bill out of pocket. Pay-for-performance and pay-for-quality schemes are in their infancy.

Academic hospitals get extra funding from the Ministry of Health, Welfare, and Sport to support their academic functions. In aggregate these payments amount to roughly $680 million USD (€600 million) annually, or 2.3% of total hospital spending. Furthermore, highly specialized surgical procedures, such as organ transplantation and neurosurgery, are performed in only a few hospitals and are paid separately. These payments are regulated by the Act on Specialized Clinical Services (*Wet bijzondere medische verrichtingen*).

Payment to Physicians

Primary care physicians and specialists are paid very differently. Since 2006, there has been a significant move away from specific fee-for-service reimbursement for primary care physicians. General practitioners are paid based on 3 segments. Segment 1 is a capitated rate that is adjusted for only 2 factors: the patient's age and socioeconomic status. This capitated rate covers about 70% of total GP compensation. GPs can also bill on a fee-for-service basis for office consultations and home visits, although these fees are quite low. For instance, the fee for a short office visit is $11 USD (€10). Finally, GPs can receive fees for employing nurses for mental health care. Nonetheless, as one professor put it, payment for GPs is "more or less based on how many patients they have [in their panel]."

Segment 2 payments incentivize care integration. They include payments for chronic care nurses and bundled payments for participation in regional care groups dedicated to chronic-disease management, such as for diabetes, COPD, and asthma. Regional care groups that receive bundled payments contract directly with networks of providers. Care groups are legal entities formed by multiple providers, typically led by GPs. For the diabetes bundle, care groups are financially responsible

Figure 4. Payment to Physicians (Netherlands)

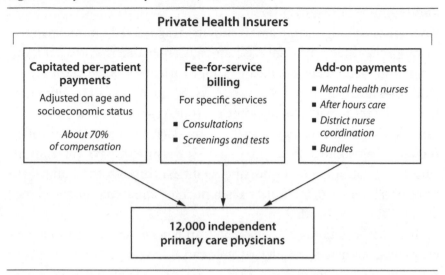

Private Health Insurers

Capitated per-patient payments	**Fee-for-service billing**	**Add-on payments**
Adjusted on age and socioeconomic status	For specific services	■ *Mental health nurses*
		■ *After hours care*
	■ *Consultations*	■ *District nurse coordination*
About 70% of compensation	■ *Screenings and tests*	■ *Bundles*

12,000 independent primary care physicians

for assigned diabetes patients in the program and can either deliver services directly or subcontract them. The price of bundles in segment 2 is freely negotiated, but the range of services that need to be provided in the bundles is set nationally. Contracts include mandatory record keeping for evaluation purposes. In 2018, additional payments for organization and infrastructure were added to pay for cooperation with district nurses and secondary care.

Segment 3 payments are pay-for-performance programs largely focused on increasing access, improving appropriate drug prescribing, and incentivizing appropriate specialist referrals. These pay-for-performance programs are voluntary. As part of Segment 3 payments, GPs also receive hourly fees for participating in after-hours care cooperatives that provide nighttime and weekend coverage. Segment 3 is the smallest fraction of GP income.

Medical specialists are paid differently. About 40% of specialists, including pediatricians and psychiatrists, are salaried employees of hospitals. Similarly, within academic medical centers all medical specialists are salaried employees. About 60% of specialists are organized into specialist-owned partnerships (MSBs). The MSB of each specialty negotiates fees with hospitals. The physician fee component of DBCs is paid from hospitals to MSBs, which then pay each member specialist.

Payment to Long-Term Residential and Home Health Providers

Payment for long-term care is highly fragmented. Municipalities, through their Regional Care Assessment Center, determine what long-term, home-based custodial care is appropriate for beneficiaries to be paid for under the Social Support Acts. Municipalities are ultimately financially responsible for at-home custodial care and social supports. Conversely, private insurers pay for home-based nursing care through the Health Insurance Act. The federal government pays for 24-hour care (either at home or in nursing facilities) through the Long-Term Care Act. Long-term institutional support for children is financed separately under the Youth Act.

For custodial home care, patients can receive services from a government-contracted provider, or they can receive a personal budget to organize the care themselves. In the past, personal budgets were paid directly to patients and families, but fraud forced a change to have the Social Insurance Bank manage these budgets. However, not all long-term care services are paid for through the Long-Term Care and Social Support Acts. For example, district nurses who coordinate care and provide health care services at home are reimbursed through the compulsory health insurance system. In 2015, the reorganization of long-term care cut funding for municipalities to provide social support.

Negotiations and Selective Contracting

Fostering competition remains a challenge within the Dutch system. Although insurers can selectively contract, it exists more in theory than in practice. Price negotiation between insurers and hospitals and other providers is less thorough and detailed than might be imagined. Insurers have little capacity to steer enrollees toward specific hospitals. As one researcher noted, "Even if there is selective contracting, people will tend to ask their GP which hospital they should go to." The penalties for going out of network are not sufficiently high to induce patients to scrupulously adhere to networks. Insurers have been unwilling to raise incentives and penalties for going out of the network. One professor noted the risk-averse nature of negotiations: "Most of the negotiations are incremental. . . . [The insurers and hospitals] have to work together next year too, so negotiations are usually pretty friendly."

Because negotiations between insurers and hospitals have been ineffective at reducing costs, the Ministry of Health, Welfare, and Sport has resorted to establishing a national Health Care Budget to set target cost growth to restrict cost increases.

Bundled Payments

Since 2010, the government has introduced a nationwide bundled payment system for diabetes, vascular risk management, and COPD. The Dutch government determines which services are included in each bundle. For example, services in the diabetes bundle are codified nationally in the Dutch Diabetes Federation Health Care Standard (DFHCS). The diabetes bundle includes checkups, eye and foot exams, dietary counseling, lab tests, and consultations with referred specialists, but they exclude medications and hospitalizations.

Insurers freely negotiate prices with entities known as care groups that are financially responsible for the cost of all services in the bundle for a fixed period. In 2011, the latest year for which pricing data are available, bundle prices were between $428 USD (€381) and $516 USD (€459). Care groups are new legal entities in the Dutch system, and they are primarily made up of GPs that contract with other providers such as dieticians or podiatrists.

DELIVERY OF HEALTH CARE SERVICES

The Dutch health care system enshrines free choice of physicians, but GPs act as strong gatekeepers for access to specialists and hospitals. Except in cases of direct admission through an emergency department, a GP referral is required for specialist care and more complex mental health care.

Hospital Care

For a population of 17 million, there are 120 hospitals, organized into 79 hospital systems. Of these 79 systems, 8 are academic medical centers. All hospitals are not for profit. Hospitals run themselves; they are free to expand or close units as they see fit. Capital costs are folded into the payments from insurers (DBCs).

As in most other countries, utilization of hospitals in the Netherlands is declining. From 2002 to 2015 the total number of hospital beds fell from roughly 48,000 to just under 41,000. About 33,000 beds are in general hospitals, and just over 7,500 beds are in university hospitals. With 3.6 hospital beds per 1,000 people, the Netherlands is about average in terms of hospital beds for the OECD, but it has more beds than the United States (2.6 per 1,000 people). Similarly, the number of overnight admissions has declined as well, as has the average length of stay, from 7.8 days in 2002 to 5.2 days in 2012. Just over half of hospitalizations are one-day admissions. There is still room to shrink hospital capacity. Acute care bed occupancy rates are under 50%—even lower than the United States, where it is about 62%. In addition, as of 2018, there were 134 hospital-affiliated outpatient clinics to deliver specialist care.

There are 2 ways to access hospital care in the Netherlands. When a GP provides a patient with a referral to see a specialist in a hospital, the patient typically has free choice of specialist, unless their insurer has selectively contracted. Specialists can see patients both as inpatients and outpatients in hospitals. About 40% of specialists are employed by hospitals, and the remainder are independent contractors, organized through specialist-owned partnerships (MSBs).

Alternatively, patients can be directly admitted through an emergency department. In urgent situations, such as vomiting blood, patients cannot call an ambulance directly. Either patients call an emergency call center (akin to 911 in the United States) or their GP office. The GP or the emergency services can then call an ambulance. Although emergency departments are supposed to be reserved for emergencies that require ambulance transportation, nearly half of presentations to EDs occur without referrals, and just over half of those (25% of all emergency department visits) are ultimately deemed nonemergent.

Upon arrival in an ED, patients first encounter a triage nurse, who can direct patients to a special GP ward, which is typically adjacent to the ED to handle the less acute problems. If a patient insists on being admitted through an ED for a nonurgent condition, their insurer may not cover the care, and the patient may pay a penalty.

There are also roughly 230 private, for-profit independent treatment centers (ZBCs), and these provide selective, nonacute treatments for up to 24 hours. ZBCs can only provide care that is freely negotiated between insurers and providers (i.e., nonemergency care). Almost all ZBCs specialize in same-day procedures, such as orthopedic surgeries and ophthalmological procedures. From a legal and regulatory standpoint, the ZBCs are classified with general hospitals.

Outpatient Primary Care

According to the Dutch government, there are about 12,000 GPs in the Netherlands, representing almost a quarter of all doctors. According to the OECD, an additional 12,500 physicians are nonspecialized or in generalist fields, such as internal medicine. Overall there are 8.8 physician visits per capita per year in the Netherlands, most of which occur in primary care settings.

GPs are self-employed, and over the last decade there has been a significant shift away from solo practice and toward group practice. Today, 28% of GPs work in solo practice, 39% in 2-person practices, and 33% in groups of 2 to 7 physicians. A typical GP panel size is 2,300 patients.

In many countries patients expect to leave a physician's office visit with some intervention: a prescription, an order for a laboratory test, or an imaging service. Not so in the Netherlands. Dutch GPs have a strong professional ethos to be efficient, intervene less, and not overtreat. As one health policy expert described it: "[Primary care] is a strong profession. They are well organized. You know, our foreign students always complain, they say, 'When I go to my GP, I expect to get some drug or referral, but instead he says, 'Well, go home. If you're still ill in 2 days, come back. Most diseases just disappear.'"

Since 2012, nurse practitioners are allowed to prescribe medications within their area of expertise. Dutch GPs use and employ nurse practitioners extensively, and these nurses have significant autonomy.

Using a personal story, one professor vividly illustrates how the Dutch delivery system works and the important role of nurses in primary care:

GP care is very well developed, and patients are quite satisfied with their GP. For example, I had this nasty cut on my finger. It had to be stitched and things like that. It was on a Sunday evening. I went to the out-of-hour cooperative of GPs, which is, by the way, next to the ER of the hospital. So, if it is too complex, you will move next door. But there is a GP and nurses at the cooperative. GP comes, stitches in, and he says, come back to your own GP in a week.

Last Monday I went to my GP. In a lot of countries, probably a specialized doctor is going to remove stitches. In this case it's a practice secretary [a nurse with secondary vocational training]. He removed the stitches and said, 'It looks good.' That's it.

GPs are responsible for providing mild mental health care, such as for situational depression. Consequently, over 80% of GP practices employ a mental health nurse.

Dutch GPs provide extensive after-hours care—nights and all weekends. Typically this care is not provided by the patient's GP office but through an organized system of GP cooperatives. About 120 primary care cooperatives, each with 50 to 250 physicians, serve the entire Dutch population. These cooperatives follow a nationally uniform model. They use telephone triage, typically performed by nurses, to decide whether a patient needs an on-site consultation, phone consultation, or home visit. The cooperatives are accessible through regional phone numbers. These cooperatives have reduced the use of emergency departments, especially given recent integration with local hospital emergency departments. Physicians who participate are paid hourly for after-hours care.

Specialist Care
There are 33,000 specialists, representing over half of all Dutch physicians. All Dutch medical specialists are based at hospitals or institutions. Therefore, most specialist care is provided in hospital settings either as inpatient or outpatient offices. Recently, some specialist care has moved toward the for-profit ZBCs.

In order to see a specialist, patients must get a referral from a GP, and at times specialists complain about a lack of referrals. Without a referral, insurers only pay 75% of the average national fee to out-of-network providers. Although it is technically possible to see a specialist without a referral, having a patient walk in and see a specialist without going through a GP is essentially unheard of. Many physicians will not see patients without a referral because of the added administrative burden. Once a patient receives a referral to see a specialist, the specialist has the ability to refer to other physicians freely. As with many countries, coordination of chronic care becomes unorganized when specialists refer to each other. However, GPs have generally proven capable of managing specialist care plans for patients with multiple comorbidities.

The Dutch system has successfully cut down on waiting times for specialists over the last decade. Since 2009, Dutch hospitals and specialists have been subject to new regulations governing wait times. The Dutch Healthcare Authority sets target wait times for consultations, diagnoses, and other services. Physicians and hospitals are obliged to publish wait times. In 2009, nearly a quarter of outpatient consultations, treatments, and diagnoses exceeded national standards. By 2014, the data showed that fewer than 15% of care instances exceeded target wait times.

Care Groups for Chronic Conditions

Since 2010, regional care groups that receive bundled payments from insurers have organized care for patients with specific chronic conditions, such as diabetes and COPD. One much-cited example is the diabetes care group, Diabeter. It was established in 2006 and acquired by Medtronics in 2015 as part of the company's strategy to make inroads in value-based care. The Diabeter model includes a multidisciplinary team of physicians, nurses, dieticians, psychologists, and an administrator who are collectively responsible for a group of diabetic patients. Diabeter's approach is focused on education to promote self-management; continuous monitoring with digital technology, such as wireless insulin pumps and glucose monitors; and wrap-around services to prevent hospital utilization. A care coordinator organizes all care for the patient. Patients and families are educated about self-management, linked electronically—email and Skype—to the clinic, and have team visits on average 4 times per year. Real-time data from patients' insulin pumps and glucose monitors as well as data on complications, hospitalizations, quality of life, and psychosocial outcomes are regularly collected and analyzed. The clinic's percentage of children with HbA1c less than 7.5% (58 mmol/mol) is 56%, compared to the national average of 31%. It also has a very low rate of hospitalizations—about 3%—compared to a national average of 8%. In 2017, the clinic network received the Value-Based Healthcare Prize from the Value-Based Healthcare Center of Europe. Diabeter has 2,000 attributed patients in 5 locations across the Netherlands.

Mental Health

Like most countries, the Netherlands has shifted from institution-based mental health care toward community-based care. Since 2010, the number of mental health contacts per 1,000 patients in primary care settings has almost doubled. While the number of integrated mental health institutions has remained steady at about 30, the number of general mental hospitals decreased from 12 to 2 between 2000 and 2014.

Mental health service delivery is divided into 3 levels. The first level of mental health care occurs in the GP's office. This care is initially managed by a mental health practice nurse who works in the GP's office. If the nurse and GP suspect that the patient suffers from a more severe mental condition, such as bipolar disorder or difficult-to-treat depression, they refer the patient to the 2nd level of care, which is short-term mental care provided by psychologists and psychiatrists in hospital-outpatient settings. The 3rd level of care is for even more severe cases requiring specialist care for complex conditions and may include inpatient care. If prolonged inpatient care is necessary, it is provided at specialized mental health institutions and financed through long-term care mechanisms.

Long-Term Care

Because of an aging population and overreliance on institutionalization, long-term care costs have been rising rapidly. Prior to the 2015 reforms, nearly 7% of the Dutch population lived in residential care facilities, such as nursing homes. Nearly 450 residential care companies provided care in about 2,000 facilities. Subsequently, policies have encouraged deinstitutionalization of long-term care. While 24/7 long-term care is financed and administered federally, municipalities are financially and administratively responsible for the organization of social support services and at-home custodial care, such as cooking and light house work, in order to keep people living in their homes and communities. These social supports are paid for through the Social Support Act and are fully organized by municipalities. If seniors living at home need some home-based nursing care, those services are organized by private health insurers through the Health Insurance Act.

The central government is responsible for 24-hour home health care and institutional care. To do this, individual insurers receive a license from the government to manage regional care offices called *Zorgkantoors*, which coordinate 24-hour home-based or institutional long-term care in cooperation with municipalities and negotiate contracts with long-term care providers.

To receive long-term support, a senior or family member must contact the government's Care Assessment Agency (CIZ), either directly or through a doctor. The CIZ determines the person's care profile and informs the regional care office (the Zorgkantoor) if the person qualifies for care under the Long-Term Care Act. Individuals can also choose to be allocated a personal budget to purchase and coordinate their own long-term care independently.

There are some social disparities in long-term care. As one expert put it: "It depends on how much information you give them. In day-to-day practice, it is not a free choice. . . . For people at a higher income it is easier for them to organize it themselves." Personal budgets used to be a source of considerable fraud, as they were paid directly to patients. Since 2015, budgets have been deposited into the SVB, which can be drawn down by beneficiaries.

Public Health and Preventive Medicine

The central government sets overall goals for public health, but municipalities are responsible for the actual public health activities. Municipalities provide vaccinations and preventive care services in schools. Municipalities also can launch campaigns for preventive screening for cancer as well as community mental health initiatives. Five regional screening organizations manage population-based screening programs for breast and colon cancer. Although regional and local offices are responsible for promoting and coordinating public health programs, the actual care occurs in GP offices. For example, most influenza vaccines and cervical cancer screenings occur in GP offices.

PHARMACEUTICAL COVERAGE AND PRICE CONTROLS

Pharmaceutical Market

The Dutch pharmaceutical market is relatively small in both absolute and relative terms. In 2017, according to the Dutch government, retail pharmaceutical sales were only $6.4 billion USD (€5.7 billion), accounting for only 7.6% of health care–specific spending. In reality, the level of spending on pharmaceuticals is likely higher because many expensive medications, such as new targeted cancer drugs, are considered part of hospital spending and not broken out in the statistics. Regardless, prescription drug spending as a share of overall health care spending is much smaller than the 14% spent in Germany and Australia or the nearly 17% in the United States. According to the OECD, on a per capita basis, in 2017 the Netherlands spent $410 USD (€360) on retail pharmaceuticals, less than Germany ($780 USD, or €686), France ($662 USD, or €582), or Switzerland ($1,080 USD, or €951) and much lower than the nearly $1,200 USD per capita spent in the United States. This places the Netherlands near the bottom of the OECD in terms of per capita spending. Approximately 68% of pharmaceutical spending is covered by compulsory health insurance, 31% is out of pocket, and 1% is financed by voluntary supplementary health insurance.

Market Access, Coverage Determination, and Price Setting

The first step to get insurers in the Netherlands to cover newly approved drugs is marketing approval based on European Union regulation and domestic laws, specifically the Medicines Act and Pharmaceutical Prices Law. All new drugs must be registered with and authorized for sale by the Medicines Evaluation Board, which is the Dutch analog of the US Food and Drug Administration. Market authorization can also occur through the European Medicines Agency authorization procedure. However, approval by the Medicines Evaluation Board does not mean that insurers will pay for a drug; it simply means the manufacturer is legally allowed to sell the drug in the Netherlands.

After receiving approval from the Medicines Evaluation board, the drug manufacturer must submit a dossier to the Ministry of Health, Welfare, and Sport in order for the drug to be listed on the Pharmaceutical Reimbursement System (GVS). Within 90 days of receiving

Figure 5. Regulation of Pharmaceutical Prices (Netherlands)

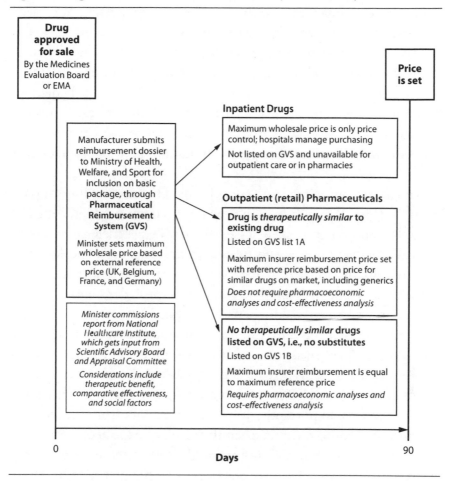

Drug approved for sale
By the Medicines Evaluation Board or EMA

Price is set

Manufacturer submits reimbursement dossier to Ministry of Health, Welfare, and Sport for inclusion on basic package, through **Pharmaceutical Reimbursement System (GVS)**

Minister sets maximum wholesale price based on external reference price (UK, Belgium, France, and Germany)

Minister commissions report from National Healthcare Institute, which gets input from Scientific Advisory Board and Appraisal Committee

Considerations include therapeutic benefit, comparative effectiveness, and social factors

Inpatient Drugs

Maximum wholesale price is only price control; hospitals manage purchasing

Not listed on GVS and unavailable for outpatient care or in pharmacies

Outpatient (retail) Pharmaceuticals

Drug is *therapeutically similar* to existing drug

Listed on GVS list 1A

Maximum insurer reimbursement price set with reference price based on price for similar drugs on market, including generics
Does not require pharmacoeconomic analyses and cost-effectiveness analysis

No therapeutically similar drugs listed on GVS, i.e., no substitutes

Listed on GVS 1B

Maximum insurer reimbursement is equal to maximum reference price
Requires pharmacoeconomic analyses and cost-effectiveness analysis

0

90

Days

the application from the manufacturer, the Ministry is required to set a maximum wholesale price to distributors. The maximum price is set using an international reference price calculated from the average price of the same drug or a similar product in neighboring countries: Belgium, Germany, France, and the United Kingdom. The Ministry can use drugs with the same active ingredient, including generics. The maximum price can only be calculated if at least 2 of the comparison countries have a comparable drug on the market.

Within 90 days, the Ministry of Health, Welfare, and Sport must also determine whether the new drug may be included in the basic insurance package. Drugs in the basic insurance package must be reimbursed by health insurers for use in outpatient settings—that is, in sales at retail pharmacies or from a dispensing GP. There are 2 drug lists in the GVS. List 1A is composed of drugs that have interchangeable therapeutic equivalents already available in the Netherlands, such as statins for lowering cholesterol. List 1B is composed of drugs without substitutes—that is, they have significant added therapeutic benefits to be unique. Placement on the GVS may carry additional restrictions on prescribing and use, such as limiting targeted cancer treatments to specific subpopulations based on genetic mutations in tumors and disease progression.

The maximum reimbursement price paid by insurers for drugs on the GVS depends on which list a drug is placed on. In general, the National Health Care Institute assesses the new drug's medical necessity, clinical effectiveness, cost effectiveness, and side effects. The Scientific Advisory Board assesses the therapeutic benefit and cost effectiveness of the drug, while the Appraisal Committee provides a needs assessment. For list 1A drugs—drugs with an available therapeutic equivalent—the minister sets a maximum reimbursement rate based on the average of prices of all medicines in the group, including generics. Conversely, because there is no equivalent for List 1B drugs, the maximum reimbursement is equivalent to the external reference price for wholesale distributors. Importantly, drugs can be exempt from the required pharmacoeconomic analysis when they are not expected to cost over a set yearly budget threshold and are unlikely to increase national drug costs. This mainly applies to orphan drugs with high prices but small numbers of patients. There is no governmental price setting for over-the-counter drugs.

Individual hospitals establish what drugs they will use and negotiate prices directly with drug manufacturers. These negotiations are limited by the maximum price set by the Ministry of Health, Welfare, and Sport. Recently there has been a push for more government involvement in regulating hospital drug prices, especially for high-cost specialty medicines. If the Ministry decides that a new, expensive drug should not be available in hospitals, it can exclude the drug from inpatient settings.

The delineation of reimbursement controls between inpatient (where hospitals are expected to negotiate) and outpatient settings has generated controversies. From 2012 onward, several especially expensive classes of drugs were removed from the GVS and placed onto hospital budgets, causing hospitals to bristle at having to pay. As a compromise, hospitals were compensated for expensive medications and orphan drugs, including many new cancer drugs, growth hormones, and TNF inhibitors such as Humira used for rheumatoid arthritis. Therefore, although prescription drug prices and spending appear to be low, the reality is that a significant portion of drug spending has been shifted onto hospital spending.

Over the last decade, the government has attempted to expand access to new, expensive drugs. From 2006 to 2012, the Netherlands experimented with several types of managed entry agreements (MEAs), or *conditionally allowed specialist medicines*. These MEAs provide temporary coverage contingent on the generation of additional evidence of therapeutic benefit. However, the Ministry of Health, Welfare, and Sport found that even with the MEAs, access to drugs that were ultimately deemed cost effective was not achieved. Consequently, the Dutch are reforming the process.

Prescribing Controls and Bulk Purchasing

Dutch insurance companies also play a role in controlling drug spending. The most important tool is the "preferred medicine" policy, or insurer formularies. Insurers are allowed to select a specific brand of preferred medication from a cluster of pharmaceuticals with the same active ingredients. Pharmacies are obliged to only provide the preferred medication to the insurer's patients. Alternatively, insurers can set a maximum reimbursement price for a specific active compound. If pharmacists buy a drug for less than the maximum price, they keep the savings. The use of bulk purchasing and competitive bidding has been effective for controlling generic prices.

Although generic substitution is not mandatory in the Netherlands, the Dutch electronic prescribing system automatically substitutes generic for brand-name drugs when they are available. Physicians must medically justify prescribing a brand-name drug when there is a generic alternative available. At the pharmacy level, pharmacy fees are fixed per dispensation, regardless of the drug's price, obviating an incentive to dispense higher-priced brand-name drugs.

Prices Paid by Patients

Several policies insulate Dutch patients from high out-of-pocket drug costs. First, many high-cost drugs have been shifted to the hospital formulary, and patients have no co-pay for these once they meet their deductible. Second, list 1A drugs are essentially free after the mandatory deductible is met. However, there is still a small problem of surprise costs before deductibles are met because although GP services are exempted from the deductible, prescribed drugs are not. Third, insurers can waive cost sharing for preferred medicines. For drugs on list 1A that are priced above the maximum reimbursement, patients must pay the difference between the reimbursement price and the retail price. However, because over 90% of drugs on list 1A are fully reimbursed, these drugs are typically free to patients. Finally, the Netherlands also has reduced taxes on drugs. The standard VAT rate is 21%, but for drugs the VAT is just 9%.

HUMAN RESOURCES

Physicians

According to the OECD, there are roughly 60,000 practicing Dutch physicians, including 27,500 generalists—such as GPs, pediatricians, and internists—and 33,800 specialists. The Netherlands has just over 3.5 practicing physicians per 1,000 people, an average rate among European countries. Because of its relatively small size, highly urban population, and high population density, the Netherlands does not have a severe rural-urban maldistribution of physicians. Only the remote and sparsely populated northern islands have a physician shortage. In addition, nearly all citizens live within a 25-minute drive to a hospital, and 99% of the population can reach an emergency department within 45 minutes.

Dutch GPs and specialists are compensated fairly well, but they are not as highly paid as US or Swiss doctors. In 2016, the average salary of GPs was $123,000 USD (€108,000), and for specialists the average salary was $190,000 USD (€168,000). The range of salaries for physicians is fairly narrow, as one researcher noted,

I believe a specialist salary goes from 180,000 to 240,000 or something.... It is a different culture. I know that I was [in the United States],
and there was some orthopedic surgeon who earned $4.2 million just
from Medicare.... In the Netherlands if you would earn $4.2 million,
you will be shamed.... Everybody in the Netherlands would say, "It's
our money! What's the guy doing?"

Medical education is provided at 8 domestic medical schools. Initial undergraduate medical education lasts 6 years. The first 4 years
consist of an undergraduate preclinical bachelor's program, and the
final 2 years focus on clinical training, conferring a doctorate of medicine. Medical education is subsidized. The mandatory annual fee is just
$2,400 USD per year (€2,083) as of 2019.

Recently medical education has shifted toward competence-based
training in which promotion to the next stage is not dependent upon
time but upon mastering a set of skills. Graduation times, residency
start dates, and completion have become nonstandardized. Students
complete their training on an individualized timeline.

Most physicians take a one-year internship before starting post-
graduate (residency) training. The College of Medical Specialists (CGS)
regulates specialty training. Training to become a GP lasts 3 years, while
training for specialties ranges from 4 to 6 years. There are work-hour
limits. Dutch residents may not work more than 60 hours per week,
with a maximum shift of 12 hours. The government pays hospitals to
cover residents' salaries and training.

Nurses

There are approximately 200,000 practicing nurses in the Netherlands, or 10.5 per 1,000 people, fewer than in Germany but more than
the United States. Like many developed countries, the Netherlands is
dealing with shortages, particularly for some specialist services. The
average salary of nurses is roughly $62,000 USD (€55,000), about 17%
higher than the average national wage.

The Netherlands has a high number of advance practice nurse practitioners (NPs). An ever-larger number of tasks, particularly mental
health and primary care, have shifted to nurses. In the Netherlands

advance practice NPs have a large scope of practice and prescribing authority, as one researcher noted,

> I think the strong point is the increasingly good and independent position of nurses, which is, for instance, compared to Germany, really a world of difference. In the Netherlands nurses are much more an independent profession. We have nurse specialists who have advanced degrees and who also have rights of prescription in certain areas. That is something for which in Germany you couldn't even think of it.

Nurses are also important for long-term care as coordinators between municipalities and patients. The same researcher went on to explain, "District nurses work in teams [for long-term care], and they are the ones with a bachelor in nursing and a one-year extra education in district in nursing. The district nurse is again allowed to assess the patient and decide how [many services and what kinds] the patient needs. Most home health care is provided by certified nurse assistants, who only require 3 years of training.

Dental Care

There are 8,500 dentists in the Netherlands, or 0.5 per 1,000 people. All dentists are private. For children under 18 dental care is covered under the basic benefits package. For adults, dental care, except oral surgery, is not covered. Most insurers offer partial dental insurance under the private supplementary insurance, but a significant amount of dental care is paid out of pocket. Consequently, some of the largest socioeconomic disparities in the Netherlands relate to the utilization of dental care.

CHALLENGES

The Dutch health care system is in the middle on cost and is efficient at providing high-quality care. As one observer succinctly noted, "Most of the parties dealing with the system are fairly happy with it. . . . The grand design of the system is workable." Indeed, there are many virtues of the Dutch system. The Netherlands has achieved universal coverage.

The government covers universal health care for children at no cost to families, regardless of household income or number of children. The private health insurance system is stable through a well-managed system of compulsory, community-rated premiums and an effective risk adjustment program that redistributes pooled funds to plans based on expected costs. The governance of the risk adjustment system and sophisticated academic modeling appear to prevent gaming by insurers, thereby preventing adverse consequences for higher-risk patients.

The Dutch system also does a fairly good job of steering patients toward higher-touch, lower-cost care in GP settings. Task shifting has been well instituted, with nurse practitioners providing significant primary care and care for mild mental health conditions. Consequently, the use of hospitals and specialists for chronic and routine care is not high. Finally, like the Germans, the Dutch have a mandatory, tax-financed national insurance program for long-term care that can be provided at home or in institutional settings. Providers are well compensated, and the quality of care delivered is high.

It should also be said that the Dutch have a way of getting through thorny systemic problems. There is a national ethos to make things work and prevent crises. Hospitals, physicians, and insurers are willing to work together to develop patchwork fixes to systemic problems. Negotiations over prices and utilization tend not to be aggressive and confrontational. This muddling-through ethos prevents crises from developing but can also postpone addressing problems and allowing some large flaws to fester without comprehensive reform. For example, by moving specific high-cost drugs from outpatient to inpatient settings and compensating hospitals with specific add-on payments from insurers, hospitals, insurers, and the government have routinely changed how expensive pharmaceuticals are paid for in order to keep out-of-pocket costs low at the point of service.

Nevertheless, there are 3 important long-term challenges for the Netherlands. The first is cost and cost growth. The Dutch are attuned to cost control and instituted the current system of managed competition in response to growing cost problems. Nevertheless, there is a sense that managed competition has not restrained costs effectively. Insurers' negotiations with hospitals have not reduced costs, and attempts at lowering cost increases of drugs have not worked well. Although cost growth is not excessive in the Netherlands, many observers think the current level is high, and it will require vigilance to keep growth low.

The 2nd and related challenge concerns long-term care. Unlike most countries, the Netherlands created a dedicated, mandatory tax system financing long-term care. Even as it provides funds, this benefit is seen as a major factor driving up health care expenditures. As a former politician put it:

> The first and biggest problem is cost. The rate of health care expenditures tends to grow at least twice as fast as the rate of national income. We know that if you look deeper into the Dutch system, that we do spend a lot more on long-term care than other countries. . . . You can't explain the difference by demography.

To address the long-term cost problem, the government has tried to transition from an "open ended entitlement" to one in which municipalities receive a budget and oversee the provision of long-term care. As the former politician explained, the transition has been politically problematic, and policy has veered back and forth:

> We talk about the elderly, you talk about the handicapped, and basically if everybody says more money should go in to it . . . the previous government made a serious cut in the expenditure on long-term care, basically by decentralizing a lot of it . . . and the next government in power basically put the money back into the system, and everything that was being cut 5 years ago is now being put back in. I see it as a waste, but you know, who dares be a politician that says you shouldn't put [more] money towards the elderly?

Complicating these changes has been the fact that many municipalities lack the technical capacity to manage long-term care. One policy analyst noted just how daunting the task was for small local governments: "We have way too many municipalities—400 or something. There is no knowledge, and nobody understands what they are doing." In response, there is a trend toward regional organizations rather than local ones to manage long-term care. Whether this can help address the problem is unclear.

Another problem is that although municipalities have responsibility for long-term care, they do not have authority over home health nursing services; these services are provided under the Health Insurance Act. This creates the perverse incentive for municipalities to shift care to home health nursing when possible. Simultaneously, insurers want to shift more care to social supports financed by the municipalities. This financing arrangement undermines coordination and seems to lead to escalating costs rather than efficiency.

Finally, there is an underlying social challenge posed by long-term care that inhibits solving the problem. The welfare-state model has long been ingrained into the Dutch culture. The state should provide for the elderly. As one Dutch observer noted, "In the Netherlands children are not financially responsible for their parents—that makes a difference. . . . From the 1950s onward the responsibility was taken from children for their old parents and taken over by the state." The recent reforms aim to shift responsibility for care of the aged from the state to local governments and the family. Many Dutch experts suggested that trying to change from a state-based delivery model to one that placed responsibility on municipalities and families met with a lot of inaction, slow walking, and passive resistance.

A 3rd challenge is the Dutch desire to have both managed competition and cooperation. The tension between the 2 often inhibits solving problems of the health system. For example, managed competition should work in part because of selective contracting with highly efficient physicians and hospitals. But selective contracting contravenes cooperation and, thus, has not reached any significant threshold. As a researcher put it, "We introduced this managed competition, but next to that we have this municipal system, and the municipal system is much more based on cooperation. The managed competition is based on competition and not based on cooperation." The Netherlands has generally reverted to a reliance on large-scale national agreements such as the Health Care Budget set by the minister as the main tools of cost control. The Health Care Budget may run counter to the principles of managed competition, but ultimately it has been necessary to keeping the system affordable.

The Dutch government, insurers, and providers have all been able to make do under what is essentially a compromise system between neoliberal ideals of competition and a historical welfare-state–based approach. Because the overall health system generally works well, there is little appetite for additional large-scale health reform. As a former politician put it, "Everybody is dead scared of losing 5 years to changing laws and in augmenting your system. They would rather try to work within the system that we have."

CHAPTER EIGHT

SWITZERLAND

The Swiss love their health care system. They can choose any doctor and any hospital in the country. There are no wait times. And there is a sense that the system delivers "Swiss quality." Yet over and over, in side comments and undertones, everyone—from physicians to health policy experts to government officials to average citizens—expressed an uneasy feeling best summarized by one health expert this way:

> [Every year] the canton has to pay more and more and more. Somehow, sometime, the system will crack because nobody will be able to pay the premiums and costs anymore. . . . Sooner or later the system will crack, but nobody cares as usual. We are on a comfortable train running fast toward the wall, and nobody cares because everything is running fine—now.

The Swiss health care system is often lauded as one of "the best" in the world. Its universal health insurance mandate satisfies liberal goals of universal coverage, while its reliance on private insurance, decentralized regulation through cantons (akin to states or provinces), and extensive patient choice appeal to more conservative beliefs. Patient satisfaction is impressively high, and the system performs well on various public health and quality metrics.

However, the system's most appealing characteristics—including the requirement for insurance, the canton-level regulation of most activities, and extensive choice with limited gatekeeping and care management—are also responsible for its most serious problems: high costs, complexity, lack of focus on chronic care coordination, and impediments to systemic reform.

Everyone I interviewed in Switzerland agreed that Swiss health care is too expensive, but no key player—insurers, physicians, or patients—seems willing to give up their advantage or access in order to reduce costs. Additionally, the system's complexity is also becoming its most well-known attribute. As one physician explained, "Every time I speak about the Swiss system, everyone says, 'Oh my god, it's so complicated. How can you work with that?'"

Even though these challenges are all known, reform is still proving hard to achieve. In its Health 2020 report the Swiss federal government acknowledges that "in the coming years, our health system will be confronted with numerous challenges which could call into question what has been achieved so far."

HISTORY

The history of the Swiss health care system is one of progressive federalization. Until the late 19th century, regulation of what few health care services existed rested almost entirely with the 26 cantons. The first Federal Constitution of 1848 mentioned only sanitary measures during epidemics as a federal—or Confederation—responsibility; all other services fell under the jurisdiction of each canton.

After a cholera pandemic in the mid-19th century, the federal government decided that something more had to be done. In rapid succession a myriad of federal laws was passed to begin improving health care services. In 1877, a federal law standardized the qualifying examinations for doctors, pharmacists, and veterinarians. In 1893, the predecessor to the Federal Office of Public Health (FOPH) was founded. And in 1890, the Confederation was given a constitutional mandate to create sickness and accident insurance. However, the first attempt to do so in 1900 failed, when a popular referendum rejected a draft law.

At the turn of the 20th century fewer than 15% of the population was insured. The existing insurance was based on trade union membership, employer, or religious affiliation. Most insurers were very small, with fewer than 100 members, and half operated in just one municipality. These insurance schemes were less health insurance than mechanisms to provide financial support for lost wages due to illnesses, occupational accidents, or death. Given most insurers' small and selective nature, there existed little coordination between groups and practically no consistent method for establishing premiums.

In 1911, the Swiss Confederation successfully passed the first Federal Law on Sickness and Accident Insurance (KUVG/LAMA). The law required health insurance funds that wished to receive federal subsidies to: (1) register with the Federal Office for Social Insurance, (2) be not for profit, (3) provide a standardized benefit package, and 4) calculate individual premiums based on members' age of entry and sex. Cantons were empowered with the responsibility to mandate insurance.

LAMA did not standardize premiums across the cantons, nor did it prohibit discrimination against preexisting conditions. Consequently, premium prices varied greatly. For instance, women paid up to 10% more than men. In addition, there was substantial adverse selection. Insurers with a higher proportion of high-risk members charged higher premiums, creating death spirals that forced many insurance companies to merge or file for bankruptcy. Health insurance could also not be carried over if a member switched their canton of residence or employment.

Beginning in the 1960s, health care costs increased significantly. All attempts by the Confederation to amend LAMA failed. Finally, in 1994, the Confederation successfully passed the new Federal Health Insurance Law (abbreviated LAMal in French and KVG in German). LAMal was then implemented in 1996 as Switzerland's principal health insurance framework. LAMal had 4 aims: (1) achieve universal coverage, (2) ensure affordability via premium subsidies for low-income individuals, (3) curb health care costs, and (4) expand the benefit package.

In April 2014, a proposal to amend the Federal Constitution was accepted by public referendum, thereby explicitly listing health care provision as a federal co-responsibility with cantons. This was the first time the Confederation was constitutionally empowered with the responsibility of providing health care. This legislation embodied Switzerland's increasing federalization of health policy.

Today, at the federal level, the Federal Department of Home Affairs (FDHA) is the final authority for decisions concerning the Swiss health care system's daily functioning. Within the FDHA the Federal Office of Public Health (FOPH) is responsible for the development of health policy, insurance regulations, and mandatory health insurance supervision. The FOPH specifies which services mandatory health insurers cover, provides federal premium subsidies to cantons, and drafts laws regarding the training of health professionals. The FOPH is also involved in consumer protection, infectious disease control, and disease surveillance. The FDHA also has a role in determining reimbursement levels for services and the pricing of pharmaceuticals.

Swiss patients have an almost unrestricted choice of insurer, hospital, and physician. Oversight and decision-making power are shared in complex ways among the Confederation (federal government), cantons (states), and municipalities as well as recognized associations of insurers and providers. In addition, the Swiss public can veto health care legislation or demand reform through the public referendum process. This has created a system that is not well coordinated at any level and is slow to change and innovate. For instance, only within the last few years has Switzerland adopted DRG-type payments for hospitals, something almost every other developed country has long since instituted.

COVERAGE

Switzerland is a country of 26 cantons, with 8.4 million people, and has 99.5% health coverage through private, not-for-profit health insurance companies.

Mandatory Basic Health Insurance

Enacted in 1994, the Federal Health Insurance Law (LAMal) created an individual mandate for health insurance. Every Swiss resident and nonresident with regular income-generating activity is required to be enrolled in a health insurance plan. Individuals are free to choose any insurer operating in their canton. They can switch insurers up to twice a year. Individuals who do not select a health insurance plan or do not pay their premiums face severe repercussions. The government can withhold wages to pay the premium—and charge up to a 50% penalty. In addition, cantons can enroll individuals who do not purchase insurance in a plan and force them to pay the premiums.

Figure 1. Health Care Coverage (Switzerland)

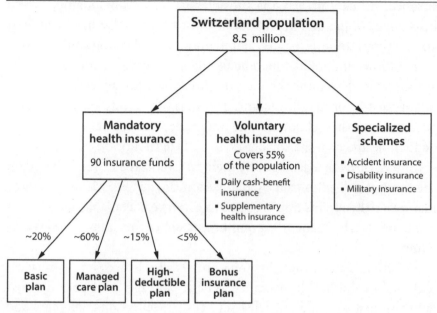

Recently, however, Switzerland has mitigated the financial stress that mandatory enrollment might cause. In 2010, cantons began paying 85% of unpaid premiums and other debts to insurers on behalf of their beneficiaries. Individuals who forgo paying their insurance bills are asked to refund insurers as soon as possible, but they do not need to give up their health care services.

When the Swiss choose a health insurance plan, they have 4 options. They can choose a basic plan, which typically has low deductibles and co-pays but higher premiums. Just over 20% of the insured opt for this. Alternatively, they can choose a managed care plan, in which they will receive a reduced premium in exchange for restrictions on their choice of providers. Managed care plans now dominate the insurance market, with more than 60% of the insured opting for them. Third, they may choose a high-deductible plan for a lower premium. High-deductible plans cover just over 15% of the insured. Finally, the Swiss can choose a bonus insurance plan that allows individuals who do not make a claim in a particular year to obtain a premium reduction the following year. Bonus insurance plans represent a negligible percentage of the market.

By law cantons must subsidize low-income individuals to buy insurance. All cantons pay the subsidies directly to mandatory health insurance companies. In addition, cantons must subsidize by at least 50% of the premiums for all children under 18 and young adults aged 18 to 25 of low- and middle-income families. However, cantons have the authority to determine the income thresholds for which households qualify as low or middle income. The sum of a family's out-of-pocket payments for their children must not exceed the cap set for an adult's deductible and cost sharing of $1,020 USD (CHF 1,000).

Since 2001, the federal government has allocated its funds based on the level of subsidies paid by the canton. It makes 7.5% of estimated mandatory health insurance costs in a given year available to each canton to be used to finance the premium subsidies for children and young adults.

All mandatory health insurers are required to cover all services included in the health insurance benefit package. This package covers most primary and specialist services as well as inpatient care and any physician-prescribed services unless explicitly excluded from the benefit package. With respect to hospital services, the benefit package covers the cost of treatment received in a shared ward. Drugs and devices must first be added to a "positive" list to qualify for payment by insurers. Some preventive measures, such as vaccinations for children and mammograms for women over 50, are covered free of cost. As is typical in many countries, dental care, eyeglasses, and prosthetics are not covered as part of the basic benefits package.

Several different government bodies decide which services are included in the benefit package, though final decisions rest with the FDHA. First, the Federal Commission for Medical Benefits and Basic Principles establishes criteria for the inclusion of benefits. The Federal Drug Commission advises the FDHA on pharmaceutical services to be included, and the Federal Commission for Analyses, Products, and Devices advises the FDHA on inclusion of medical devices. Finally, the FDHA decides the actual contents on the mandatory health insurance benefit package.

Although all services LAMal covers are expected to meet criteria of effectiveness, appropriateness, and efficacy, most (excluding drugs and devices) are not formally assessed. This has resulted in some services being included in the LAMal benefit package that have little scientifically proven value. For example, homeopathy and herbalism are covered only if qualified doctors perform them. Claudine Burton-Jeangros, a professor at the University of Geneva, argues that inclusion in the benefit package is more based on political influence than scientific evidence. She cites the inclusion, then removal of alternative medicine as an example, noting that when the lobbying winds shifted against alternative medicine, it was quickly dropped as a covered benefit.

Voluntary, Private Supplemental Insurance

Since 1996, insurers have supplemented their mandatory basic plans with voluntary, private supplemental products. By 2011, over 1,000 different supplementary health insurance products existed. Private insurance companies offered three-quarters of them, and mandatory health insurance companies offered the rest. The last available data (2012) suggests that nearly 55% of the Swiss population had a voluntary, private supplemental insurance plan.

There are 2 main types of voluntary supplemental health insurance: daily cash-benefit insurance and supplementary health insurance. Employers purchase daily cash-benefit insurance on behalf of employees to help them pay their employees' wages during an illness or accident for a limited period of time. Supplementary health insurance, meanwhile, is usually purchased by individuals seeking enhanced benefits, such as private hospital rooms, dental care, or eyeglasses. Beginning in 2001, private voluntary health insurance plans have been prohibited from helping to cover the cost-sharing obligations of the mandatory basic insurance plans.

Insurers

There are about 90 insurers in the 26 Swiss cantons offering mandatory health insurance plans. These health insurers must be not for profit— that is, they cannot profit from the sale of their mandatory basic plans. However, these companies can be financially and legally affiliated with a for-profit insurer, and these "sister" companies can offer—for a profit—private supplementary health insurance policies that cover single rooms, choice of specialist, vision care, and the like. Thus, the public and private health insurance marketplaces frequently comingle.

All mandatory health insurers are members of at least one of the following 3 associations: Santesuisse, Curafutura, and RVK. Of the 3, Santesuisse is the largest organization and represents all mandatory health insurers' political interests. It has significant clout, as it is a shareholder of Swiss DRG SA, the company responsible for developing the hospital reimbursement system. It is also a partner with TARMED Suisse, a company responsible for developing the ambulatory physician fee schedule. Curafutura was founded in 2013, when 4 large mandatory health insurers left Santesuisse and banded together to create a new organization. Finally, RVK represents small and medium insurers; members of RVK are usually also members of Santesuisse.

In 2014, the Federal Law on the Supervision of Mandatory Health Insurance (KVAG/LSAMal) gave the FOPH the power to oversee insurers and intervene on premium pricing. However, in a country known for its financial secrecy, little transparency is actually required of insurers. Hence, neither the government nor the citizenry know much about the flow of resources, which services are turning a profit, the extent of insurers' financial reserves, or whether margins come from the nonprofit or for-profit arms of insurance companies. There is little political will to force insurers to be more transparent in their finances, as over 35% of politicians also serve on the boards of the health insurance companies.

Switzerland's LAMal coordinates with 3 other social insurance schemes: accident insurance, disability insurance, and military insurance. All workers receive employer-sponsored accident insurance under the Federal Law on Accident Insurance (LAA). Disability insurance is provided under the Law on Disability Insurance (LAI). Cantons administer benefits for the elderly and the disabled. Military insurance was established in 1852 and covers all individuals employed in defense or security positions. These plans cover disability insurance, compensation for loss of income due to accidents or illness, and retirement accommodations.

FINANCING

In 2016, the last year with reliable data, Switzerland spent over $82 billion (CHF 80 billion) on health care, or 12.2% of GDP. This translates to about $9,700 USD (CHF 9,500) per capita. Importantly, per capita

Figure 2. Financing Health Care: Statutory Health Insurance (Switzerland)

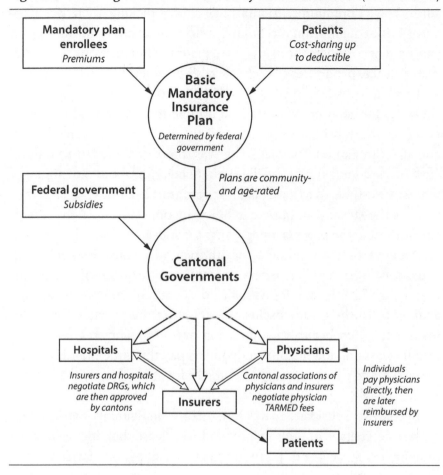

spending varies twofold from canton to canton. Switzerland has one of the highest levels of out-of-pocket health care spending in the world.

Mandatory Basic Health Insurance

Funding for mandatory health insurance in Switzerland comes from 3 sources: (1) individual insurance premiums, (2) canton subsidies for individuals, and (3) individual out-of-pocket costs.

All individuals must purchase mandatory basic health insurance. The premiums for these plans are community rated with age banding. Progressively higher premiums apply to the following 3 age cohorts: 0–19, 19–26, and 26-plus. Although all mandatory health insurers must offer the exact same benefit package, there exist large variations in premiums between cantons and between insurers within cantons. Insurers collect premiums. To minimize cherry-picking, there is a mandatory risk-equalization mechanism among all insurers within a given canton that considers the age, gender, prior hospitalizations, and pharmaceutical expenditures of each insurer's beneficiaries.

In 2012, $4.05 billion USD (CHF 4.00 billion) was paid in premium subsidies for children and low- and middle-income individuals. Fully 54.2% of the subsidies were financed by the Confederation's budget and 45.8% by cantonal budgets. This was then distributed to 2.3 million (27% of the country) subsidy-eligible beneficiaries, about 0.6 million of whom are estimated to have paid no premiums at all. Several factors—such as the subsidy amount, eligibility, income thresholds to receive subsidies, and the process for applying for subsidies—vary by canton.

All government funding of health insurance subsidies and health care services comes from general taxes. There are no specific taxes earmarked for health care. Individuals do not receive any tax benefits—analogous to the US tax exclusion—to offset the purchase of health insurance. Thus, health care financing overall remains regressive: the middle class and low-income individuals pay the same premiums, deductibles, and co-pays as high-income individuals, despite their different incomes.

Even with subsidies, many low-income individuals contribute a greater percentage of their income to health care than higher-income individuals. Since 2000, premiums have doubled, but Swiss salaries have increased by only 22%. Estimates suggest that by 2030 the average Swiss household may spend 11% of its monthly income on health insurance, compared to just 6% today. Over one-quarter of the population needs governmental assistance to pay their premiums. In 2016, nearly $860 million USD (CHF 843 million), or 1%, in premiums was not paid. In 2016, 22% of all Swiss residents went without needed care because of costs; this rate increased to 31% among low-income people. This has become an increasingly serious barrier to accessing care.

Voluntary, Private Supplemental Insurance

Individuals pay for voluntary supplementary health insurance themselves, with no subsidies or tax incentives. Voluntary health insurance represents 7.2% of total health care expenditures.

Cost Sharing

Besides premiums, individuals pay directly for services not included in the basic benefits package, such as vision and dental care. This amounts to nearly two-thirds of all private expenditures on health care. In addition, cost-sharing payments—deductibles and co-pays—contribute to 5.5% of total health expenditures.

For basic plans of mandatory health insurance, beneficiaries must pay the full cost of their health care until they reach their deductible, which varies from $306 USD (CHF 300) for the basic plan with greatest choice to $2,550 USD (CHF 2,500) for the high-deductible plan. Beyond deductibles, beneficiaries pay 10% of costs up to an annual cap of $357 USD (CHF 350) for children and $714 USD (CHF 700) for adults. They must also pay a fixed co-payment of $15 USD (CHF 15) for each day of inpatient care to cover meals, which one physician described as "a ridiculously small amount compared to what you really eat." They are also responsible for a 10% coinsurance for all other services. Total out-of-pocket payments are capped at $1,020 USD (CHF 1,000) for the basic mandatory plans or $3,264 USD (CHF 3200) for high-deductible plans.

By international standards out of pocket payments in Switzerland are high, at $2,300 USD per capita and 28% of total health care expenditures. This is significantly higher than the average per capita out-of-pocket payment of $860 USD (CHF 840) in other developed countries.

Long-Term Care

Unlike the Netherlands and Germany, Switzerland has no mandatory long-term care insurance; rather, custodial care for the elderly is viewed primarily as a familial or individual responsibility. Municipalities, with some cantonal contribution, are primarily responsible for the public financing of long-term care. Overall, either public financing or social insurance covers about 40% of long-term care, with households paying for the remaining 60%.

The mandatory health insurance plan pays for nursing-home care at $9.14 USD (CHF 9) per day, with additional payments depending on the degree of care dependency. The maximum daily mandatory health insurance payment, for the highest degree of dependency, is $110 USD (CHF 108). If this does not cover the total costs, the patient pays up to

20% of the mandatory health insurer's fixed daily contribution. The individual's canton usually pays for any remainder.

Long-term care benefits may also be paid for by the federal law on Old Age and Survivors Insurance (AVS) or the federal law on Disability Insurance (AI) for the disabled elderly. Cash benefits are calculated based on prior salary level and cover the costs of rehabilitation, medical, and nursing services.

Nevertheless, because LAMal is a universal plan, it does cover some of the costs associated with long-term care. The insurance plan pays for medical costs incurred in nursing homes as well as some home health care expenses, though it does not pay for care with activities of daily living, such as assistance bathing, dressing, or eating. Reimbursement depends on the intensity of care and the out-of-pocket contributions of the individual.

Finally, living expenses provided to the elderly and the disabled under federal law may be used to subsidize the medical costs of care. These *prestations complémentaires* are means-tested benefits that correspond to living expenses, such as nursing homes and some home care costs, that are considered unaffordable for the individual. The monthly amount per individual is fixed by cantons for local nursing homes.

Public Health

As of 2012, 2.1% of all public expenditures on health went toward public health and prevention, a proportion that has declined recently. The responsibilities to oversee public health initiatives are split between the federal government and cantons. The FOPH develops national public health policy. At the cantonal level the Conference of the Cantonal Ministers of Public Health (GDK/CDS) coordinates the public health officials representing all 26 cantons.

Some public health and screening measures are covered under the mandatory health insurance benefits package. These include Pap smears, HIV tests, colonoscopies, mammograms, genetic counseling, and certain vaccines.

In 1989, the Conference of Cantonal Ministers of Public Health and the federal government created Health Promotion Switzerland, a foundation to run and evaluate health-promotion activities. It is financed through a mandatory annual deduction of $2.45 USD (CHF 2.40) from each insured person's insurance contribution. In addition, public health services are often performed by nonprofit organizations contracted by cantons.

Mental Health

Because mental health services are provided by psychiatrists, psychotherapists, psychiatric day care units, specialized psychiatric hospitals, and psychosocial treatment centers, the data is relatively fragmented. Mandatory basic health insurance finances ambulatory psychiatric care, which is defined as psychiatric care provided by independent physicians. Ambulatory psychiatrists can provide care without a primary care physician referral, and mandatory health insurance reimburses them. However, a patient can only see a psychotherapist if a physician first refers them to a psychotherapist who practices in the same organization as the physician.

Cantons organize mental health care services and are responsible for funding about 50% of inpatient psychiatric care costs as well as most costs of long-term psychotherapy institutions.

PAYMENT

Payment for hospital inpatient care accounts for 32.9% of all health expenditures. The next largest spending area is for independent physician practices, at 22.0% of total expenditures, followed by long-term care (13.3%), retail medical drugs and devices (11.0%), hospital outpatient care (8.6%), prevention and administration (6.5%), and dental care (5.7%).

Hospitals

Hospital payment was reformed in 2012. Under mandatory basic health insurance, cantons must cover at least 55% of the cost of each inpatient case, with insurers providing a maximum of 45%. Hospital payment for mandatory health insurance is based on DRGs. The DRG rates are the result of a step-by-step process. First, the Swiss DRG—a joint institution of providers, insurers, and cantonal representatives—develops national recommendations for DRG reimbursements based on the

Figure 3. Payment to Hospitals (Switzerland)

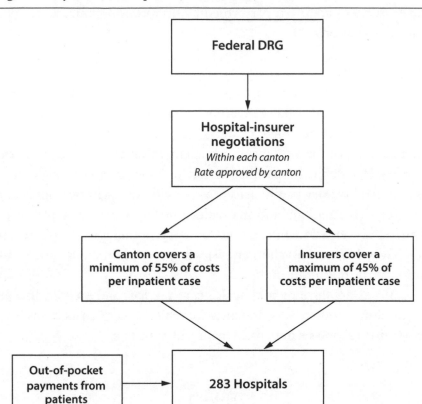

data from 42 Swiss hospitals. These recommendations are then used as a starting framework in negotiations between hospitals and insurers within cantons to determine canton-based reimbursement rates. Finally, cantonal governments approve these rates.

For private hospitals the government does not provide any funding. Instead, the mandatory health insurance pays the cantonal DRG for a patient's care, and private, supplementary insurance pays all additional fees for the room, the surgeon, the food, and so on. Consequently, the majority of private hospitals' revenue comes from supplementary health insurance.

Since 2012, patients can now choose any hospital outside their home canton so long as that hospital is included in the list of hospitals covered in the canton of treatment. Complicating the issue, reimbursement for the cost of treatment must not exceed the cost expected in the canton of residence. Thus, if a patient from a low-cost canton, such as Uri, receives treatment in a hospital in a high-cost canton, such as Geneva, the Geneva hospital gets paid a low amount.

There are no hospital budgets or limits on how many services a hospital can provide and, thus, how much revenue a hospital can generate.

Cantons are the owners of most public hospitals and determine hospitals' capital costs for new buildings and equipment. Consequently, many cantons have a dedicated portion of their budget set aside for hospital infrastructure and equipment.

In 2018, the Swiss government introduced TARPSY (for "tarif" and "psychiatrique"), a new reimbursement scheme, known as a tariff structure, for inpatient mental health care. TARPSY is based on DRG and condition complexity is an attempt to increase comparability of services.

Ambulatory Physician Payment

As of 2012, approximately 22% of total health expenditures were for ambulatory care either in office-based practices or in physician offices affiliated with hospitals.

For all but managed care plans, insurers operate within their canton and are required by law to contract with "all willing providers" in that canton. This precludes creating any kind of network of providers based on lower negotiated fees or higher quality except for managed care plans, where the beneficiaries agree to only use insurer-designated providers.

Since 2004, within mandatory health insurance plans, physicians have a nationally agreed-upon payment level—called a tariff structure—that determines the insurance payment for services provided. Analogous to RVUs in the United States, this unified tariff system, known as TARMED (Tarif Médical), specifies a number of points for each type of service. The number of points is based on the resources that the service is expected to consume. For mandatory health insurers the monetary value of each point—namely, how many Swiss francs each point is worth—is negotiated at the canton level between associations of insurers and associations of physicians. In 2010, Tarifsuisse SA was created; it represents 75% of mandatory health insurers in these

Figure 4. Payment to Ambulatory Physicians (Switzerland)

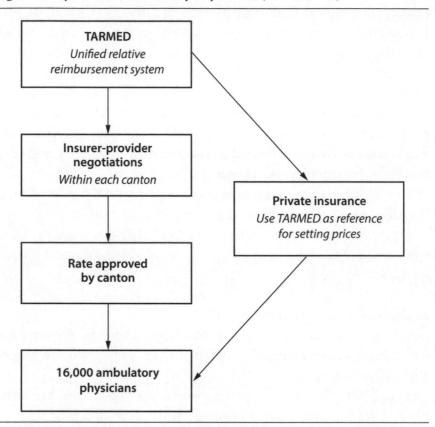

insurer-physician negotiations. For instance, under TARMED the rate for a primary care physician visit is $15.30 USD (CHF 15.00) per 5 minutes, not including any procedures or medications.

Because of rapid cost increases, the Swiss government announced in 2017 that it would change the ambulatory care payment structure. Payments for specific high-volume specialty procedures—such as cataract operations, colonoscopies, and radiotherapy—will be reduced by 10%. This is projected to save over $408 million USD (CHF 400 million).

Hospital-based providers represent about 45% of Swiss physicians. They are salaried; their hospital determines their pay. Pharmacists and other providers, such as nurses, dentists, and midwives, are paid on a fee-for-service basis by both mandatory health insurers and voluntary supplemental health insurers.

Physicians and other providers freely set their fees for private insurers. However, most usually use the TARMED structure.

Individuals usually pay both non-hospital-based primary care providers and specialist physicians directly, and their insurance company later reimburses them.

Long-Term Care

Long-term care institutions receive 13.3% of total health expenditures. A sixth of this funding comes from mandatory health insurance; another sixth comes from the Swiss Confederation. The mandatory health insurance pays nursing homes a flat per-day rate of $9.15 USD (CHF 9), though this payment can increase up to $110 USD (CHF 108) per day depending on the intensity of care needed and the degree of dependency. In 2017, some 149,000 people were residents in long-term institutions.

Long-term home care, meanwhile, is provided by Spitex, a nonprofit organization that sends nursing and caregiving staff to care for the elderly and disabled in their homes. In 2017, nearly 350,000 people used Spitex services. Spitex spends approximately $608 USD (CHF 600) per patient per month. In 2016, the public sector covered 42% of Spitex expenditures, mandatory health insurance covered 39%, and patients themselves paid for the remaining 19%.

Mental Health

It is estimated that Switzerland spends $6.5 billion USD (CHF 6.3 billion) annually on mental health care. More than half of this goes to acute psychiatric inpatient care and long-term institutional psychiatric care. Payments for outpatient behavioral health services are determined using TARMED. TARMED rates differ based on the provider's profession—physicians are paid more than mental health social workers—and the services provided. Patients have a 10% coinsurance for outpatient mental health services, which is capped at $714 USD (CHF 700) per year.

Inpatient mental health care is paid using a per-diem rather than a DRG rate. Importantly, the inpatient rates decline with length of stay, incentivizing shorter hospitalizations. The canton and mandatory health insurance share the cost of mental health hospitalizations, with the amount paid by the federal government varying by canton. The patient has a 15% co-pay for psychiatric hospitalizations, without caps for food and other services.

DELIVERY OF HEALTH CARE SERVICES

Hospital Care

Currently there are 293 hospitals in Switzerland, which vary in size from 2 to over 2,000 beds. Switzerland has 2.9 acute care beds per 1,000 population, compared to the EU average of 3.6 beds per 1,000. Since 2000, the number of acute care hospitals has fallen by 50% and the number of acute care beds by 20%. Of the 293 hospitals, 21% are publicly owned and managed, either by the cantons or by public companies, and non-profit companies run 25%. Cumulatively, public or nonprofit hospitals operate nearly 65% of all hospital beds. More than half of all Swiss hospitals are privately owned and tend to be smaller-specialty hospitals for ophthalmology or psychiatry. In Switzerland 5 hospitals are university affiliated. Unusually, public hospitals in Switzerland are expected to generate a positive margin, which, as Jacques-Andres Romand, chief medical officer for the Canton of Geneva, notes, "is totally ridiculous, because it's a public service, but we ask them to be for profit." Yet to generate revenue, even public hospitals may require patients to dip into their private insurance to get the best room or specialist, generating additional revenue.

A patient is free to access care in any hospital they wish, even if it is outside the canton in which they live or work—so long as that hospital is on a list of partner hospitals with their own canton. The hospital would then be reimbursed according to their cantonal rates.

To coordinate their health care activities, the cantons work together in the Conference of the Cantonal Ministers of Public Health (GDK/ CDS). This organization also makes decisions regarding specialized care. For instance, it works to determine which hospitals will deliver the 39 highly specialized medical services, such as stroke, neurosurgery, severe trauma, and organ transplantation. A board consisting of 10 cantonal ministers of health makes all decisions regarding these fields, and those decisions are binding for all cantons. For instance, only 6 hospitals—the university hospitals of Geneva, Lausanne, Bern, Basel, and Zurich as well as the Cantonal hospital of St. Gallen—have been designated to provide liver transplantation.

Ambulatory Care

Independent primary care physicians and specialists working in solo or group practices are the primary providers of ambulatory care. Approximately 53% of physicians work in ambulatory care settings. Cantons license independent physicians to practice in their canton. Unless patients are enrolled in a managed care plan, they are free to choose any licensed ambulatory provider in their canton—whether primary care physician or specialist. There is no real gatekeeper model, as referrals to specialists are typically not required. Physicians are paid on a fee-for-service basis. There are currently no monetary incentives for care coordination or chronic care management.

Interestingly, acute care hospitals are beginning to encroach on private practices' ambulatory care services. Specialists at acute care hospitals are now seeing more patients who previously would have gone to private practitioners.

There are no real waiting times in Switzerland. Approximately 68% of adults can see a physician the same day when they are sick, and over 80% of Swiss patients wait less than a month to see a specialist.

Mental Health

Cantons are responsible for organizing mental health care, which is covered by mandatory insurance if it is provided by physicians. Few primary care physicians provide substantive mental health care. Instead, most behavioral health services are provided by psychiatrists, the vast majority of whom work in private practice. Nonphysician behavioral health services, such as psychotherapy, may be covered if it is prescribed by a physician and provided in his or her practice. Public hospitals, public and private psychiatric hospitals, and residential facilities provide inpatient behavioral health services.

Long-Term Care

Formal long-term care is provided in old-age homes, medical nursing homes, and in patients' homes. The cantons generally subsidize the construction, maintenance, and operational costs of public nursing and old-age homes, which constitute two-thirds of all long-term care institutions. Total occupancy of these facilities is 95% to 97%, resulting in waiting lists for many nursing homes. There is currently no standard for assessing need; different institutions use different metrics for deciding which patients to accept.

Home health care is primarily provided by the Swiss Association of Home Care Services, also known as Spitex. This is an umbrella organization for 24 cantonal Spitex associations that provide domestic aid and care services, primarily for the disabled and elderly living at home. About half the costs of Spitex are covered through public funding. Outside of Spitex, informal caretakers, such as family members, perform most of the custodial care at home, and this represents a significant part of the total burden of care.

As the population ages, experts predict that needs will go unmet. As Burton-Jeangros explains, "It is impossible to imagine that we will provide enough places in nursing homes for the aging population."

Preventive Care

Some preventive services—including vaccinations, general health exams, and cancer screenings for at-risk populations—are delivered by primary care physicians and specialists. These are paid for under mandatory health insurance.

Since the 1980s the Confederation has introduced population-based prevention programs for AIDS, drug abuse, tobacco, and alcohol. Cantons, however, are responsible for implementing these prevention efforts. This decentralized and diffuse responsibility, characteristic of the Swiss health care system, has limited the effectiveness of national prevention strategies.

Quality Controls

The Confederation's Health 2020 strategy has made expanding the measurement and quality of care a top priority. In 2008, the Swiss Inpatient Quality Indicators were introduced to monitor and evaluate the quality of acute care hospitals. In 2012, the FOPH and the Foundation for Patient Safety initiated 2 national quality programs to reduce surgical and medication errors. The National Association for Quality Improvement in Hospitals and Clinics (ANQ) publishes quality indicators for inpatient, psychiatric, rehabilitative, and geriatric facilities. In 2011, ANQ members signed a national quality contract that created financial incentives for adhering to ANQ quality initiatives. Hospitals that join the contract must provide data to an ANQ database for performance evaluation. By 2013, almost all hospitals in Switzerland had joined the contract and were participating in quality initiatives.

Physicians are not routinely evaluated on their quality of care. The fact that many physicians have no electronic records for data collection further challenges evaluations. For instance, in Geneva 30% of physicians keep only handwritten records. However, an ongoing project called BAGSAN is exploring the possibility of using routine ambulatory care data to develop quality indicators for providers.

One grassroots initiative to improve the quality of care is Smarter Medicine, a program based on the Choosing Wisely campaign in the United States. Because the current fee-for-service payment system for physicians incentivizes high-volume care, nearly 25% of all care is deemed inappropriate. Choosing Wisely has begun listing interventions that should be avoided, primarily for ambulatory and hospital care. The organization also helps educate physicians, though there are no penalties or rewards to bind physicians to providing high-value care.

Patient Satisfaction

Switzerland has comparatively high rates of patient satisfaction with the health care system. Even for the majority of Swiss enrolled in managed care plans, access and choice are considered plentiful. Fully 54% of Swiss interviewees in a Commonwealth Fund survey believed the system was working well. The fact that only 3% to 5% of individuals switch insurers each year seems to confirm a high satisfaction rate. As one expert explains, "I still say most people are happy with the system because you get access to a lot of things. People complain about their premiums, but that makes sense, because all their care is expensive. No, on average, I think people are still happy."

PHARMACEUTICAL COVERAGE AND PRICE CONTROLS

Pharmaceutical Market

Switzerland is home to 2 major pharmaceutical companies: Novartis and Roche. Yet the Swiss pharmaceutical market is tiny, totaling approximately $5.7 billion USD (CHF 5.6 billion) in 2016. However, Switzerland has the world's 2nd-highest drug expenditures per capita, at $939 USD (CHF 919).

Mandatory health insurers reimburse drugs included in the mandatory health insurance basket. Drugs excluded from the basket are paid for either by private supplemental health insurance or by patients out of pocket.

Market Access and Coverage Determination

The 2002 Federal Law on Therapeutic Products (HMG/LPTh) transferred responsibility for drug and device market authorization from the cantons to the Confederation and created the Swiss Agency for Therapeutic Products (Swissmedic), a public institution affiliated with the Federal Department of Home Affairs (FDHA). Fees paid by companies applying for market authorization, payments from the federal government, and services rendered to 3rd parties finance Swissmedic. It approves market entry for new pharmaceuticals based on quality, safety, and effectiveness. Applicant drugs must have information on purported benefits and potential side effects, laboratory tests, and clinical trials. Although normal assessments can take over a year, companies can pay a fee to fast-track their assessment, which can cut the review time in half. Drugs that have been approved for the first time are granted protection from competitors for 10 years; after that, market authorization lasts for 5-year periods.

After Swissmedic approves a new drug for market entry, it must then go to the Federal Office of Public Health (FOPH), which determines its efficacy and appropriateness. These 2 qualities are assessed using material provided by the drug manufacturer as part of their original application to Swissmedic. Next the Federal Drug Commission (FDC) reviews the information collected by the FOPH and provides recommendations on the drug's effectiveness, appropriateness, and cost effectiveness.

Figure 5. Regulation of Pharmaceutical Prices (Switzerland)

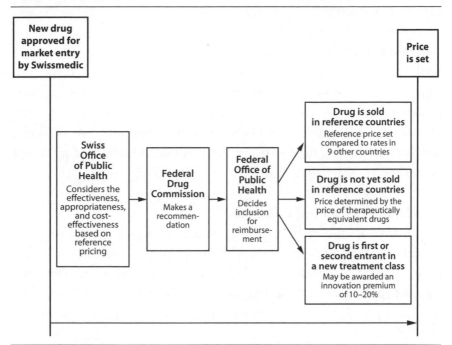

FOPH decides whether a drug should be included on the positive drug lists. Only pharmaceuticals explicitly included on the positive lists are reimbursable by mandatory health insurance. The FOPH will also determine the drug's cost based on the manufacturers' prices in 9 reference countries: Austria, Belgium, Denmark, Finland, France, Germany, the Netherlands, Sweden, and the UK. If the drug is not yet sold in any reference country, its price is determined by that of therapeutically equivalent drugs. If the drug is the first or 2nd entrant in a new treatment class or adds therapeutic value, it may be awarded an innovation premium of 10% to 20%.

The FOPH decision on a drug's qualification for mandatory health insurance reimbursement is reevaluated every 3 years. At the 3-year mark, FOPH must reaffirm that the drug still fulfills its conditions for inclusion in the mandatory health insurance benefit basket and whether the price of the drug is still cost effective. If the price is 3% higher than the expected cost-effective price and if this has led to greater than $20,400 USD (CHF 20,000) in surplus earnings for pharmaceutical companies, then FOPH can mandate the companies to pay back those earnings to insurers.

Generic Pricing

Switzerland uses significantly fewer generic drugs than other European countries. Generics represent just 23% of the total drug purchases, compared to 85% in the UK. The prices for generics are much more expensive in Switzerland than in other countries. For example, the cheapest generic drug in the Netherlands costs just 15% of what that same drug costs in Switzerland.

Physician Prescribing Controls

Physicians can prescribe any drug that has received marketing approval—there are no limits on what drugs physicians can prescribe. Drugs can be prescribed off label—that is, for indications the drug was not approved for. If the drug is not on the specialty list covered by mandatory health insurance, however, then patients need to pay out of pocket.

Importantly, Switzerland has few pharmacists compared to other developed countries, just 0.54 pharmacists per 1,000 people, compared to the EU average 0.82 per 1,000 people. To compensate, some cantons rely on self-dispensing physicians, who can both prescribe and distribute pharmaceuticals. In 2017, about 15% of all physicians were self-dispensing. Clearly these physicians have a conflict of interest because they earn profits from the very drugs they prescribe. Such self-dispensing physicians are responsible for nearly 25% of all pharmaceutical sales in Switzerland, and some people believe these physicians are contributing to the high rates of national spending on drugs. The persistence of these self-dispensing physicians, despite their role in high pharmaceutical spending, is indicative of the slow nature of health care reform in Switzerland.

Prices Paid by Patients

Typically, patients must pay for prescription drugs out of pocket at the time of purchase; their health insurer then reimburses them. For certain high-cost drugs, however, the insurer may be able to pay directly. There is also a 10% coinsurance rate for pharmaceuticals. This increases to 20% if the patient chooses a brand-name drug when a generic is already available. Pharmaceutical cost sharing is included under the annual coinsurance cap of $357 USD (CHF 350) for children and $714 USD (CHF 700) for adults. Maternal health care is exempt from deductibles, co-payments, and coinsurance, which includes coinsurance for drugs.

HUMAN RESOURCES

Physicians

In 2016, there were 35,592 total physicians practicing in Switzerland. This amounts to 4.2 physicians per 1,000 Swiss residents. By comparison, France has 3.2 physicians per 1,000 people, the UK has 2.8 per 1,000, and the United States has 2.6 per 1,000. Of all physicians, nearly 60%—about 21,000—are specialists.

In 2014, the last year with reliable data, the median wage for a GP was quite high, at $242,000 USD (CHF 237,000). Specialists earn significantly more. Swiss neurosurgeons had the highest median salary of any specialty, roughly $711,000 USD (CHF 696,555). A total of 118 Swiss physicians earned more than $1.02 million USD (CHF 1 million) in 2014.

Switzerland is expected to face a physician shortage within the next decade. In the next 10 years over 60% of practicing primary care physicians are expected to retire, leading to a shortage of 2,000 physicians. In 2016, the Federal Council announced that $102 million USD (CHF 100 million) would be allocated to increasing the number of graduating medical professionals. In the short term, Switzerland has attempted to augment its workforce by recruiting foreign physicians, and nearly 30% of physicians in Switzerland were trained in another country.

There are 6 medical schools in Switzerland. Swiss medical education is a 6-year process. The bachelor's in medicine is obtained after 3 years and must then be followed by the master's in medicine, which requires 2 years in university and 1 year of clinical training. Even though the federal government regulates medical curriculums' content, medical education varies between the French- and German-speaking parts of the country. In Zurich, for example, the application process is exceptionally competitive, but once a student is enrolled in a medical training program, they are expected to complete the program. In the French-speaking parts anybody can apply for medical training, but there is a very strict paring down of students based on academic performance at the end of the first year. According to experts, only about a third of students continue to the 2nd year. After medical school, graduates enter residency, which generally lasts between 5 and 7 years, depending on the specialty. The national association of doctors determines specialty curriculums.

Following residency, physicians must decide whether to enter public practice—university practice—or private practice. As one physician explains, "Most public physicians, they like power. They like to be valued as teachers, but the income is quite low. Conversely, in private practice, most physicians do not do any research or teaching; they like to earn money." Most physicians tend to prefer working in private urban hospitals, where the pay and volume of patients are both high. Indeed, physicians have tended to cluster in urban areas so much that cantonal governments started regulating the creation of new private practices. Although primary care practices may open as usual, specialty practices need to be approved by the government of the canton in which they wish to operate before they can open. This will be particularly relevant in big cities such as Geneva.

Nurses

In 2015, there were about 9 nurses per 1,000 people in Switzerland. This is much higher than in the United States but lower than the Netherlands, at 10.5 per 1,000 population, and Germany, at 13.8 per 1,000. Switzerland has also seen one of the fastest increases in the number of nurses since 2000.

For nurses, training has become more formalized in the past 20 years. Today a bachelor's or master's degree in nursing may be obtained from a professional school.

CHALLENGES

Many conservative commentators highly praise the Swiss health care system. Swiss citizens and residents have totally free choice of health insurer, the type of plan they can enroll in, and their physicians and hospitals. Almost all parts are private and nongovernmental. All insurers, all physicians, and the vast majority of hospitals are private. And even public hospitals are managed like private institutions that generate a margin.

However, there are distinctly non-free-market elements to Switzerland's health care system. Getting health insurance is not a free choice that individuals can refuse. Switzerland has an individual mandate to purchase private health insurance, and it is scrupulously enforced. The government can—and does—enroll people in an insurance plan and require them to pay the premium as well as penalties. In addition, the Confederation regulates mandatory insurance plans, the standard benefit package, and drug pricing through inclusion in the specialty list and set reimbursed prices. Insurance products are standardized, and costs—at least for those services and treatments included in the basic benefits package—are controlled.

Overall, the Swiss are very satisfied with the service they receive from their system. The dominant recurring complaint is about the high—and increasing—costs. There are 6 challenges in the Swiss system: quality of care, regressive cost distribution, chronic care coordination, mental health services, payment reform, and data collection.

The first challenge relates to quality. Traditionally the cantons are delegated responsibility for assuring quality of reimbursable medical services. However, the existing lack of quality metrics and the paucity of routine and rigorous measurement as well as public disclosure of quality data are serious problems. Swiss hospitals perform well on avoidable hospital admissions, which account for only 3.1% of all inpatient stays, and on 30-day mortality rates for acute myocardial infarctions (5.9%) and ischemic heart disease (7.0%). However, Swiss hospitals have higher rates of 30-day mortality for strokes compared to peer countries, with a 16.5% mortality rate. Hospital stays are also longer than the OECD average.

The availability of data on the quality of services and interventions is especially poor. One problem seems to be cultural. The Swiss have a long tradition of privacy and nontransparency, symbolized in the Swiss banking system but pervading its culture. This inhibits data collection. Another problem is the system's structure: so much is organized at the canton level, and there is no centralized data collection. Yet another barrier to the availability of data is the lack of EHRs that would make data collection from physicians more systematic and routine. Seemingly, few physicians know the value of different procedures—or the costs. Insurers hold tightly to most quality data, leaving providers to make poorly substantiated judgment calls when deciding how to treat their patients. As a physician explains,

> We do not have any data—none. It's very, very difficult to gather data and to do some good, real, evidence-based studies. What we would like to know is very difficult to find out . . . sometimes we're in the gray [areas]. We don't know if an intervention is useful, but the patient wants to do it. So I don't want to tell the physician, "Don't do that."

I ran into similar messages often in my interviews. Professor Burton-Jeangros said that "people believe the system delivers high-quality care . . . there is no data [proving this]. It's an impression, because people think access or choice equals quality."

Given that insurance coverage is mandatory, patients' feelings of deserving *any* care they desire exacerbates this issue. Having been forced to pay high premiums, many patients think that they should "get their money's worth." If a doctor does not provide them with a treatment they want, the patient can easily switch providers, so few physicians are willing to deny patients services, even if the services are unnecessary or the benefits unproven.

A 2nd challenge relates to high costs that disproportionately burden low-income individuals. Switzerland spends 12.2% of its GDP on health care, one of the highest rates of spending worldwide. Health insurance premiums are the same regardless of income. Although there are subsidies for lower-income adults, it varies by canton and does not cover the middle class. Because neither premiums nor deductibles and co-pays are adjusted for income, the burden of both premiums and out-of-pocket payments is much larger for middle- and lower-income households. Thus, as one Swiss physician noted, "My premium is the same as the guy who takes care of my car . . . don't ask me why." Furthermore, out-of-pocket spending is especially high, at 28% of health care expenditures. The bottom income quintile pays 22% of their disposable household income for health care. Many experts noted that low-income households pay essentially as much on health care as they do on rent.

Premiums also vary by insurer, depending on the type of plan chosen. Although logically it would benefit patients to shop around and switch to lower-priced plans, few do so. Omar Kherad, a physician, explains, "People are very afraid of insurers because a large portion of the Swiss population has voluntary supplemental insurance. If you want to switch, insurers can decide if they will cover your supplementary insurance or not." To keep their supplemental insurance plans, many Swiss residents choose to stick with their current plan, even if this means forgoing savings.

Because each insurer must cover the same basic benefit package, all willing providers in a canton, and all hospitals in the country, there is no real difference in access to services, specific physicians, or hospitals among the insurers. In addition, the broad range of insurance-covered services gives consumers little incentive to shop around and hospitals and providers no real motivation to control costs.

The Confederation has not implemented any budgets for care nor any legislation to ensure high-value care. Swiss economists now predict that when the basic plan premium reaches $816 USD (CHF 800) per month—which is not much more than the premium today—the whole system will collapse. Jacques-Andres Romand compared the issue to gas prices in the United States: "It's like asking how much the price of a gallon of fuel in the United States would have to rise before the United States begins to use less. . . . We don't know exactly what the premium level would have to be here for change to happen."

Although the Swiss system's original aim was to have many insurers offering the same services, thereby competing with each other on lower costs and higher quality, in reality the system has not achieved this. As Romand explains, "The system doesn't work at all. Over the last 20 years we have seen a yearly increase in costs, which means a yearly increase of your premium. . . . In Geneva, we are heading to around $600 USD (CHF 590) [per person, per month] mean premiums, which is quite expensive." Keeping in mind that a middle-class family of 4 in

Switzerland pays roughly $1,840 USD (CHF 1,800) for health insurance and $2,040 USD (CHF 2,000) for rent, and adding in food, taxes, and transportation, there is little left at the end of the month.

Another factor complicating cost inefficiency is physicians' salaries. Because they are much higher than in surrounding countries, an increasing number of physicians from Germany, Italy, Greece, and France have come to Switzerland to practice. Consequently, many private practices have opened, driving up costs.

Third, there is no chronic care coordination. Switzerland's population is older than in most other OECD countries, and the rates of chronic conditions are increasing. Care coordination remains a serious deficiency. For example, although cancer organizations have pushed for national guidelines on mammography, there remains no such legislation, and approaches vary by canton. There is some interest in managed care, primarily among the younger physicians; however, the population in 2014 voted to reject a managed care initiative, with an overwhelming 75% voting against. The general sentiment was this: "I want to choose my physician, and managed care will take that away from me." Ironically, in Geneva over 60% of residents are already enrolled in managed care systems. The messaging—not so much the actual content—of managed care seems to be scaring voters off.

Many physicians I talked to cited the lack of coordination as one of the system's biggest issues. Pilot projects that are introduced in one canton have no hope of being rolled out nationally. Kherad noted that although managed care initiatives have been successfully implemented in the German parts of the country, they have never worked in the French parts. He posits, "We are more, you know, flexible. People in the Latin part of the country don't want to be forced into anything. But in the German part, it works quite well, actually."

For now, "while there has been discussion about chronic care management, that's where it stays" as mere discussion. Until the issue becomes pressing, it seems unlikely that policymakers will initiate any new programs, payment reform to incentivize chronic care coordination, or any other changes. Until then, coordination of care will remain patients' responsibility.

A 4th challenge is mental health care. Although mandatory insurance covers mental health care, few primary care physicians provide substantive services. Instead, psychiatrists provide most behavioral health services. There are no current efforts to integrate behavioral health services with primary care, even though integrated models have been shown to improve care coordination and patient outcomes.

The lack of mental health integration with primary care has hindered patient access. The average wait time for an appointment regarding an acute psychiatric issue is 6 days. Although in 2008 the Conference of the Cantonal Ministers of Public Health made recommendations to integrate mental health services, cantons have made almost no progress in doing so.

Fifth, Switzerland must confront its use of fee-for-service payments and the perverse incentives it creates. Switzerland is well known for its impressively high physician salaries. Various calls for reform have been met with outrage by physicians—and then stymied. An initiative has been proposed to move the current multi-insurance system to a single-payer model. Interestingly, the general populace has already voted down the reform several times at the federal level; it is now being proposed at the cantonal level.

Swiss residents seem, at best, to have mixed feelings about a single-payer system. When I asked experts whether they thought the reform was a good idea, the responses varied widely. One reason may be that, as one expert explained, "The only comparison we have of the single-payer system is France. The access is just perfect, but, my god, you have to wait so long to see a physician. I don't want that. I like my system." Proposals for a single-payer system will be reintroduced at the national level again in 2020. If premiums continue to rise as projected, experts predict that the Swiss may view reform more favorably.

Finally, there is a paucity of reliable data by which to benchmark and reform the system. There are currently no nationally consistent data measuring provider performance or health inequalities. As Samia Hurst, a Geneva physician, notes, "We often lack even basic data, let alone a benchmark to measure it by."

Although certain forays into data collection and measurement at the hospital level have been made—such as the publication of hospital performance information online by the FOPH—these data do not allow for direct comparisons and are not considered completely reliable. No payments on the basis of quality for either physicians or hospitals have been implemented. Several physicians I spoke to seemed to distrust the idea of publicly reported data. One described such attempts as "very, very, very fancy, and I'm quite afraid of that. . . . We have to be very careful of which quality indicators you choose."

CONCLUSION

Future reforms will need to focus on these issues. There must be nationally established standards of care as well as evaluations of providers in delivering such care. Cantons would do well to require more stringent data reporting from their hospitals and insurers. A federal budget should be created to at least *begin* incentivizing cost-control measures. Inevitably the federal role in health care must be strengthened. As appealing as it may be to leave health care regulation to the cantons, this decentralization has led to fragmented, inefficient care. The system's standardization, price control, and performance measurement all lie with an increasing incorporation of the Confederation into health care.

CHAPTER NINE

AUSTRALIA

A 64-year-old Australian patient made headlines with his medical bill: $12,200 USD ($18,000 AUD) for robotic prostate cancer surgery from a private practice surgeon in Sydney. The bill did not even cover additional fees for an assistant surgeon, anesthesiologist, the operating room, or extra tests. Altogether, the patient was staring down a $17,000 USD ($25,000 AUD) out-of-pocket bill.

Although surprise medical bills are no shock to Americans with private insurance networks, in Australia they occur because of what one health policy expert called the "untidy," overlapping public and private health insurance systems. All Australians can use public hospitals free of charge, but they will need to endure waiting times and have no real choice of a hospital-based physician or surgeon. Consequently, about half of Australians have private insurance, which facilitates treatment in private hospitals, with free choice of physician and no queues—although there can be waits for services such as cancer chemotherapy.

Surprisingly, the government promotes this jumbled system, with penalties for the well off and subsidies for middle- and low-income people to buy private insurance. Even patients who do not have private insurance can still be treated at private hospitals by private physicians, and Medicare—Australia's public insurer—will pay 75% of the usual public charge, with the patient responsible for the rest.

While Americans have little recourse when stuck with a surprise bill, the Australian patient had a guaranteed backup: the public health care system. Rather than undergo robotic prostatectomy in a private practice setting, he got the surgery at a public hospital—for free. And although waiting times for elective surgery and emergency room visits are growing in

Australia, he got his operation just 5 weeks after his initial consultation—
well within international guidelines for treatment. "I went from being out
of pocket something like [$17,000 USD ($25,000 AUD)] to paying next
to nothing."

HISTORY

Established in 1901, Australian Commonwealth is a young federation,
with responsibilities for health split between the Commonwealth (federal) and state/territory governments. For most of the 20th century,
political power in Australia oscillated between the center-left Australian Labor Party and the center-right coalition of Liberal parties. Generally the Labor Party supported universal public health insurance and
free public hospitals. Conversely, the Liberal coalition preferred mar-
ket-oriented approaches, such as private insurance paying for privately
organized care. Because of the historical seesaw between these 2 coalitions, the Australian system is an amalgam of both frameworks.

Medical Insurance Before 1954

The precursors to modern health insurance in Australia were voluntary "Friendly Societies." These began in the 1840s as associations that
insured members for sickness and unemployment. For an annual fee,
members were entitled to reimbursement for a portion of medical costs
from a list of contracted physicians and pharmacists. Most physicians
charged additional private fees for certain services, such as childbirth.

In 1938, Prime Minister Joseph Lyons's center-right United Australia Party (UAP) government first proposed a national health insurance
scheme that would provide medical benefits and pensions financed by
payroll deductions. Because of opposition from both physicians and
trade unions, the UAP abandoned the proposal. UAP dissolved in 1944,
succeeded by the center-right Liberal Party.

In 1944, the Labor-led government proposed the Hospital Benefits
Act and the Pharmaceutical Benefits Act, which established the Pharmaceutical Benefits Scheme (PBS). But the Australian High Court ruled
the Pharmaceutical Benefits Act unconstitutional, prompting the Parliament to amend the constitution. At the time, Labor was so politically

dominant that the amendment passed easily, with a minor concession to the Liberal coalition: a clause barring conscripted medical service. With new constitutional power, Labor passed the National Health Service Act of 1948, which expanded the Commonwealth's ability to manage hospitals and health clinics. The government also enacted the Pharmaceutical Benefits Act of 1947 that created a new Pharmaceutical Benefits Scheme (PBS). This new PBS was more limited than the original legislation and allowed for Commonwealth reimbursement of pharmaceuticals prescribed by physicians. Physicians generally opposed the PBS, and early adoption was low.

In 1949, political power shifted back to the Liberal Party (the conservatives), led by Robert Menzies. The Liberal coalition immediately attenuated the PBS, limiting the benefit to "life saving and disease preventing drugs" and introducing a patient co-pay. The Liberal coalition also passed a market-based approach to national health insurance, including a Medical Benefits Scheme that was voluntary, relied on not-for-profit insurers, and provided government subsidies to help people pay premiums. In 1953, the Liberal Party passed the National Health Act, which consolidated the Pharmaceutical Benefits program, Hospital Benefits Scheme, Pensioner Medical Service Act, and Medical Benefits Scheme.

The National Health Act also created the Pharmaceutical Benefits Advisory Committee (PBAC) as an independent body that approved drugs to be placed on the PBS formulary. Unlike insurance for hospital and physician services, pharmaceutical benefits were less controversial *and* less dynamic over time. For hospital coverage, the Menzies government reintroduced means testing for public hospitals and required people above an income threshold to purchase private hospital insurance. The government provided premium subsidies for private insurance to prop up the industry. People above the financial threshold who were uninsured were responsible for all hospital costs out of pocket.

Development of Medicare and the Modern System

The ascendency of the Liberal Party (the conservatives) created a system that protected private practice and doctors' setting of rates, although public funds paid much of the bill. By 1954, Australia had its first draft of a national insurance scheme, but the structure was unstable. The private system was voluntary, and by the 1960s a third of the population still lacked private insurance. In addition, there was no fixed fee schedule, so physicians, who were paid by fee-for-service, regularly raised rates, forcing the government to endlessly increase its subsidies.

After decades in opposition, the Labor Party regained power in 1972. Prime Minister Gough Whitlam immediately set about enacting Medibank, Labor's plan for compulsory, public, universal insurance. It created universal medical insurance: physicians billed patients, and the Commonwealth reimbursed 85% of the federally established fee, or physicians billed the government Health Insurance Commission directly and received 85% of the federally scheduled fee—a practice called bulk billing. For hospital care, the Commonwealth mandated free access to public hospitals. This was financed by the states with generous subsidies by the Commonwealth. Medibank polarized physicians. The Australian Medical Association opposed it, but many physicians, aligned with the General Practitioners Society of Australia, supported it, leading to a significant decline of support for the Australian Medical Association.

In 1976, the government flipped. The (conservative) Liberal coalition returned to power under Prime Minister Malcolm Fraser, who tried to privatize Medibank incrementally. The government made health insurance voluntary, allowing some Australians to opt out of Medibank entirely and purchase private insurance. The government also reduced Medibank's physician reimbursement rates. In 1981, Medibank was formally repealed and replaced with a scheme reminiscent of the one created by the Menzies government in the early 1950s.

In 1983, the Labor Party returned to power and enacted a universal, tax-funded national health insurance scheme—Medicare. The experience with Medibank and the fact that many state governments were under Labor's control facilitated implementation. Initially, Medicare was financed by a 1% income tax. It also included incentives to get physicians to bill the government directly so patients would not see a bill. Private insurers were prohibited from insuring the gap between fees charged by non-bulk-billing physicians and the Medicare fee schedule, a strategy enacted to discourage physician fee increases. Specialists could only be paid a Medicare rebate if patients had received a GP referral, strengthening the gatekeeper role of GPs.

By the 1990s, modern Medicare had bipartisan support. Subsequent debates over reform to Medicare have centered on levels of means testing, support for private insurance, and whether to increase Medicare-earmarked taxes to support long-term care. Any talk of repealing the system in favor of an out-of-pocket or publicly supported private insurance system is dead on arrival.

The swings between Labor and Liberal governments shaped the Australian health system's structure into one in which financial and care delivery responsibilities are divided between the Commonwealth, states, private providers, and private insurers. Although the Medicare system itself may have a beauty in simplicity, it is only part of a patchwork system of private and public payers, government subsidies, and both private and public delivery systems. States devote a considerable share of their budgets to financing free public hospitals, and private insurers negotiate fees with private hospitals and private providers. No single payer or institution is actually responsible for the total cost of care for the entire population.

COVERAGE

Australia has a 2-tier system of public and private insurance, each of which pays for both publicly and privately delivered care. About half of Australians are covered by some form of supplemental private health insurance, but most middle- and lower-income Australians use the public system exclusively. Most affluent Australians pay for private insurance. The government subsidizes the purchase of private insurance and, by extension, private hospitals.

Australia has 25 million citizens and permanent residents. Australian residents are automatically enrolled in Medicare—Australia's universal, publicly funded, and government-administered program. Medicare pays for physician visits and free hospital care in public hospitals.

In addition, about half of the population has some supplemental private insurance covering: (1) services not covered by Medicare, such as speech and occupational therapy as well as most dental care; (2) greater choice of doctors when they are admitted to public hospitals; and (3)

Figure 1. Health Care Coverage (Australia)

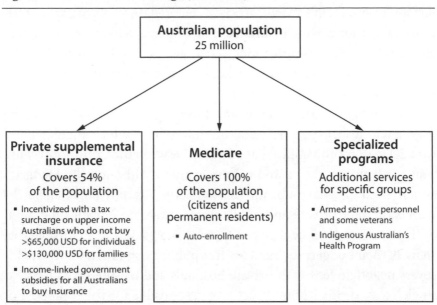

access to private hospitals. The government provides fairly generous, income-linked subsidies to incentivize the purchase of private insurance. The Department of Veterans' Affairs covers all hospital and physician services for veterans. The Department of Health also has specific programs, such as the National Aboriginal and Torres Strait Islander Health Plan, to meet indigenous populations' health needs (about 3.3% of the population), who have severe disparities in access and health outcomes due to historical marginalization and rural geography.

Medicare
Medicare covers hospital care and physician services listed on the Medicare Benefits Schedule (MBS) and pharmaceuticals through the Pharmaceutical Benefits Scheme (PBS). The MBS benefits package is extensive, covering most physician visits, diagnostic tests, surgical procedures, optometry, some dental surgery, and dental care for chronically ill persons. However, a number of routine services are not covered, including ambulance services, physical therapy, podiatry, routine dental care, and eyeglasses. Patients with chronic conditions can receive

additional subsidized health services through the Medicare Enhanced Primary Care program.

The Medical Services Advisory Committee (MSAC) advises the Commonwealth's Department of Health about which services should be subsidized. MSAC uses an evidence-based health technology assessment (HTA) approach that considers the strength of evidence regarding the service's safety, care effectiveness, and cost effectiveness. It also considers the total cost of a new medical service to the system. The minister of health appoints MSAC committee members—physicians, health economists, and researchers. Two MSAC subcommittees, the Evaluation Sub-Committee (ESC) and PICO Advisory Sub-Committee (PASC), provide additional expertise.

Once a service is added to the MBS, there are rarely any utilization limits so long as the service is ordered for appropriate uses. The MBS has grown over time. Currently there are more than 5,700 items on the MBS list, and in 2015 the Department of Health established the MBS Review Taskforce, which is charged with reviewing the MBS to identify obsolete or outdated services.

The PBS provides subsidized drugs to Australian citizens. The Pharmaceutical Benefits Advisory Committee (PBAC), composed of about 20 experts, makes recommendations to the minister of health on whether a new medicine should be included on the PBS. Overall the pharmacy benefit is generous. As a member of the PBAC summarized, "There's a very heavy subsidy of pharmaceuticals, and about 90% of prescriptions [for] pharmaceuticals in Australia are written on the PBS."

Private Supplemental Health Insurance

There are 2 types of private health insurance: coverage for private hospitals and coverage for services not provided by Medicare, called general treatment. Insurers offer combined hospital and general treatment coverage, but both types of insurance can be purchased separately. In 2018, about 54% of Australians (13.5 million people) had private insurance, nearly all of which was for hospital and general treatment. Overall, about 45% of Australians (11.2 million people) had private hospital coverage that included some extra services. Only 9% of Australians (2.3

million people) had private insurance only for extra services. Hospital-only coverage is extremely rare.

Private hospital coverage allows for greater choice of physicians as well as access to private hospitals, which usually have shorter waiting lists for elective procedures. Patients with private insurance can elect to be treated as a public patient in public hospitals, but in that situation they have limited ability to choose doctors. Patients opting to use their private health insurance in a public hospital get greater choice of hospital accommodations—such as single rooms—and which physicians will treat them.

General treatment coverage for services not reimbursed by Medicare, such as ambulances and physical therapy, cannot pay for out-of-hospital services covered by Medicare. Additionally, private insurance may not cover the gap between physician charges and Medicare reimbursement levels for services not delivered in hospitals. Since 2018, these supplemental private insurance plans are required to offer packages in 4 tiers—gold, silver, bronze, basic—each with specified services.

The Australian government offers several carrot-and-stick incentives to promote private health insurance. First, private insurance beneficiaries must wait 12 months to claim benefits for many preexisting conditions and up to 2 months to claim benefits for other services, such as psychiatric care. Second, high-income Australians who do not take out sufficient private insurance are subject to the Medicare Levy Surcharge, an additional 1% to 1.5% income tax. Third, there is a continuous coverage provision known as Lifetime Health Cover (LHC), which penalizes people through higher premiums if they purchase private insurance after age 30. For example, the premium for a person who takes out private hospital insurance for the first time at age 40 is 20% higher than someone who takes out hospital coverage at age 30. The maximum premium penalty is 70%, and it is removed after 10 years.

Long-Term Care Insurance

Long-term aged and disability care are not considered part of the health insurance system. Based on the Aged Care Act of 1997, the Commonwealth government covers long-term care for Australians over the age of 65 as a welfare entitlement—a social service. This includes coverage for both in-home and institutional long-term care. Coverage extends to home-based social supports, such as grocery shopping, intensive at-home nursing care, and residential nursing homes.

Coverage for disabled care for people under 65 is paid for through the relatively new National Disability Insurance Scheme (NDIS). NDIS is reserved for Australians with a permanent and severe disability, such as cerebral palsy and autism. NDIS is administered by the National Disability Insurance Agency (NDIA) and is jointly funded by the Commonwealth and states. The NDIS broadly supports people with disabilities to find and pay for "reasonable and necessary" services, such as occupational therapy and mobility assistance. The NDIS can either pay providers directly or give recipients (or their families) a fund to manage and pay providers.

FINANCING

Health care financing in Australia reflects the political history of the Labor and Liberal coalitions. The Labor coalition's legacy is embodied in the federally financed Medicare program and free public hospital system. The federal government, through Medicare, is the only insurer for office-based care. Conversely, public hospitals are primarily a state responsibility. In contrast, the Liberal coalition's legacy is in the continuation of private insurance for services in private hospitals and allowing physicians to freely set fees. Taken together, the result is a system that is mostly publicly financed but with essential roles for private insurance, private hospitals, and out-of-pocket payments.

According to the Australian Institute for Health and Welfare, in 2017 Australia spent $130 billion USD ($181 billion AUD) on health care for about 25 million people. This translates to about $5,200 USD ($7,400 AUD) per person, accounting for 10.3% of GDP.

Fully 68% of total spending, $87.9 billion USD ($124 billion AUD), is public. The Commonwealth—federal government—contributes 41%, or $53 billion USD ($74.6 billion AUD), of total spending. States account for 27%, or $35 billion USD ($49.6 billion AUD). On the private side only 8.8%, or $11.3 billion USD ($15.9 billion AUD), of total spending is funded through private insurance. Out-of-pocket spending

Figure 2. Financing of Medicare and Private Health Insurance (Australia)

A. MEDICARE

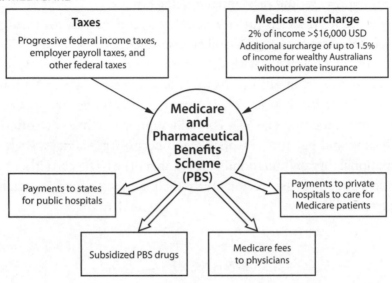

Taxes
Progressive federal income taxes, employer payroll taxes, and other federal taxes

Medicare surcharge
2% of income >$16,000 USD
Additional surcharge of up to 1.5% of income for wealthy Australians without private insurance

Medicare and Pharmaceutical Benefits Scheme (PBS)

Payments to states for public hospitals

Payments to private hospitals to care for Medicare patients

Subsidized PBS drugs

Medicare fees to physicians

B. PRIVATE HEALTH INSURANCE

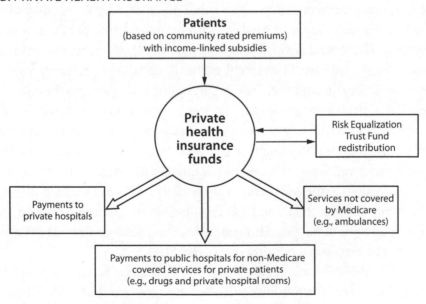

Patients
(based on community rated premiums) with income-linked subsidies

Private health insurance funds

Risk Equalization Trust Fund redistribution

Payments to private hospitals

Services not covered by Medicare (e.g., ambulances)

Payments to public hospitals for non-Medicare covered services for private patients (e.g., drugs and private hospital rooms) is relatively high: 16.5%, or $20.5 billion USD ($29.8 billion AUD). The remainder comes from other sources, such as workers' compensation.

From 2006 through 2017, GDP grew by an average of 2.6%, while health care expenditure grew by an average of 4.6%. Consequently, from 2006 to 2017 health care spending as a share of GDP rose from 8.8% to 10.3%.

These Department of Health statistics do not include the cost of long-term care for the elderly at home and in nursing homes or the cost of long-term support for disabled Australians, all of which are considered social welfare services. Long-term care for the elderly constituted an additional $15 billion USD ($22 billion AUD) in 2017. If it were counted as health care spending, long-term care would account for nearly 11% of total health care spending. Three-quarters of long-term care for the elderly is paid for by the Commonwealth and financed by taxes. The remainder is paid out of pocket. Long-term disability services cost about $15 billion USD ($22 billion AUD) in 2019, as the new National Disability Insurance Scheme continues to be rolled out and more Australians are enrolled in the program. Its financing is evenly split between the Commonwealth and the states.

Public Health Insurance

In 2017, the Commonwealth spent $53 billion USD ($74.5 billion AUD), or 41% of all spending, on curative health care in 4 primary ways:

- Funding Medicare payments by the central government to physicians (30% of Commonwealth spending)
- Funding the Pharmaceutical Benefits Scheme (14% of Commonwealth spending)
- Sending money to individual state and territory governments to help them pay for public hospital care (28% of Commonwealth spending)
- Incentivizing wealthier people to purchase private insurance through levying a Medicare surcharge on eligible, well-off Australians who do *not* buy private insurance and subsidizing private insurance premiums (8% of Commonwealth spending)

The remainder of Commonwealth spending is for the Department of Veterans' Affairs (4%) and other services, such as community and public health.

Medicare has no premiums. It is paid for by a Medicare levy—a 2% income tax—and general taxation. Individuals with incomes under $15,100 USD ($22,000 AUD) are exempt from the levy, and Australians with incomes between $15,100 and $18,900 USD ($22,000 and $27,475 AUD) only pay a portion of the tax. In 2013, the Medicare levy was increased from 1.5% to 2% to fund the National Disability Insurance Scheme, but the increase failed to fully fund the program's expansion. In 2018, plans to increase the levy to 2.5% were abandoned. The general taxation revenue comes from a combination of progressive income tax, employer payroll taxes, property taxes, and a 10% goods and services tax (GST). General taxation funds the Pharmaceutical Benefits Scheme.

Additional Medicare levy funding comes from a high-income Medicare surcharge for wealthy people who fail to purchase private insurance. The surcharge applies to individuals earning over $62,000 USD ($90,000 AUD) and households earning over $123,000 USD ($180,000 AUD). The additional tax begins at 1% of income and rises to 1.5%. In 2017, the total Medicare levy (including the surcharge) raised $11 billion USD ($16 billion AUD).

Australian state governments contributed just over 27% of total health care spending in 2017. Most state spending is for services in public hospitals (55%), primary care (19%), and community health (14.7%). Each state receives a share of tax revenue from the Commonwealth through the goods and services tax (GST).

Private Supplemental Insurance
Private health insurance accounted for about 9% of spending, about $11 billion USD ($15.9 billion AUD) in 2017, and it is financed through premiums. The private health insurance system is community rated, meaning insurers cannot charge different rates based on health status, gender, race, or use. To incentivize private insurance and reduce inequality, the Commonwealth provides premium subsidies. These subsidies range from 0% to just over 30% of premiums, depending on age, income, and type of plan selected.

To prevent the community-rated system from falling into adverse risk selection and a death spiral, the Australian Prudential Regulation Authority manages a Risk Equalization Trust Fund, which redistributes funding across all private health insurers. The overall regulation of private health insurance falls under the purview of the independent Private Health Insurance Administration Council (PHIAC).

Long-Term Care

In 2017, total spending on long-term care for the elderly was about 10% of total health care costs—$15 billion USD ($22 billion AUD). From a budgetary standpoint, though, such costs are considered welfare, not health expenditures. A little over three-quarters was paid for by the Commonwealth government and 22% by patients. Long-term care falls into 3 categories: home supports (12% of overall spending), intensive home-based care (9.3% of overall spending), and residential—nursing home—care (74.5% of overall spending). The remainder goes toward "flexible spending" for people who transition between the different types of services frequently.

The government finances a much greater share of home-based supports and health care (about 92% and 91.4%, respectively) compared to institutional care (72.5%). In 2017, the average Commonwealth expenditure per patient was about $2,030 USD ($2,893 AUD) for home supports, $11,420 USD ($16,264 AUD) for home care, and $34,900 USD ($49,724 AUD) for institutional long-term care. The remainder is covered by patients out of pocket.

The DisabilityCare Australia Fund, which is earmarked for NDIS, is expected to cost over $15.5 billion USD ($22 billion AUD) in 2019, and its solvency has been a politically contentious issue. Financing is split evenly between the states and the Commonwealth through a series of intergovernmental agreements.

Public Health/Preventive Care

Funding for public health is split between the Commonwealth and states and territories. Spending on public health accounts for about 1.5% of total health care spending. In 2017, the Commonwealth and states each contributed about 47% of total public health spending, with the remainder coming from private sources.

Out-of-Pocket Costs

For public hospital care and physician services, Australia does not have deductibles and coinsurance in the American sense. There are some co-pays for pharmaceuticals. Nevertheless, about 17% of total health care spending is paid out of pocket for 5 types of services. First, because Medicare pays only a portion of the MBS fees to physicians, patients often pay the rest. These are called "gap payments" to primary care and specialist physicians, and they account for about 13% of out-of-pocket expenses. Second, flat co-pays for pharmaceuticals on the PBS and payments for noncovered pharmaceuticals account for just over 33% of out-of-pocket costs. Third, about 11% goes toward private hospital care. Fourth, dental care accounts for 20% of out-of-pocket spending. Finally, there are out-of-pocket costs associated with privately insured care. A professor of pediatrics, Gary Freed, described a typical scenario:

> Let's say I want to see a cardiologist. I can go private and pay large sums of money out of pocket to be seen quickly, or I can go to the public hospital system, and there can be a queue.

Over time, Medicare has established multiple safety net programs to limit out-of-pocket costs. The oldest is the Greatest Permissible Gap (GPG) amount, a dollar threshold that is the difference between the Medicare Benefit Schedule fee and the 85% Medicare payment for specialist services. In 2018, the maximum gap was $57.20 USD ($83.40 AUD). Second, the Original Medicare Safety Net (OMSN) applies to all out-of-hospital Medicare services. It limits the total annual out-of-pocket costs to cover gap payments to physicians. In 2018, this limit was roughly $316 USD ($461 AUD). After that threshold is reached, the Medicare payment for all outpatient physician services is raised to 100% of the MBS fee, and the patient is not responsible for any additional gap payment.

Finally, the Extended Medicare Safety Net (EMSN) was introduced in 2004. EMSN applies to all out-of-hospital Medicare services, but it considers the total out-of-pocket costs for all services. Once the EMSN threshold is met, Medicare pays for 80% of future out-of-pocket costs for the remainder of the calendar year. The 2019 EMSN thresholds were about $1,460 USD ($2,133 AUD) for individuals and families and $470 USD ($680 AUD) for specific classes of public benefits recipients, called *concession cardholders*—for example, pensioners. There are caps on EMSN benefits for certain services, including assisted reproductive therapy, obstetrics, and some surgeries. Recent work suggests that the EMSN program disproportionately benefits higher-income Australians.

PAYMENT

Physicians and private hospitals are mainly paid through a fee-for-service model, while public hospitals are paid through activity-based funding. In the public sector, value-based and capitated payments to providers are almost nonexistent. Some private health insurers have capitated contracts with private hospitals. The federal government, through Medicare, is the only payer for outpatient physician services. States, Medicare, and private insurance all pay for hospital care.

Public Hospital Payments

According to the Australian government, in 2017 29.7% of health care costs, or about $36.7 billion USD ($53.5 billion AUD), went to public hospitals. About 40% came from the Commonwealth, 51% from states and territories, and the rest from private insurers and individuals.

Historically, Commonwealth payments to hospitals were based on fixed global budgets. The Australian government gave block grants to states, which in turn set capped budgets for hospital networks. However, the system is in the process of transitioning to an activity-based funding system using DRGs.

Public hospitals must provide free care to all Medicare patients, so payment to public hospitals occurs through governmental funding. The actual mechanism for funding hospitals is different in each state, and the process is being reformed because constrained hospital budgets generated significant waiting lists for elective procedures. As one researcher described the problem:

> Our public-sector waiting lists are caused because we have had prospectively capped funding of the public hospitals. If you get a fixed

Figure 3a. Payment to Public Hospitals (Australia)

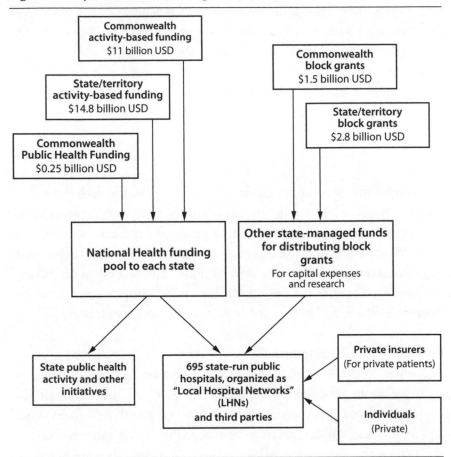

amount of money determined in advance, then you naturally end up with waiting lists.

[Conversely], Australian private hospitals have prospectively un-capped funding. . . . You do more operations, you get more money. So if they have a waiting list, they just open another [operating] theater and build some more beds.

So our biggest reform in Australia that's going on at the moment is the shift from retrospective capped funding of public hospitals to pro-spective uncapped funding. . . . I'm hopeful that over a 10-year period this will allow managers of public hospitals to build the capital stock to provide the supply of services to meet demand.

Additional block grants are given to smaller regional hospitals that do not have enough activity to earn sufficient payments. Block grants are also available to hospitals for both teaching and research activities.

The Independent Hospital Pricing Authority (IHPA) plays a crucial role in determining unit costs by determining the National Efficient Price and National Efficient Cost for public hospital services. The National Efficient Price (NEP) is based on the average cost of an acute care episode provided in a public hospital. First, each episode of patient care is assigned a National Weighted Activity Unit (NWAU). One NWAU is the average intensity of a hospital service; more intensive care is assigned a higher NWAU. In 2018–2019 the NEP for one NWAU was $3,440 USD ($5,012 AUD). For example, in 2018–2019 a tonsillectomy had a weight of 0.7158 NWAUs and NEP of about $2,460 USD ($3,588 AUD). A coronary bypass had a weight of 5.157 NWAU and NEP of roughly $17,700 USD ($25,848 AUD). In effect, NWAU is a reference price for an average inpatient cost of sufficient quality. The amount of funding a local hospital network (LHN) receives is based on expected NWAUs.

Because of low service volume in rural hospitals, the Independent Hospital Pricing Authority provides supplemental payments to these hospitals based on a National Efficient Cost pegged to the average cost of hospitals across Australia. Public hospitals must apply to state governments for additional capital expenditures. Private hospitals have no limits on capital investments and can expand their bed supply freely.

Public hospitals may also admit privately insured patients. Medicare does not cover certain services within public hospitals for privately insured patients, such as private rooms and use of operating rooms. For private patients treated in public hospitals, private insurers negotiate directly with public hospitals to pay for those services. Those charges must be paid by private insurance or by the patients out of pocket. Public hospitals thus have a financial incentive to admit private patients because they earn more money.

Private Hospital Payments

For privately insured patients treated in private hospitals, Medicare pays 75% of the MBS rate for services covered under the MBS, with pri-

Figure 3b. Payment to Private Hospitals (Australia)

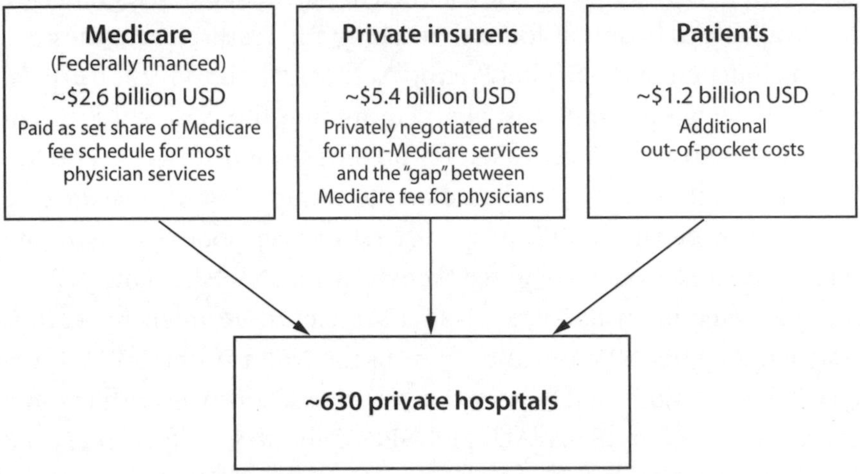

Medicare (Federally financed) ~$2.6 billion USD Paid as set share of Medicare fee schedule for most physician services	**Private insurers** ~$5.4 billion USD Privately negotiated rates for non-Medicare services and the "gap" between Medicare fee for physicians	**Patients** ~$1.2 billion USD Additional out-of-pocket costs

~630 private hospitals

vate insurance paying the remaining 25%. Medicare does not pay for rooming fees, operating room fees, or medications. Private insurers must negotiate directly with private hospitals for services that Medicare does not cover in private hospitals. In addition, private insurers negotiate regarding how much they will pay above the minimum 25% of the MBS fee schedule.

Physician Payment

In the outpatient setting Medicare is the sole payer.

Physicians can directly bill Medicare—what is called "bulk bill"—and receive a set fee from the government—100% of the MBS fee for primary care and 85% for specialist care. However, physicians are allowed to balance bill patients directly, and Medicare reimburses patients at a set rate. Thus, as one physician put it, "You can charge what you like. It is the Wild West."

For each service Medicare pays a fixed rate. For outpatient primary care it pays 100% of the MBS fee. Primary care physicians can either bulk bill Medicare directly and collect 100% of the MBS fee or set their own fee above the MBS fee, in which case patients need to cover the gap. The payment to specialists depends on their practice setting. In the outpatient setting specialists either can bulk bill Medicare directly and collect 85% of the MBS fee schedule or charge above the Medicare fee

Figure 4. Payment to Outpatient Physicians (Australia)

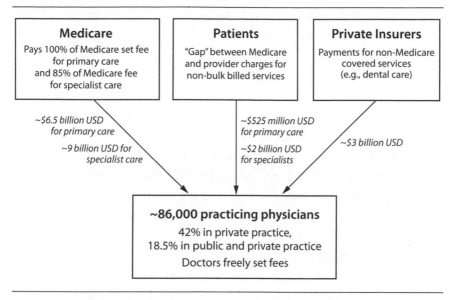

Medicare	Patients	Private Insurers
Pays 100% of Medicare set fee for primary care and 85% of Medicare fee for specialist care	"Gap" between Medicare and provider charges for non-bulk billed services	Payments for non-Medicare covered services (e.g., dental care)

~$6.5 billion USD for primary care

~9 billion USD for specialist care

~$525 million USD for primary care

~$2 billion USD for specialists

~$3 billion USD

~86,000 practicing physicians
42% in private practice,
18.5% in public and private practice
Doctors freely set fees

schedule. In this case Medicare will still only reimburse at 85% of the fee, and patients are responsible for the remainder of the cost. Like primary care physicians, specialists may set their own fees—and charge different rates to different patients. Whereas over 85% of primary care physicians bulk bill, only 31% of specialty visits are bulk billed. This varies dramatically by specialist type.

The average gap payment for specialists was roughly $21 USD ($31 AUD) in 2018. These rates also vary across and within states. As one researcher explained, "In the state of Victoria [home to Melbourne], you could pay anywhere from $100 to $500 USD for an outpatient cardiology visit. And you don't know because no one talks about what the fees are ... there's no competitive aspect to this at all."

For care in public hospitals, specialists are employed on a salary they negotiate with the hospital. However, when they care for privately insured patients in the public hospitals, they bill those patients separately. Specialists from public hospitals can also act as Visiting Medical Officers (VMOs) in private hospitals and bill private patients. Individual specialists determine how much time they spend in public hospitals caring for public patients, how much time they spend at private hospitals, and how much time they spend in their private outpatient offices.

A physician described a typical time split: "Most doctors may spend half a day a week or a day a week in public hospital settings because there's prestige associated with that . . . then they spend the rest of their time in private settings."

In private hospitals both Medicare and private insurance pay for physician services. Physicians may choose to be employed and paid a salary or practice as a VMO and receive payments on a fee-for-service basis from insurers. From a VMO's perspective, they may bill Medicare at 75% of the MBS fee schedule, with private insurance covering at least the remaining 25% of the fee. Private health insurers and hospitals directly negotiate how much the insurer pays above the minimum benefit. Physicians may own part of a private hospital as well.

Payment to Long-Term Providers

Long-term care is federally subsidized through several complex payment mechanisms for custodial care at home, home health care, and institutional care. The government regulates the number of long-term care providers and pays them based on assessed needs, which is managed through the My Aged Care portal. For minor custodial supports at home paid for through the Commonwealth Home Supports Program (CHSP), the government provides subsidies for low-level, home-based support services. Government subsidies are paid directly to CHSP providers, which may also charge means-tested fees. The average out-of-pocket payment is just under $210 USD ($300 AUD) per patient.

More intensive home-based care is paid for through the Home Care Packages Program. Each patient is assigned a home care package based on needs. Patients may then direct their package to registered home care providers. Packages range from a maximum annual subsidy of roughly $5,610 USD ($8,000 AUD) to $34,390 USD ($49,000 AUD). For nursing home care the government uses a tool called the Aged Care Funding Instrument to calculate subsidies that are paid directly to nursing homes.

There is a byzantine system of out-of-pocket spending for long-term aged care in patients' homes and in nursing facilities. The government's Aged Care Assessment Team determines each patient's specific out-of-pocket contribution. There are 3 types of means-tested, out-of-pocket costs. First, there are basic daily fees. All home care recipients must pay a basic daily fee (BDF) of up to 17.5% of the basic pension, which equals $2,500 USD ($3,700 AUD) per year. For care in residential facilities residents are charged 85% of the basic pension—$12,500 USD ($18,300 AUD) per year for the basic daily fee.

Second, elderly patients must also pay an income- and asset-tested contribution for home and institutional care. For home-based care, consumers with incomes under roughly $18,950 USD ($27,000 AUD) will only pay the basic daily fee, but means-tested care fees will rise with income. For institutional care, people with assets under about $33,300 USD ($48,500 AUD) and incomes below about $18,500 USD ($27,000 AUD) only pay the basic daily fee. However, as income or assets rise, beneficiaries must pay a means-tested care fee in addition to the basic daily fee.

Third, nursing home recipients can be asked to pay a portion of accommodation costs (i.e., rent) in a lump-sum amount or in a rental-style arrangement.

There are annual and lifetime caps on out-of-pocket payments for income-linked care and accommodation fees. In 2018, the annual cap for home care was about $3,900 USD ($5,400 AUD) for part-pensioners (middle income) and a little under $7,700 USD ($10,800 AUD) for non-pensioners (higher income). The lifetime cap for home care contributions was just under $44,000 USD ($65,000 AUD). For institutional care the annual cap for means-tested care fees was approximately $18,000 USD ($27,000 AUD) in 2018, and the lifetime cap was roughly $44,000 USD ($65,000 AUD).

DELIVERY OF HEALTH CARE SERVICES

Australian health care is oriented around primary care. Patients have free choice of primary care physicians. Although Australians are not required to select a GP, referrals are required for admission to public hospitals and to see specialists, except in emergencies. Without a primary care physician referral, Medicare will not reimburse specialists. Patients on Medicare do not always have free choice of specialists once admitted to public hospitals. Privately insured patients generally have free choice of providers within public and private hospitals.

Hospital Care

In 2017, Australia had 695 public hospitals with 62,000 beds, or 2.5 beds per 1,000 people. There were also 630 private hospitals with a total of 33,000 beds, or an additional 1.4 beds per 1,000 people. In total there are 3.9 hospital beds per 1,000 people. This places Australia between the United States, which has only 2.4 beds per 1,000 people, and Germany, which has just over 8 beds per 1,000 people.

Like most countries, average inpatient length of stay has been slowly decreasing, from 6.3 days in 2003 to 5.3 days in 2017. Length of stay on average is slightly higher at public hospitals than private ones. In 2017, average lengths of stay for public and private hospitals were 5.7 and 5.6, respectively, excluding same-day discharges.

However, unlike in most other countries, hospitalization rates are high—and rising. According to the government, in 2014 the overall admissions rate was 395 per 1,000 population. By 2017, that number increased 423 per 1,000. For comparison, in the United States hospitalization rates are declining and hover at about 100 per 1,000 population, and in Germany, the European country with the 3rd-highest hospitalization rate, it is 255 per 1,000 people.

Upon referring patients to hospitals, primary care physicians indicate how urgently an admission is required, and hospital administrators enter the details onto a waiting time register to create priority queues. For public patients hospital administrators assign a physician to the patient and arrange which outpatient clinic will provide any follow-up care. Privately insured patients can generally choose their own specialist physician, and specialists usually provide follow-up care in their private offices after discharge from the hospital.

The bifurcated public and private hospital system is the result of an uneasy merging of the 2 political visions. Private hospitals offer services paid for by both private insurers and Medicare for most inpatient care, as well as outpatient physician services. However, private hospitals rarely offer outpatient services directly. More often independent physicians in private offices provide services; the private hospital bills Medicare using the physician's provider number. Specialist physicians can work on salary at public hospitals while also receiving private fees in private hospitals and clinics.

Public hospitals mainly provide free care for middle- and lower-income Australians who rely on Medicare. However, the line of demarcation is not as strict in both directions. Privately insured patients purchase the right to use both the public and private systems, and many use public hospitals for services not generally available in private hospitals. Publicly insured patients, however, are essentially shut out of private hospitals unless they choose to pay out of pocket.

In general, public hospitals provide more emergency care, childbirth, and acute care services, while private hospitals provide elective surgery, rehabilitative care, and mental health services, although the majority of acute inpatient mental health care is still provided in public hospitals. In 2017, public hospitals provided nearly all emergency department services, accounting for 43% of public admissions. In contrast, only 5.6% of private hospital admissions were for emergencies, while 82% of private hospitalizations were for elective or planned care.

Part of the explanation for Australia's high hospitalization rate may be the financial incentive to admit private patients. In public hospitals the division between public and private beds can be illusory. As one Australian physician put it,

> The larger public hospitals have a separate private wing where private doctors will admit private patients so that the [physicians] can charge whatever they want. And then the public hospital can bill the [private] insurance company for the occupancy of those beds. So it's extra money for the public hospital . . . if it was a public patient, then it would come out of their activity-based budget.

Having separate private wings in public hospitals appears to have become less common in recent decades.

There is little data to effectively compare the quality of care of private and public hospitals. According to the Australian Institute of Health and Welfare, in 2017 approximately 5.5% of all hospitalizations had an adverse event, with public hospitals having higher rates—6.6% compared to 3.7% for private hospitals. This *may* be due to differences in the patient mix or that public hospitals admit emergency patients while private hospitals tend to admit patients receiving elective procedures.

The government also publishes data on waiting times for elective surgery in public hospitals. Waiting times tend to vary by geographic area, procedure, and socioeconomic status. In 2017, the waiting time for elective surgery for patients with Medicare was 42 days, compared to 21 days for patients with private health insurance. Median waiting times ranged from 28 days in the Northern Territory to 54 days in New South Wales (Sydney). Waiting times can be much longer for some procedures. For example, average waiting times for knee replacements are much higher in public hospitals than in private ones: 211 days versus 57 days. In theory, the transition from capped hospital budgets to activity-based funding was supposed to alleviate waiting times in public hospitals, but it is not clear whether the transition has been successful.

Outpatient Care

Outpatient care mostly occurs in primary care physicians' offices. According to the OECD, there are over 29,000 general practitioners (1.2 per 1,000 population). Primary care physicians are the backbone of the Australian health system, acting as care coordinators and gatekeepers to specialist care. Nearly all (92%) primary care physicians are in private practice, and nearly 88% are in group practices. Access to primary care physicians is good for most. In 2018, 85% of Australians reported seeing a primary care physician within the last year. However, there still appear to be some access barriers. In 2017, about a quarter of Australians reported delaying seeing a primary care physician, and 16% reported cost as the primary barrier.

Since the 1990s primary care physicians' scopes of practice have focused more on chronic care for adults. For instance, 40% of primary care physician appointments entail managing at least one chronic condition, and 12% of appointments involve managing mental health conditions. Because Australian primary care is based on the general practitioner model, internal medicine and primary care pediatrics are virtually nonexistent. Children receive primary care from general practitioners. As a result, pediatric primary care is less effective than in other countries. An academic pediatrician I spoke to noted that, compared to countries with dedicated pediatric primary care, Australian children are more likely to be referred to emergency departments for nonurgent care.

For all the focus on GPs for adults, surveys show that about half of patients in need of treatment had difficulty getting after-hours care without going to the ER. For patients with one chronic condition, the primary care physician gatekeeper model is effective. But once there is a primary care physician referral to a specialist, the specialist can refer patients to other specialists. Thus, a pulmonary physician can refer a patient to a cardiologist or rheumatologist. This specialist-to-specialist referral system leaves patients lost in a sea of specialists. One researcher outlined the coordination challenge:

> The gatekeeper role gives general practitioners a structural position to be care coordinators . . . but once you get into a specialist practice, the specialist can refer you to their other specialist colleagues. . . . So for the multimorbid patients the specialists start referring to each other, and they often leave the GP out of it . . . so the specialist referrals undercut the care coordination role of the GP.

Consequently, among patients with chronic conditions, 36% reported care-coordination problems in the past 2 years. Similarly, 41% of Australian patients with chronic conditions were dissatisfied with their care quality.

There are 2 government initiatives that address care coordination for the chronically ill. First, in 2007 a primary care physician Super Clinic program provided over $440 million USD ($650 million AUD) in capital funding to over 400 primary care physician practices for multidisciplinary, GP-led Super Clinics. Super Clinics are expected to have consulting rooms for specialists, psychologists, and diagnostic services. Second, in 2015 the government established 31 Primary Health Networks (PHNs) to improve links between local hospital networks and community-based services. Councils of local primary care physicians, nurses, and other staff lead PHNs. They conduct local needs assessments, fund or provide after-hours care and mental health services, and coordinate with primary care physician offices.

According to the OECD, Australia had a little over 44,000 medical specialists, or 1.8 per 1,000, in 2017. Nearly all specialists practice in inpatient and outpatient hospital settings. Because Medicare is the only payer for office-based outpatient care, there are no referral networks, such as PPOs or HMOs; rather, referral networks tend to be organic and locally organized.

As in many other countries, rural patients face access problems. A 2017 report from the Australian Institute of Health and Welfare found that the overall rate of employed medical practitioners was 4.1 per 1,000 in major cities, compared to 2.5 in remote and very remote areas. Although there are more primary care physicians per 1,000 people in remote areas than in major cities—1.37 per 1,000 people in rural settings, compared to 1.1 per 1,000 people in urban ones—people in remote areas were less likely to see a primary care physician in the previous year and reported longer waiting times for appointments and less access to after-hours services. Furthermore, emergency hospital admissions rates for surgery are significantly higher in very remote areas compared to major cities (22 per 1,000 versus 12 per 1,000).

Mental Health
About 20% of Australians have some mental health issue, and between 2% and 3% have a severe mental illness, such as schizophrenia. In 2011, the total disease burden attributable to mental disorders was below only cardiovascular diseases and cancer.

Australia has 3,200 psychiatrists (1.3 per 10,000 population), 24,500 clinical psychologists (8.8 per 10,000 population), and 21,500 mental health nurses (8.5 per 10,000 population). There is a significant urban-rural maldistribution of mental health professionals. Rural areas had 1.3 full-time psychiatrists per 10,000, while very remote areas had 0.33 per 10,000. As a physician noted, "The access problem is nationwide. We don't have enough psychiatrists."

The first line of mental health care is GPs. Medicare pays for mental health care provided in GPs' offices as well as consultations with psychiatrists and psychologists. Prescription medications for psychiatric conditions are covered under the Pharmaceutical Benefits Scheme. An estimated one in 8 primary care physician encounters were related to mental health issues, accounting for 30% of all Medicare-subsidized mental health services.

The 2nd line involves hospital outpatient specialist psychiatric care. Finally, there is hospitalization. The division between public and private health insurance manifests itself in different specialization across hospitals. Public hospitals admit more patients with severe mental illness, such as schizophrenia, and private hospitals admit patients with less acute mental illness, notably depression and personality or behavioral disorders. Even patients with private insurance are often cared for in both sectors because most private health insurance packages frequently limit the number of inpatient bed days.

As in other countries, there has been a push to deinstitutionalize Australia's psychiatric services, moving as much care as possible to community-based settings rather than inpatient or residential facilities. The Better Access initiative is a national health policy aimed at improving community-based mental health care and improving coordination between primary care physicians and mental health professionals. Since 2006 this initiative has added several mental health benefits to Medicare, including compensating primary care physicians for managing mental health conditions as well as broader rebates for psychiatrist consultations and for a specified number of clinical psychology sessions.

Long-Term Care

Australians who need long-term elder care must work through the My Aged Care system. A My Aged Care Assessment Team evaluates a person's needs and determines which one of 3 broad categories of benefits they qualify for. First, the CHSP provides basic social and domestic support for about 785,000 people at home. CHSP is like an à la carte system, where recipients can choose from a mix of services, such as nutrition and meal preparation, transportation, and light nursing care. Second, the Home Care Packages Program provides care packages for more intensive home-based care for about 100,000 Australians. Finally, about 240,000 Australians with the highest needs live in long-term residential facilities. A small number receive what is called "flexible care" packages, which involve cycling between home-based and institutional care. In 2017, there were 1,523 CHSP companies, 702 providers of home care, and 902 residential care facilities. There is significant overlap—that is, many companies provide both residential care and home-based care.

Public Health and Preventive Medicine

Public health programs include national screening initiatives for breast, cervical, and colon cancer as well as antismoking and obesity campaigns. Australia has been an international leader in antismoking campaigns, pioneering packaging with disease imagery and defending those practices in court. These can be run by the Commonwealth or in collaboration with states. There are also state-specific educational initiatives. In reality, primary care physicians deliver a significant amount of preventive care. Clinicians are expected to discuss lifestyle risk factors with patients. About 60% of patients report having had discussions about healthier behaviors with their doctor.

PHARMACEUTICAL COVERAGE AND PRICE CONTROLS

Despite using a lot of drugs per capita, overall spending on drugs in Australia is much lower than in the United States, largely because the government negotiates value-based prices for all drugs covered through Medicare's Pharmaceutical Benefits Scheme (PBS). Australians have good access to all Medicare-subsidized drugs, with small co-payments and low limits on total out-of-pocket spending.

Pharmaceutical Market

Australia's market for drugs is tiny. According to the government, in 2017 Australia spent just about $15 billion USD ($22.5 billion AUD) on drugs, or roughly $620 USD ($900 AUD) per capita. This is 66% of Switzerland's level and 40% of the United States'. Pharmaceuticals account for about 12.4% of total national health expenditures. Unlike the United States, drug expenditures are driven by volume, not higher prices. For instance, according to the OECD, rates of antibiotic consumption are about 18.5 per 1,000 people per day, higher than German (14.1) and Dutch (9.7) rates.

Coverage Determination

The Therapeutic Goods Administration (TGA) is the Australian equivalent of the US Food and Drug Administration. TGA must approve all drugs before they can be sold. First, drug manufacturers must submit

Figure 5. Regulation of Pharmaceutical Prices (Australia)

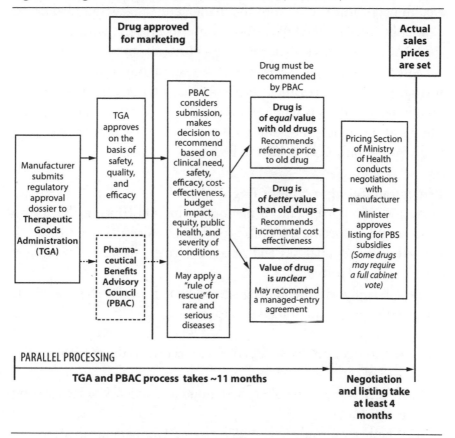

a dossier on medicines' quality, safety, and efficacy. Then, if the TGA approves a drug for sale, the new medication is listed on the Australian Register of Therapeutic Goods (ARTG) and may be sold freely.

Importantly, TGA approval does not immediately confer coverage by the PBS. Whether PBS reimburses a drug—that is, provides the drug to patients at a government-subsidized price—is up to the minister of health, who takes formal advice from the Pharmaceutical Benefits Advisory Committee (PBAC). Unless the minister of health approves the drug, consumers pay the full price. Historically, drug companies could only submit a funding approval dossier to the PBAC after receiving approval from the TGA. But recent reforms allow drug makers to parallel process, submitting requests for funding approval immediately upon submitting a dossier to the TGA. If the PBAC recommends that a new drug be listed on the PBS, the Commonwealth Department of Health negotiates a price with the manufacturer. New branded drugs cannot be listed on the PBS without a positive recommendation from the PBAC, but generics do not require a PBAC recommendation.

After submitting a dossier, the TGA takes about 11 months for approval. The PBAC assessment process usually takes 4 months, and an additional 4 months is required for the PBS to negotiate a drug price. Thus, under parallel processing it takes about 15 months for a new drug to go from submission to TGA to listing on the PBS.

Prices and Reimbursement Regulation

Price and reimbursement regulation occur both during the listing process and at specific intervals after listing. Australia relies on both cost-effectiveness analyses and reference pricing to set limits on new pharmaceutical prices.

In evaluating whether a drug should be part of the PBS, the PBAC considers 5 specific quantitative factors:

1. The comparative cost-effectiveness relative to the current standard of care
2. If the new medicine offers better outcomes compared to existing treatments
3. Whether a subsidy from PBS is required for patients to afford the new drug
4. The expected volume of use and impact on the PBS budget
5. Possible reductions or increases of health spending in other sectors, such as hospitalizations

As part of the application for subsidy for new medicines, companies must provide a cost-effectiveness analysis, and PBAC typically distributes those analyses to independent university-based committees for review. There are 2 PBAC advisory subcommittees: the Economics Subcommittee (ESC) reviews the pharmacoeconomic analyses of manufacturers, and the Drug Utilization Subcommittee (DUSC) analyzes the expected use of new drugs and measures actual use after drugs are approved.

New drugs' cost effectiveness and economic evaluation are done differently depending on the drug. For drugs that are clinically equivalent, or "noninferior" to existing therapies—that is, no worse than existing drugs but not an improvement—the PBAC uses a cost-minimization approach. In this case, the new medicine is reference priced based on existing therapies. Consequently, the new competitor is incentivized to lower its price to take market share from drugs currently on the market.

Conversely, if a new drug claims to be therapeutically superior to existing medications, the PBAC requires companies to submit a more comprehensive cost-effectiveness analysis. There is no formal maximum cost per QALY threshold, though the PBAC tries to get drug prices under $34,000 USD ($50,000 AUD) per QALY—which is approximately the threshold in both the UK and Norway. For drugs expected to cost the health system up to about $14 million USD ($20 million AUD) per year, the minister of health can accept the recommendation for listings on the PBS with an expectation that they will be funded from within the existing health budget. Drugs expected to cost more than $14 million USD ($20 million AUD) per year require a full cabinet vote for listing on the PBS, as it may require additional budget allocation.

In addition to these quantitative measures, the PBAC considers social factors, including the severity of the medical condition being treated, equity concerns, and public health effects of reimbursing a new drug. For example, the PBAC applies a "rule of rescue" when a drug is for an uncommon and deadly condition for which there are no alternatives. The rule of rescue can generate a positive recommendation for a drug even when the cost-effectiveness data are significantly above the informal threshold. The PBAC can recommend covering a new drug at the manufacturer's price or at a reduced price.

After the Department of Health receives the PBAC recommendation, the Pricing Section of the Department of Health negotiates with the manufacturer. Drugs with a noninferiority claim are internally reference priced. The Pricing Section sets the price charged in Australia at the level charged for the least expensive drug within the comparison group.

The process for drugs with multiple indications is more complicated. The Pricing Section will use weighted pricing, where the final price of a drug is a weighted average of the cost-effective price for each disease, weighted by burden. The Pricing Section can also enter risk-sharing agreements with the manufacturer, typically at the PBAC's recommendation. These so-called managed entry agreements can set mandatory price reductions after a certain spending threshold is hit, or they can offer provisional coverage on the PBS while more data on clinical effectiveness are gathered.

Although managed entry agreements may seem attractive because they offer accelerated access to drugs based on a provisional approval, according to one member of the PBAC, drug makers often see them as a way to introduce a drug without lowering the price: "We might agree on a certain number of patients, and that will be treated at 100% of the price, and then a reduced price for patients above that threshold . . . so that's a very common mechanism for giving a discount without reducing the price. And it can be a frustrating process because it leads to so much obscurity around the pricing arrangement."

After a price is negotiated, new drugs can be placed on one of 3 different formularies. Formulary 1 (F1) consists of single-brand medicines on patent. Drugs on F1 have a mandatory price cut of 5% after 5 years. Additionally, drugs on F1 may have additional price reductions levied by the government if a new, comparable drug is placed on F1 at a lower price.

Formulary 2 (F2) consists of drugs with multiple brand-name equivalents, generics, and biosimilar drugs. If a 2nd branded version of a drug on F1 enters the market, both drugs are automatically moved to F2, which carries an automatic 16% price drop. Once a drug is placed on F2, the manufacturer must disclose the ex-factory prices to the Department of Health. If the ex-factory price is more than 10% below the PBS price, then the PBS price will be reduced to meet the ex-factory price. Furthermore, F2 drugs' prices are based on sets of similar medicines. For example, if the price for one statin drug decreases, prices for all other statins must also fall.

The Combination Drug List (CDL) consists of drug combination products, which can include drugs on both F1 and F2. Prices of drugs on the CDL formulary are linked to the price of the component drugs on F1 and F2.

Prescribing Controls

Once a drug is listed, the government monitors usage. The prices for all drugs are reviewed 24 months after PBS approval. At that point PBAC may recommend a revised listing or postmarket review to change the price or its prescribing limitations.

The PBAC may mandate additional controls on physician prescribing. Unrestricted Benefit has no requirements for documentation from a prescribing physician. However, when drugs are classed as having Restricted Benefit, physicians must provide a reasonable explanation for prescribing to the PBS. Finally, Authority Required obliges physicians to provide a significant amount of documentation to explain why the prescription is required.

In practice, physicians have significant latitude. A member of the PBAC noted that the process for restricting prescribing still needs some reform: "There's very little compliance monitoring. Virtually none. We provide doctors with feedback on the patterns of use, but we don't actually monitor compliance."

Prices Paid by Patients

For drugs not covered by the PBS, patients are responsible for the full cost at whatever price the manufacturer sets. For PBS-subsidized drugs patients are subject to mandatory co-payments, but there are several caps on total out-of-pocket expenses. Mandatory co-payments are income linked. In 2019, the normal drug co-payment charge was about $28 USD ($40 AUD) for most PBS medicines but dropped to $4.50 USD ($6.50 AUD) for concession-card holders—that is, pensioners. If the cost of a drug is under the co-payment, then the patient pays the full cost.

The income-linked maximum out-of-pocket limit for drug co-pays insulates patients from budget-busting drug spending. In 2019, the maximum out-of-pocket payment was about $270 USD ($390 AUD) for concession-card holders and $1,060 USD ($1,550 AUD) for all other patients. Payments at both community pharmacies and public hospitals count toward the limit.

HUMAN RESOURCES

Physicians

According to the OECD, in 2017 Australia had a total of 90,000 practicing physicians, or 3.7 per 1,000 population, with specialists exceeding generalists—about 44,000 versus 40,000, with another 6,000 physicians "not further defined," such as residents and internists. Women made up just under 41% of the workforce. The government provides data on the geographic distribution of physicians. In 2016, there were 4.2 physicians per 1,000 people in major cities, compared to 1.8 per 1,000 in very remote areas. As a researcher succinctly put it,

> Australia is a geographically large country, and Medicare does not impose limits on how many doctors can practice in a geographic area. There are many rural and remote areas with almost no access to specialists. Specialist and medical workforce distribution is a serious problem, with clustering around Sydney Harbor, where doctors want to live.

The average physician works just over 42 hours per week. About 37.3% practice exclusively in the public sector, 42.2% exclusively in the private sector, and 18.5% in both the public and private sectors.

Similar to most countries, GPs are paid less than specialists. Compared to international counterparts, Australian GPs are relatively low paid. GPs make an average of about $103,000 USD ($150,000 AUD) per year, or 1.9 times the average Australian wage. However, many GPs receive a tax benefit targeted to small businesses, such as deducting a greater number of practice-related costs, such as office supplies and travel expenses, which offsets some of their lower income.

In contrast, specialists make an average of about $206,000 USD ($300,000 AUD) per year. Of course, specialties based in private practice have high incomes. The Australian Tax Office notes that the average salaries of surgeons, anesthesiologists, and internal medicine specialists ranged from $202,000 to $266,000 USD ($299,000 to $395,000 AUD), making them the highest-paid professionals in Australia.

Physician training is a blend of the UK and American medical education models. Medical school can begin either immediately after graduating high school or after getting an undergraduate degree. For students beginning medical school as undergraduates, the degree program typically lasts between 5 and 6 years. Graduate programs for students who already have an undergraduate degree last 4 years. Most medical schools offer an MD or bachelor's of medicine and bachelor's of surgery (MBBS) degrees.

The Commonwealth subsidizes and controls medical education. Nearly all medical students are in Commonwealth-supported universities, in which the Commonwealth funds each university for a set number of student places. Students pay approximately $7,200 USD ($10,500 AUD) per year. To remedy urban-rural physician maldistribution, about 30% of Commonwealth-supported places are bonded through the Bonded Medical Place Scheme, which requires students to sign a contract with the government to work in a workforce-shortage area for at least one year after completing their medical degree.

After a one-year internship, most junior doctors spend an additional year or 2 working in a public hospital before beginning training to become a GP or specialist. For students seeking to become primary care physicians, training occurs in GPs' private practices for a minimum of 2 years. Aspiring specialists work for 4 to 7 years in a public hospital to gain specialty training. This period is known as *registrarship*.

Nurses

There are about 305,000 active nurses and midwives registered in Australia, and just over 275,000 are employed as clinicians. The overall supply of employed nurses is 11.4 per 1,000 people, a slight increase over the last decade. About 3,500 are solely midwives, while about 30,000 are both RNs and midwives. Moreover, 90% of nurses in Australia are female. Especially in rural areas, there are persistent nursing shortages, which are expected to grow over time.

Nurse practitioners (NPs) may function without physician supervision in clinical roles. Becoming an NP requires 2 additional years of master's-level education after being an RN. NPs can prescribe medications, refer patients to other practitioners, and receive payments through the MBS, but specific scopes of practice are context dependent.

Dental Care

According to the government, there are just over 16,000 dentists, or about 0.57 per 1,000 people. Except for Australians with qualifying conditions, Medicare does not pay for most dental services. The government subsidizes routine dental care up to $700 USD ($1,000 AUD) over 2 years for children under age 18 in families with under $56,200 USD ($80,000 AUD) in income. Consequently, more than three-quarters of dental care is privately financed, and over half is paid for out of pocket. This results in significant disparities in access. Just under half of Australians report going to the dentist in the past year, and 32% of people aged 5 and over delayed dental care due to cost. Among people who went to the dentist, one in 5 did not get follow-up treatment, also due to cost.

CHALLENGES

There are many positive features of the Australian health care system. First, there is universal coverage for most services. This includes universal access to free or heavily subsidized hospital care, primary care, and specialist physician services. No patient is turned away from public hospitals for want of insurance, although there may be long waiting lists for some elective procedures. Second, patients have free choice of primary care physician. Third, prescription drugs are affordable at the point of service, and the Pharmaceutical Benefits Scheme effectively limits drug prices. Out-of-pocket costs are capped and income-linked. Finally, the financing structure is quite progressive. With no premiums, Medicare, the PBS, and long-term care are almost universally financed through national progressive income taxes, and a very small fraction of patients forgo care because of cost.

Nevertheless, Australia confronts at least 5 serious challenges over the next decade.

First, there is poor coordination across the continuum of care arising from how care is financed. Funding is divided, with states paying the bulk of hospital care, the Commonwealth government paying for physician services, and private payers covering physicians and select elective procedures. This creates significant barriers to care coordination and drives cost growth. No single payer is responsible for the entire continuum of care. There is always an incentive to push patients from one setting to another—from hospitals to outpatient or outpatient to hospitals—rather than improve the continuum of care.

While giving each Australian state latitude to experiment with different ways to pay for hospital care may produce some innovation, on balance this division creates an adversarial budget battle between states and the Commonwealth government. As Professor Freed noted, efforts to keep federal spending low almost invariably affect states adversely: "The federal government was constraining how much doctors would be reimbursed, so they were charging more and more over the federal reimbursement, which meant more people would go to the state hospitals. The federal government didn't care because it wasn't their problem."

There is a minority opinion that the division of financing and provision of care across states and the federal government allows for innovation. As one physician described the system,

> I don't see those problems of federal coordination as a major structural problem. I think they're just part of the landscape we work with. . . . I think it is a tension, and I think it's got productive and counterproductive aspects. . . . The productive aspect I think is that you get this driving of innovation. . . . There are some distortions, but I think they're offset by the benefit.

This view is analogous to arguments in the United States with regard to innovation because of diverse payers. Although having different states try new delivery models may yield some successful initiatives, that *nobody* is solely accountable for the total cost of care across the continuum of health care appears to be more of an impediment to developing more seamless coordination of care in different settings and cost-saving reforms.

The problem of care coordination is especially pronounced in long term care. Residential long-term care facilities and home-based care are federally financed. A high percentage of Australians are transferred to hospitals—paid for predominantly by the states—to die. A practicing physician put this phenomenon succinctly: "The skill set of the home care workforce around dying is not strong enough. So they tend to get fed up and call an ambulance and transfer their charge over to an acute hospital." The problem is also entrenched in the funding model for institutional long-term care, which has resulted in facilities with few fully qualified nurses. Because nursing staffing levels are low, extra care for dying patients is often beyond the facilities' capacity. Compared to the United States, far more Australians die in hospitals, receiving more care than required, rather than at home or in residential facilities.

The 2nd challenge is linked to the care coordination: Australia lacks robust health systems research to drive quality improvement or cost cutting. The quality of care in private hospitals is essentially a black box. Private payers have no economic incentive to conduct health systems research so as to document quality or identify sources of savings because they may not reap the benefits. While other countries are cutting costs by moving more services to outpatient settings, the cross-cutting payer incentives stymie such reforms in Australia. Private insurance cannot cover service in outpatient settings, so many procedures are stuck in hospitals. As a professor explained, "[A patient's] private insurance will cover inpatient care, but it's not going to cover outpatient care. So the whole notion of moving something to an outpatient setting for a [lower-cost] procedure doesn't work in [the] system." Another professor noted that there is a strong incentive for specialists to provide care in inpatient settings, leading to a growth in day procedure centers that in other countries would be considered outpatient—but in Australia are inpatient facilities. As a result, Australia is bucking an international trend with regards to hospitalizations: whereas most countries are seeing declines in hospitalization rates, Australia's use of hospitals has been increasing.

Third, waiting lists, especially for nonurgent procedures, are quite long. Physicians—especially surgeons—have no incentive to reduce them. Physicians in public hospitals have little control over their revenues. In contrast, if a physician or surgeon can see a patient in a private hospital setting, they can receive higher payments. As a result, there is little reason for physicians practicing in both public and private settings to cooperate with initiatives to reduce public waiting times. Furthermore, physicians are not paid to find ways to do more procedures in less time and clear backlogs. Indeed, a surgeon may profit by the backlog, suggesting to patients that with private insurance they would be operated on more quickly and, consequently, have private insurance compensate the surgeon more.

Fourth, there are biases in favor of wealthy Australians. Although the Medicare system is universal and progressively financed, wealthier Australians have built-in financial advantages. At upper-income levels there are 2 aspects of regressive financing. First, the Medicare surcharge flattens out as incomes rise, and the reliance on the Goods and Services Tax is a regressive consumption tax. In addition, the Commonwealth subsidizes premiums for private insurance, which is by design predominantly used by wealthier households. Although some subsidies, such as for drug costs, are income linked, the government's caps on out-of-pocket costs subsidize high-cost outpatient physician services for wealthier Australians. On the delivery side, richer Australians have systemic advantages in access to services—particularly in the choice of physicians. Public hospitals have a significant incentive to treat private patients, and the free setting of physician fees allows wealthier patients to jump the queue by paying more out of pocket. In practice, queue jumping is not totally routine, as private hospitals do have their own limits on bed availability.

Finally, the urban-rural maldistribution of resources is especially acute. Despite being one of the largest countries in the world by land-mass, almost three-quarters of the population lives in 3 states—New South Wales, Victoria, and Queensland—and those states are on the eastern seaboard, with large, urban centers. The distributional problem is especially acute for historically marginalized indigenous populations. Severe measures, including basically conscripting medical students to practice in rural environments, have not fixed the issue.

CHAPTER TEN

TAIWAN

"We go to the hospital like it's the shopping mall," said Phoebe Chi, CEO of the Taiwan Association of Cancer Patients. Indeed, the Taiwanese treat medicine much like a low-cost consumer good. Patients can go to any doctor and any hospital in the country. They can even order blood tests and an MRI scan themselves and have the system pay for them.

The inevitable corollary is that the system frequently provides impersonal and austere care. Underpaid physicians see up to 90 patients a day, all for a few minutes. Hospitals are decorated and furnished more like graduate housing, and families are expected to provide custodial care for their relatives who are hospitalized.

But care is usually timely. And the system has an exemplary electronic health card that makes payment seamless and gives government officials real-time health data. Overall, national health care costs are about half of those in other systems—and a third of the US expenditures—making Taiwan a country with an enviable health system.

HISTORY

Universal health care is a relative novelty in Taiwan.

For most of the 20th century only a fraction of the population had *any* health insurance. They got it through a handful of smaller social insurance funds tied to specific sectors of the economy, such as civil service and farming. As recently as the early 1990s, nearly half the Taiwanese population still had no health insurance. When they needed medical care, they had to rely on charity care, drain their savings, or go without needed treatment—which sometimes meant they would "just accept it [and] go home to die," as Lee Po-Chang, a kidney transplant surgeon who later became director-general for the national health insurance system, put it.

In the early 1990s Taiwan was in the midst of a dramatic upheaval galvanized by democratic ambitions and economic growth. Since declaring the Republic's independence in 1949, the nationalists had ruled through a kind of martial law, suppressing political dissent. But by the 1980s there were growing demands for more democratic freedoms. Simultaneously, there was tremendous economic growth. The economy was expanding at 10% annually, and the middle class increased substantially. These 2 trends fueled public expectations for more public political engagement and expanded government services. At the top of the list of demands was better, more affordable health care.

Nationalist leaders in the government were determined to act, in no small part because they risked losing support to an opposition party whose platform included universal health coverage. Officials studied other countries' health care systems and, based on that research, constructed one that would work best for Taiwan. As officials later told American journalist T. R. Reid, in designing their health care system, the Taiwanese consciously followed an old Chinese proverb: "To find your way in the fog, follow the tracks of the oxcart ahead."

Among the experts they tapped for advice was Bill Hsiao, a Harvard health economist who led the first planning effort. They also spoke with Uwe Reinhardt and Tsung-Mei Cheng—both Princeton economists— who argued that Taiwan was a natural candidate for a single-payer scheme: the population was not too big, and the transformation would not require dismantling a lot of existing insurance infrastructure. Above all, a single-payer system would embody the Taiwanese government's 2 most important values: equality and efficiency. The idea came to be known in Taiwan as a *single-pipe system*, a phrase Reinhardt had used. The planning committees embraced it, recommending that Taiwan collapse the country's existing social insurance plans into a single, tax-financed government health insurance program.

Taiwan's lawmakers took up the idea, igniting a political debate in which the stakeholders raised familiar, predictable objections.

Physicians worried about the effects on their incomes. The sickness funds lobbied to keep operating. Employers were unhappy about the payroll taxes to finance the plan. But the bipartisan consensus for reform—and the obvious need for it, given the large number of un-insured—meant advocates for the scheme had sufficient political support to overcome the opposition. On July 19, 1994, the new National Health Insurance (NHI) system was enacted. Less than one year later, on March 1, 1995, it commenced operation.

Taiwan could pull off the quick transition in part because NHI adopted many of the old social insurance fund operations. Reimbursement worked in the same way, except that now it was a central government agency, not the separate sickness funds, processing payments. To ensure that everyone who already had insurance felt their new coverage was equal to or better than what they previously had, the government made sure that the benefits package of the most generous fund, which had covered civil servants, was the baseline, and then they added to it. This assuaged worries that a single-payer system would be worse than what existed before.

But NHI did not include any meaningful efforts at cost control.

Within a few years expenditures exceeded revenue, prompting the government to introduce a series of modifications that quickly brought the NHI's budget back into balance and eventually led to surpluses. These reforms included legislation that brought new revenue into the NHI by increasing the existing payroll taxes and creating new taxes on income and tobacco. The government also established a global budget, introduced DRG payment for some hospital services, applied more rigorous cost-effectiveness analyses to drug prices, and experimented with pay-for-performance reimbursement schemes.

In 2006, Taiwan created its first comprehensive long-term care program. It operated wholly outside the NHI and in a wholly different way, providing income-linked assistance and with financing from general tax revenues. The program was a partial solution at best because it excluded many people and offered low benefits. In 2016, following several years of debate, the government proposed to transform the long-term care program into a social system that would operate in parallel with the NHI.

But right before the transition was supposed to take place, political control of the government changed with an election. The new regime abandoned the reform plan, which it had opposed, and chose instead to modify the existing long-term care program. The updated program offered more assistance to more people, but it still left a large swath of the population relying on their personal resources and charity for long-term care needs.

Even so, few people dispute that the NHI has largely achieved its primary goals of equity and efficiency. Taiwan has universal coverage, and its per capita spending is low by international standards. But Taiwan's system and its performance have not received significant international attention, largely because of its unusual political status. As Hsiao observed, statistics on Taiwan's health performance are not part of the usual comparative databases, such as the one maintained by the OECD, because of Taiwan's disputed status as a nation and its conflict with China. This limits study of the system.

COVERAGE

Taiwan has a population of just under 24 million. More than 99% of its residents have insurance through the government's comprehensive NHI system. Private coverage exists, but by law it cannot cover services the NHI provides. Private supplemental insurance pays cash directly to beneficiaries, who can then use the money to get amenities like private beds, fill in the NHI's small coverage gaps, or for some other purpose.

Public Insurance

NHI is administered by the National Health Insurance Administration (NHIA), which is part of Taiwan's Ministry for Health and Welfare. Enrollment is automatic. It happens at birth or, for those who arrive in the country and do not sign up on their own, at the first encounter with a health care provider. It covers all citizens as well as all foreigners who reside in the country for more than 6 months.

The NHI benefits package is comprehensive. It includes inpatient and outpatient care, prescription drugs, and mental health care, but unusually it also covers dental and vision care for both children and

Figure 1. Health Care Coverage (Taiwan)

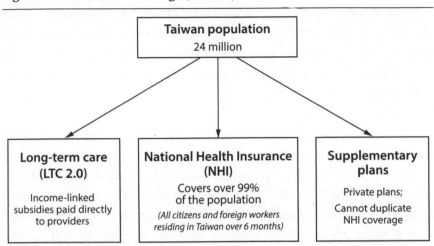

adults. Also unusually, NHI pays for Traditional Chinese Medicine (TCM) as long as the government licenses the providers and Taiwan's food and drug administration approves the medications.

There are some services the NHI does not cover, though. These uncovered services are a bit unusual by developed country standards; they include birth control, abortion, smoking cessation therapy, and drug addiction therapy. It also does not pay for certain devices or equipment such as hearing aids, artificial eyes, or wheelchairs. The NHI website offers an explanation for these exclusions: they are "not required to actually treat the patient."

The architects of NHI believed that cost sharing was important to provide some disincentives for seeking unnecessary care. As the NHI official website explains, "The main reason for requiring a co-payment is to remind the insured that medical resources are used to help people who are ill or injured and should not be wasted under any circumstance." For that reason, NHI links inpatient and outpatient care to cost sharing. But even these cost-sharing amounts are low—at a maximum of about $18 USD (550 NTD) for emergency care.

Private Coverage
Although insurance companies cannot sell insurance that duplicates, even in part, the coverage NHI provides, they can—and do—sell sup-

plemental health insurance policies. These are old-style indemnity policies in which patients just get cash when they file claims. Some of these indemnity policies are diagnosis specific—they pay only if the policyholder gets cancer, for example. Others pay whenever the policyholder incurs a major medical expense authorized by a licensed provider.

Patients can use the money to replace lost wages, cover out-of-pocket health expenses, help pay for new drugs or treatments that NHI has not provided, or pay for amenities like private hospital rooms. Patients can also use the cash benefits to pay for services from the few physicians who do not accept NHI reimbursement. They can also use the money to pay for special VIP clinics, which offer extra attention from top doctors, that some hospitals operate.

There are no official data on these plans, so it is difficult to say definitively how many people have them or how patients use the money. Anecdotal evidence suggests they are most popular with middle-class professionals and small business owners as well as the better-paid foreign workers. Individuals frequently take out multiple policies at a time because many pay out only small sums. Calculations by one industry source in Taiwan suggest that in 2019 the number of active private health policies was actually 3 times larger than the population. But that figure is a bit misleading—only a fraction of the population has the policies. Nobody really knows how big that fraction is.

Long-Term Care

Taiwan's Ministry of Health and Welfare plays an important role in long-term care—sometimes as the provider of services, more commonly as its financier. But the Ministry performs these functions through a set of programs that are largely separate from the NHI and that function in a very different manner.

In 2017, the Taiwanese government launched its long-term care plan, Long Term Care 2.0 (LTC 2.0). Its explicit goal is to help seniors age in place. It subsidizes the long-term care needs of people with disabilities or dementia as well as the frail elderly. To assess who is eligible for benefits, the Ministry uses a series of internationally recognized tests, such as the Study of Osteoporotic Fractures index for frailty and the Clinical Dementia Rating Scale.

LTC 2.0 subsidies go directly to the providers of long-term care, not the patients. LTC 2.0 also underwrites the construction and operation of a nationwide network of care centers. These centers employ counselors who can help families with needs assessments and care arrangements. In addition, the centers provide activities and services for people who live at home with long-term care needs. For example, they offer memory classes for seniors with age-related cognitive decline.

Although LTC 2.0 subsidies are income linked, they are not generous. Families still end up paying a significant fraction—sometimes the majority—of long-term care costs on their own. One reason this arrangement persists is the widespread belief that helping the disabled and elderly with their daily needs, unlike the treatment of illness and injury, is primarily the responsibility of the patient's family.

A common solution to this cost problem is for families to hire foreign care workers, whom the government has long allowed to work in Taiwan on a temporary basis. Paradoxically, these foreign care workers are required to sign up for NHI if they are in Taiwan for more than 6 months, but they are not eligible for LTC 2.0 benefits themselves.

FINANCING

Taiwan's government does not break down total health spending in ways directly comparable to the national figures that the OECD uses. Based on the Ministry's official statistics, in 2018 total health care spending in Taiwan was low: $34.6 billion USD (1,100 billion NTD)—or roughly $1,500 per capita USD (47,500 NTD)—accounting for 6.3% of GDP. The total budget for the NHI was just under $20 billion USD (approximately 600 billion NTD), or less than 4% of GDP. This is approximately $840 USD (26,600 NTD) per capita. The rate of growth was about 3% per year, comparable to other developed countries.

Finally, it is hard to compare official government health cost data to the data from other countries. The estimates may be artificially high because they include out-of-pocket spending for personal items like diapers and vitamins, which are not included in most other countries' estimates. Conversely, they may be low because there are no reliable data on the costs of private supplemental health insurance.

Figure 2. Financing Health Care (Taiwan)

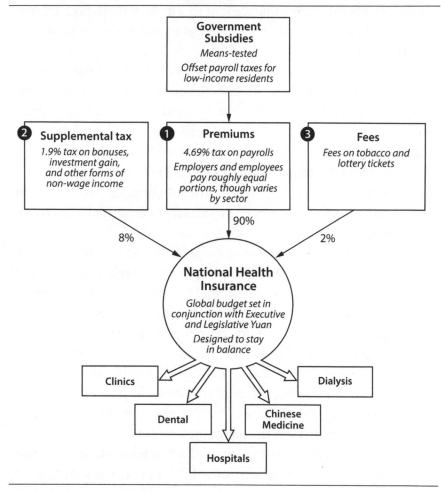

Government Subsidies
Means-tested
Offset payroll taxes for low-income residents

❷ Supplemental tax
1.9% tax on bonuses, investment gain, and other forms of non-wage income

❶ Premiums
4.69% tax on payrolls
Employers and employees pay roughly equal portions, though varies by sector

❸ Fees
Fees on tobacco and lottery tickets

8%

90%

2%

National Health Insurance
Global budget set in conjunction with Executive and Legislative Yuan
Designed to stay in balance

Clinics

Dialysis

Dental

Chinese Medicine

Hospitals

Public Health Insurance

The NHI has 3 main sources of financing: (1) premiums, which come from a combination of payroll taxes and government subsidies; (2) a supplemental tax on nonwage income; and (3) tobacco taxes and lottery fees.

About 90% of NHI funding comes from the premiums, roughly two-thirds of which come directly from the payroll taxes. The total payroll tax rate is 4.69%, with employers and employees paying about half, although the precise percentages depend on the type of employment. For instance, civil servants contribute less than private-sector employees. The typical family of 4 pays roughly $100 USD (3,200 NTD) in monthly payroll taxes, equivalent to about 2% of household income. In Taiwan these payroll taxes are considered and explicitly referred to as NHI premiums.

The government has taken several steps to mitigate the impact of these payroll taxes. The biggest step is subsidies for low-income people, people with disabilities, and the unemployed. About 3 million people receive these subsidies, which the government finances with general revenue, and they account for about one-third of total premiums.

About 8% of NHI funding comes from a 1.9% tax on nonwage income, including one-time bonuses, investment gains, and rental income. The final 2% of NHI funding comes from dedicated tobacco and lottery fees.

In 2016, the NHIA in the Ministry for Health and Welfare took another major step to help the poor and others struggling with medical bills. Previously the agency would "lock" electronic medical cards for people who had fallen behind on payroll taxes. Providers use the card to log appointments and file for reimbursement, so this effectively made it impossible for people with outstanding bills to get care until they had paid up—unless a doctor or hospital would see them for free or with off-the-books cash payments. In 2016, the government ended that practice, a step, the NHIA said, that "symbolizes a new level of protection for the human right to receive medical care."

Even with all of these protections and subsidies in place, some people still end up with unpayable medical bills. To help those people, the Taiwan government offers interest-free loans for the payment of old medical bills. In 2016, it gave out more than 2,000 such loans.

Private Health Insurance
Private insurers sell the supplemental indemnity policies directly to consumers, frequently as an add-on to life or property insurance. They also sell some policies through employers, who can offer it to employees as an optional benefit. Costs vary enormously depending, in part, on the type of insurance and who it covers. Based on anecdotal reports, monthly premiums seem to be less than $200 USD (6,300 NTD).

Global Budgeting

To limit total health care spending, the Ministry of Health and Welfare defines a global health budget each year and adjusts payments to hospitals and physicians quarterly to ensure the budget is not exceeded.

The Ministry spends nearly a full year setting a health care budget, which is the main tool it has for cost control. It examines current health care spending and adjusts it for population growth, inflation, and decisions to cover new drugs or treatments. The Ministry then develops both a high- and low-end request for what the NHI should spend the next year. That proposal goes to the Executive Yuan, Taiwan's equivalent of the cabinet, for approval. Once the Executive Yuan signs off, the budget goes back to the Ministry, where a 35-member committee—including representatives for hospitals, patient groups, and other stakeholders—finalizes the global budget. The committee determines how much of the global budget goes to each of 5 areas—hospital care, medical clinics, dental care, Traditional Chinese Medicine, and dialysis. Once that is done, the NHIA distributes money to the 6 regional health authorities, which process claims and write checks. The budget also sets aside money for risk adjustment in case the projections prove inaccurate.

Because fee-for-service is the predominant method of reimbursement, there are incentives for providers to perform more services or more expensive services. To ensure such behavior does not lead to exceeding the global budget, the NHIA adjusts how much it pays per service—that is, the price—quarterly to reflect the volume of services. "Under the global budget system," NHIA Director General Lee Po-Chang explains, "the unit price for all fee schedule items is inversely related to the service volume."

To illustrate how the system works, Lee cited a hypothetical example in which the government had set the global budget at one point per NT dollar and allocated 1 million NTD overall. If utilization came in higher—say, 1.1 million points' worth of services—then the NHIA would reduce the point value to 0.909 NTD per point. (That's the ratio of 1 million:1.1 million.) For a procedure that NHIA paid 1,000 NTD the previous quarter, it would now pay 909 NTD.

Figure 3. Payment to Hospitals (Taiwan)

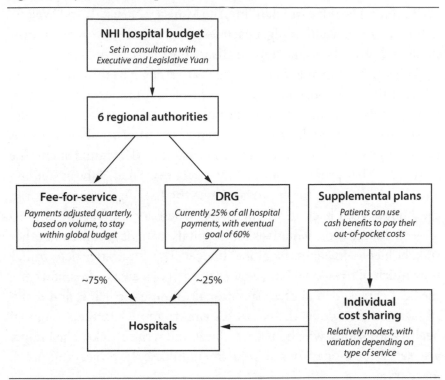

PAYMENT

NHIA distributes money for NHI to 6 regional authorities, which in turn pay hospitals, clinics, and other providers directly. Most payment is fee-for-service.

Payments to Hospitals
Roughly three-fourths of hospital payments are on a fee-for-service basis. The remainder goes through DRG payments, which the NHIA has been introducing gradually. The government's goal is for DRG payments to account for 60% of all inpatient revenue eventually. The NHI also uses pay-for-performance incentives to encourage better care for several major conditions. As of 2018 more than 50% of patients with asthma and early-stage chronic kidney disease were part of pay-for-performance programs.

Figure 4. Payment to Physicians (Taiwan)

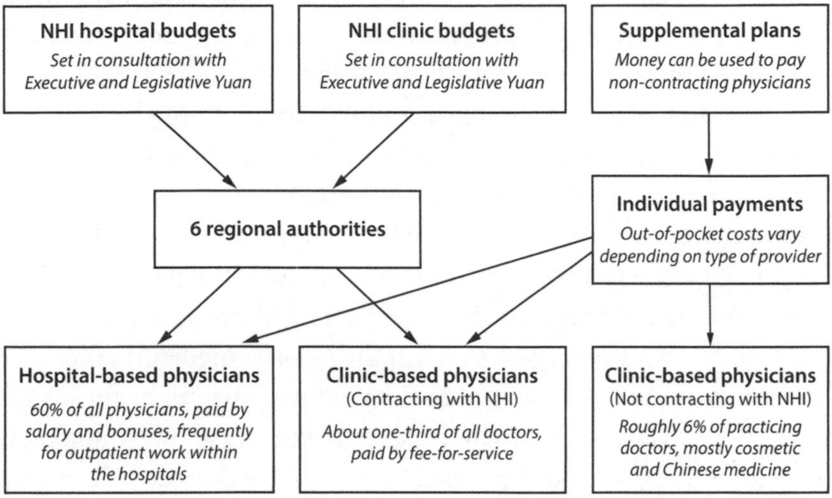

NHI hospital budgets	NHI clinic budgets	Supplemental plans
Set in consultation with Executive and Legislative Yuan	Set in consultation with Executive and Legislative Yuan	Money can be used to pay non-contracting physicians

6 regional authorities	Individual payments
	Out-of-pocket costs vary depending on type of provider

Hospital-based physicians	Clinic-based physicians (Contracting with NHI)	Clinic-based physicians (Not contracting with NHI)
60% of all physicians, paid by salary and bonuses, frequently for outpatient work within the hospitals	About one-third of all doctors, paid by fee-for-service	Roughly 6% of practicing doctors, mostly cosmetic and Chinese medicine

Payments to Physicians

There is no specific figure on how much physicians are paid.

Physicians and dentists work for hospitals or incorporate themselves into clinics—the equivalent of physician offices. The NHI pays hospitals and clinics for physician and dentist services. Thus, physicians working on their own or in small clinics are paid on a fee-for-service basis, while those working for hospitals can be paid in a variety of ways, including salary and bonus payments. Billing and payment through the fee-for-service system is relatively seamless: clinics and hospitals file claims through the electronic health cards and receive their payments electronically.

Roughly 6% of physicians do not take NHI payments and rely entirely on private payment, operating concierge-style practices for people who can afford them. A significant percentage are cosmetic surgeons and TCM doctors, although exact numbers are not available.

Out-of-Pocket Payments

Reliable and official figures on out-of-pocket spending are not available. But according to one official estimate, provided by the NHI director at the request of an outside scholar, about 12% of health care spending in Taiwan is out of pocket.

Out-of-pocket payments are explicitly meant to remind people that health care services should not be wasted but are meant for the sick and injured. Nevertheless, they are relatively low. A patient admitted to the hospital is directly responsible for 10% of charges for the first month of treatment, 20% of the next month, and 30% for anything beyond that. There are also caps on out-of-pocket inpatient expenses: 6% of average national income per single episode and 10% per year.

Co-pays for outpatient and emergency care are flat fees, which vary depending on the type of institution and whether the patient got a referral. They are generally small and have a maximum of less than $18 USD (550 NTD) for emergency care at the top-tier medical centers.

Another source of out-of-pocket spending is payment for a small group of medical devices, such as heart stents and artificial hips. The NHI reimburses these devices based on the cost of devices it deems less expensive but clinically equivalent. Patients can still get the newer devices but only by paying the price difference.

As in other countries' systems, NHI has caps, discounts, and waivers for groups the system deems vulnerable. There is zero cost sharing for patients with cancer and 29 other catastrophic illnesses as well as low-income households, veterans, and children under age 3. NHI waives prescription co-pays for treatment of diabetes, high blood pressure, and roughly 100 other chronic diseases. It waives physical therapy co-pays for certain intense therapies. It also reduces co-pays for people living in remote areas.

Payments for Long-Term Care
Payments for long-term care under LTC 2.0 are on a fee-for-service basis and go directly to care providers. LTC 2.0 payments cannot go to foreign care workers, even though they remain a major source of care for the Taiwan population.

Payments for Complementary and Alternative Medicine
NHI does not pay for complementary or alternative medicine. It does pay for TCM, including acupuncture, but only because it considers that a legitimate form of medicine. However, NHI only pays for Chinese medicines approved by Taiwan's Food and Drug Administration.

Payments for Public Health and Preventive Medicine

NHI pays for a variety of preventive measures, although some of the funding for that coverage comes through separate agencies: the Health Promotion Administration and the Taiwan CDC. NHI also pays directly for the provision of some public health measures, like vaccines, through a series of public health centers that it operates across the island. Campaigns to improve awareness and behavior—on everything from tobacco usage to better eating habits—fall under the jurisdiction of the Health Promotion Administration.

DELIVERY OF HEALTH CARE SERVICES

The Taiwanese have unfettered and radical choice. They are free to choose not only hospitals and physicians but also their own tests—without a physician's order. Patients can go to any hospital, clinic, or health center at any time. Furthermore, they can literally walk up to the counter and ask for a test such as an MRI scan. On average the Taiwanese have 14 interactions with the health system per year, yet there is no problem of queuing.

Hospital Care

Taiwan has 484 accredited hospitals, including 7 dedicated to TCM. The vast majority of hospitals are private and nonprofit. The number of hospitals has declined significantly from a peak of 750 in 1995. Today there are 5.7 inpatient beds per 1,000 population.

All but one hospital, a TCM provider, contract with the NHIA. Overall, hospital spending accounts for 68% of total NHI spending. This high number reflects that the majority of hospital payments (about 55%) is for outpatient services by physicians at the hospital. This means about a third of total payments are for hospital in-patient care.

Taiwanese hospitals differ from hospitals in other developed countries in 2 main ways. First, facilities have a reputation for crowding, which likely reflects the high demand for services. Second, by comparison to other developed countries, Taiwanese hospitals are spartan. In many Taiwanese hospitals families and friends are expected to remain at bedside and, when practical, to attend to the patient's daily needs like feeding and bathing.

Co-payments for some hospital and specialty care are higher without a referral, but the increased out-of-pocket costs remain modest by international standards—the equivalent of just a few US dollars, with exact figures depending on the circumstances.

Yet NHIA says that queuing is not an issue. Indeed, about 83% of hospital patients report getting care within 30 minutes.

Ambulatory (Outpatient) Care

In 2018, Taiwan had 22,089 outpatient clinics equivalent to physicians' and dentists' offices. Approximately one-third are dental offices.

Patients have totally free choice of physicians. They can see any doctor at any time, without a referral. The majority of physicians work in hospitals. When they provide outpatient care they do so through facilities that are part of the hospitals. In nonhospital clinics about 85% of physicians are in solo practices. For care after hours, the Taiwanese use hospital emergency rooms.

Providers and patients alike report that access to care is generally quick and accessible. This is possible only because the average physician has extended hours—until 9:00 p.m.—and sees 50 patients in a day, with the most popular ones seeing more than 100 patients. Both the medical community and NHIA officials worry that this feverish pace is leading to physician dissatisfaction and burnout. In 2017, an NHIA survey of physician satisfaction reported that 38.7% were unsatisfied and just 30.2% were satisfied.

The main appeal of private, concierge clinics is not to jump queues but to spend more time and get more attention from physicians or to see one of those handful of renowned physicians who have decided they can get enough income from private patients alone.

Although group practices are rare, some family physicians participate in a program called the Family Physician Integrated Care Project (FPICP). The FPICP, which dates back to 2003, creates networks of primary care providers (including pediatricians and gynecologists) who share patient records, provide 24-hour telephone consultations, and refer to common hospitals to coordinate care. Research suggests that patients in the program are more likely to get regular and preventive care.

Addressing urban-rural disparities is a major issue in Taiwan. One 2017 study, for example, found that three-fourths of rural communities had no dedicated pediatric clinics. To help address this, the Ministry now operates public health clinics that provide a wide variety of medical services, including both primary and preventive care. In addition, the government offers higher payment to providers who operate in underserved areas.

Mental Health Care

Taiwan has 43 major psychiatric hospitals and one teaching psychiatric hospital. After years of major shortages, the number of mental health beds increased. By 2014, there were 32 acute and 59 chronic hospital beds per 100,000 population. This is relatively high compared to other countries like China, which has approximately 32 psychiatric beds per 100,000 population, and the United States, which has under 12 beds per 100,000 population.

As in the rest of the world, Taiwan's mental health community has pushed for deinstitutionalization. Initiatives like LTC 2.0 have helped by offering more community services for people with disabilities. NHIA officials say that the vast majority of people who get psychiatric treatment do so in outpatient settings—sometimes through primary care providers, sometimes through psychiatrists, sometimes through psychologists and other therapists, and sometimes through local health centers. But experts have said community support services remain highly underutilized, suggesting that people with mental health conditions are not getting all the support and treatment they need.

Long-Term Care

Taiwan has some nursing homes for the elderly and disabled, but the majority of people receiving long-term care do so in their own or family members' homes. This heavy use of non-institutional care arises from 2 factors: (1) the government's emphasis on aging in place and (2) the traditional Taiwanese beliefs that care for the disabled and elderly should be a family responsibility. To the extent that people need to hire caregivers, they can do so through agencies or the informal market. They continue to rely heavily on foreign-born workers, whose presence in the country the government has long supported, even though hiring those workers means forgoing the subsidies from LTC 2.0.

Complementary and Alternative Medicine

According to the NHI, there are 800 clinics specializing in TCM— roughly 17% of all clinics.

Preventive Medicine

Patients can get preventive care in a variety of settings. The Ministry of Health and Welfare operates public health centers that provide basic screenings and immunizations. Even residents with regular physicians will frequently use the centers to get vaccines. They also provide services like testing for sexually transmitted diseases.

Electronic Health Records

One of Taiwan's most famous delivery innovations is its electronic medical records system. Each patient has a card that includes personal information, such as address and insurance billing number. Providers use the cards to log interventions and file for reimbursement as well as to access online medical records through 2 systems: (1) MediCloud, which includes diagnoses, allergies, vaccinations, and records from the 6 most recent visits, and (2) PharmaCloud, which includes prescription information.

The Ministry uses the information from the cards to track utilization of services as well as to give public health authorities real-time information on potential disease outbreaks and epidemics.

My Health Bank is yet another electronic records system that gives patients cloud-based access to their medical histories. It is a work in progress in part because it has been difficult to get detailed, usable hospital records into the system. Interoperability is the big obstacle. Hospitals still keep clinical information, like scans or details of specific procedures, which are in incompatible information systems. Enabling those systems to communicate and allow wider access to the information is a focus of ongoing efforts by the Ministry.

Figure 5. Regulation of Pharmaceutical Prices (Taiwan)

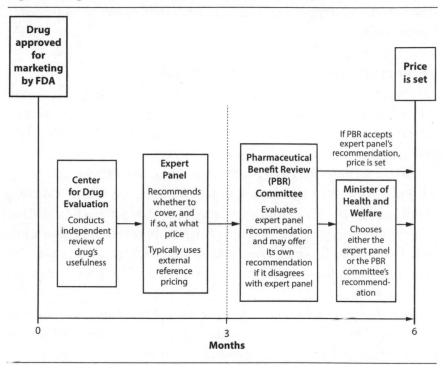

PHARMACEUTICAL COVERAGE AND PRICE CONTROLS

Taiwan uses both comparative effectiveness data and reference pricing to make decisions about drug coverage and pricing, pegging drug prices to the average of what other developed countries pay.

Pharmaceutical Market

Taiwan's overall spending on drugs in 2018 was $6 billion USD (about 190 billion NTD) or $255 USD (8,000 NTD) per capita. By the standards of developed countries, the consumption of prescription drugs is relatively high, whereas prices are relatively low.

The government does not buy drugs directly. Clinics and hospitals purchase the bulk of them and then apply to the NHIA for reimbursement. Hospitals frequently negotiate discounts, enabling them to make a profit on the "spread"—that is, the difference between what they pay and what the NHIA reimburses. The NHIA is now taking steps to limit those profits by using data about past profits to determine future reimbursements.

Coverage Determination and Price Regulation

Taiwan's Food and Drug Administration reviews drugs to make sure they are safe and effective. Once a drug is cleared, NHIA undertakes its own review process to decide whether it will go on the NHI formulary and, if so, how much the NHIA will reimburse for it.

First, the Center for Drug Evaluation (CDE), an independent agency within the Ministry, develops a report focusing on whether a drug should go on the NHI formulary. CDE assesses the drug's clinical value generally by reviewing the findings of similar bodies in Australia, Canada, and the UK. If a drug is already for sale without coverage in Taiwan, the CDE will use data from electronic records to supplement the research from abroad.

The CDE prepares a report on the drug's performance without recommendations. A panel of physicians, pharmacists, economists, and other outside experts then reviews this report and recommends both a price and a set of guidelines for reimbursement. Next, this panel's recommendation goes to the Pharmaceutical Benefit Review (PBR) inside the NHIA. The PBR committee has both experts and stakeholders, including representatives from the drug manufacturers and patient advocates. If the PBR committee accepts the expert panel's recommendation, the NHIA will begin listing and paying for the drug provisionally, subject to review by the Ministry director a year later. If the PBR committee disagrees with the expert panel, the drug company may reapply.

In making these decisions, both the expert panel and PBR committee must adhere to fixed pricing guidelines, based on their determination of the drug's value. Specifically, they must classify drugs as breakthrough drugs (category 1), drugs that offer modest improvement over existing therapies (category 2a), or "me too" drugs that offer no meaningful improvement over what is available already (category 2b). For category 1 drugs the recommended price will be the median price of the drug in 10 developed countries: Australia, Belgium, Canada, France, Germany, Japan, Sweden, Switzerland, the UK, and the United States. For category 2a and 2b drugs the expert panel and the PBR committee may choose from several pricing options, including the lowest price in those 10 countries, the price in the manufacturing country, or the cost of comparable treatments already available in Taiwan.

This is not the end of the process, though.

The director general of the NHIA has discretion to negotiate even lower prices. If drug manufacturers are not happy with the offer, they can petition for reconsideration. The NHIA director general can grant that, going so far as to commission a whole new review. Eventually, if a manufacturer is not happy with what the NHIA is offering, it can simply refuse to sell the drug in Taiwan. This happens occasionally.

An official timeline allows 3 months for the CDE and expert panel review and then another 3 months for PBR committee deliberations. In reality the process can take longer, especially if the manufacturers end up appealing the decision.

Over the years, the NHI has gradually lowered prescription drug prices. According to some estimates, in 1995, when the NHI first launched, it was paying 89% of the 10-country index. After 2005, Taiwan's reimbursement fell to around 50% of the index. NHIA officials take pride in their control of pharmaceutical costs, citing it as one reason they have run budget surpluses. Drug industry officials argue that the government manages drug pricing too aggressively, making it more difficult for people to get important treatments.

Regulation of Physician Prescriptions

Physicians can prescribe any drug approved for sale in Taiwan. Physicians can prescribe medications for off-label use, but they assume extra financial liability for adverse effects when they do. Using electronic records data, the NHIA monitors physicians' prescribing patterns. When data show physicians overprescribing, the NHIA contacts the physicians with the data and encourages them to be more judicious.

Prices Paid by Patients

Out-of-pocket costs for prescription drugs vary depending on the price of the medication. For drugs that cost less than $3.50 USD (100 NTD) there is no co-pay at all. From there co-pays rise steadily to a maximum of $7 USD (200 NTD) for any drugs that cost more than about $32 USD (1,000 NTD).

HUMAN RESOURCES

Physicians

As of 2017, Taiwan had 1.97 Western-medicine doctors and 0.28 TCM doctors for every 1,000 population. The number of Western-medicine physicians has been rising steadily since the NHI's inception.

Physicians work in 2 main types of settings. About 60% of physicians are hospital employees; the rest practice on their own in clinics or offices.

The Ministry does not keep official data on physician salaries, but annual average incomes are between $70,000 and $80,000 USD (2.1 and 2.4 million NTD), according to private-sector estimates. That is more than 4 times the median wage in Taiwan but is relatively low by international standards. Low wages and overwork have created concern over a "brain drain," with some Taiwanese doctors working in mainland China—part or even full time—because the government there, desperate to handle its own shortage of providers, sometimes pays more.

Only 5% of physicians train as primary care or family physicians, although family medicine is part of the core training for all Taiwanese medical students. The rest train as specialists, though a significant portion end up working as general practitioners to meet the demand.

Physicians go through 6 years of education, including 2 years of premedical classes, and then at least 1 year of clinical rotations. Physicians who wish to provide TCM can train in a variety of ways—by studying TCM exclusively or by first studying Western medicine and then getting an extra degree in TCM. In either case, they must go through 2 years of dedicated training in TCM once their formal studies are over—and, as with Western-medicine physicians, pass certification tests (although the tests themselves are different).

Nurses

Taiwan has 159,621 nurses. That is roughly 6.8 per 1,000 residents, much less than typical European countries, such as the Netherlands with 10.5 per 1,000 residents. Nursing in Taiwan requires a 4-year college degree. Tuition is the same as it is for any other undergraduate study. Full-time nurses earn about $45,000 USD (1.4 million NTD) a year. Shortages are an ongoing problem.

CHALLENGES

Large majorities of the Taiwan population consistently say they are satisfied with the health system's overall performance. It is not difficult to see why.

Virtually all citizens now have health insurance, enabling everybody to get the health care they need without experiencing financial hardship. They have free choice of hospitals and physicians and can even order their own tests. They get access to both Western and Chinese medicine. They do not generally have to wait for appointments or elective procedures. And they get all of this with very low out-of-pocket costs. Overall spending is low—lower than any European country per capita. Partly this is because of the system's low administrative costs and partly because cost-control efforts, including the global budget, have been successful at restraining spending, including spending on prescription drugs.

Researchers in Taiwan have not studied the NHI's effects on health outcomes as closely as researchers in the United States, but the available data offer good reason to think that the health of the Taiwanese has improved since the NHI's implementation. It appears that with NHI more pregnant women are getting ultrasounds and Rh and other screenings. Similarly, there has been a decline in deaths from causes "amenable to health care." Indeed, the most dramatic effects were among precisely those groups—the old and the young—who were most likely to gain health coverage from NHI.

The Taiwanese also developed a model for personal electronic medical records. These records do more than make the delivery of basic health care quicker and more convenient; they are also useful for both health policy and public health. The data facilitate careful tracking of utilization of services, allowing the NHIA to contact physicians whose billing patterns suggest excessive use of expensive tests or treatments. NHIA can also adjust reimbursements for Taiwan to remain within its global budget. In addition, during the SARS and H1N1 influenza outbreaks, Taiwan officials could track the disease in close to real time.

Yet Taiwan's health care system has challenges. First, doctors see patients at a frenetic pace—50 to 100 per day—and work late into the night. This raises questions about quality and burnout. There is also the worry of a brain drain, with many physicians practicing overseas and many students being scared away from the profession. Although the number of Western-medicine physicians is increasing, it is still low. Given the high demand, low numbers of physicians, low salaries, and high workload, there is a threat at the very core of the physician-patient relationship. With burnout potentially increasing, the system could be at risk. Clearly more physicians need to be trained, the number of patients seen per physician lowered, and salaries increased. But this would produce higher costs and, because physician training takes years, cannot occur quickly.

Second, advocates for patients with cancer say the government does not approve new therapies quickly enough or pay what it takes to get the most advanced treatments. They worry this creates a 2-tier system in which only wealthy people can get those treatments. They say this may be the reason why cancer survival rates in Taiwan lag behind those in other medically advanced health systems. In a 2014 self-assessment, the Ministry of Health and Welfare gave the Taiwan system an "A" grade for its breast cancer mortality rate but a "D" for the cervical cancer mortality rate. It is unclear whether the challenges regarding cancer care are related to not having the latest drugs or to the amount of time physicians spend with patients and the quality of care they provide. Patients may blame access to drugs, but the real culprit may be the problem of physician shortages and overworked personnel.

In addition, with most physicians in solo practice and seeing so many patients per day, they lack infrastructure to coordinate chronic care and mental health care. Even with electronic medical records, it is difficult to make care plans and then administer them among different providers. Recent reforms have encouraged the Taiwanese to register with primary care physicians who can oversee care and give referrals. But so far it has not had much effect. This lack of chronic care coordination will be a growing problem as chronic diseases become more pervasive.

Long-term care is another big challenge, one that has bedeviled Taiwan for some time. The LTC 2.0 initiative has made more funding available to more people and made it easier for people who need assistance to stay at home rather than in institutions. But it remains available to a limited class of people who qualify based on condition and provides a limited amount of assistance, forcing a large number of Taiwanese who need long-term care to rely on their families or pay for it themselves. Of course, even with those deficiencies, the quality of long-term care in Taiwan appears to be high. One relevant data point is a 2015 worldwide survey by the Economist Intelligence Unit of Quality of Death in different parts of the world. Taiwan ranked 1st in Asia and 6th overall.

More spending could mitigate several of these challenges. Even a modest increase in national health spending would give the NHI plenty of money to increase physician salaries, train more physicians, and cover the newest drugs more quickly. And modest increases would still leave overall spending far below the average of OECD countries. Indeed, in 2008 Uwe Reinhardt proposed that Taiwan consider increasing its spending by 1% or 2% of GDP not only to acquire those new drugs but also to wipe out some of the out-of-pocket costs that NHI enrollees still have to pay. It has not happened.

Increasing health spending would require the Taiwanese government to raise more money—either by pushing up the income-related premiums, increasing the nonwage or lottery and tobacco taxes, or finding some other new revenue source. Even in Taiwan, with its relatively low health care spending, raising taxes for health is politically challenging. In the meantime, leaders of groups representing cancer patients and other people battling serious illnesses have proposed an alternative, stopgap solution: some kind of balance-billing scheme—like the one in place for those handful of medical devices—for cutting-edge cancer drugs that the NHI is not yet ready to cover. But policymakers have not given the idea serious attention.

CHAPTER ELEVEN

CHINA

After multiple efforts to expand insurance coverage, China today is close to realizing a major achievement: providing health insurance to almost its entire population. Unfortunately this insurance is broad but not deep. Most payment for medical services—and especially for long-term care—is still out of pocket.

What's more, the delivery system has not matched the progress in insurance coverage. Chinese patients go to hospitals for almost all conditions, from simple respiratory infections and routine diabetic checks to serious cancers. There is little ambulatory primary care available, partially because of the way physicians are licensed, partially because of extremely low pay and prestige, and partially due to patient habits.

Although hospitals are considered the best place to receive care, there is deep distrust of doctors and hospital administrators because of endemic corruption. Physicians accept "red envelopes" stuffed with cash from patients as well as kickbacks from drug companies for prescribing their medications. Consequently, one physician noted that "patients do not have much trust in health professionals. When they come to see a doctor, most of the time their position can best be described as half trust and half doubt." In the extreme, this distrust results in violent attacks on physicians, nurses, and other medical personnel.

These issues are not new to Chinese officials. They have plagued the system for decades. And health policy experts acknowledge that fundamental change is needed to improve the system. And yet, despite big changes in insurance coverage, funding, and public health services, implementing innovations in how care is delivered and how physicians and patients behave has proven almost impossible.

HISTORY

China's current health care system originated in 1982, when the government overhauled the centralized, Communist health care system that had been established more than 30 years earlier when Mao Zedong and the Communist Party came to power in 1949.

Under the centralized system the national government set the budget for each sector of the health care system, fixed the income for doctors, nurses, and administrators, and implemented 2 different health insurance systems—one for urban areas and another for rural areas. There was no private insurance. In urban areas the Government Insurance Scheme (GIS) insured officials, staff, and their dependents at government agencies, schools, universities, and research institutes. The Labor Insurance Scheme (LIS) covered employees and their dependents at state-owned factories. Poverty aid programs insured unemployed urban residents. In rural areas the Cooperative Medical Scheme (CMS), a prepaid health security program, covered most of the population, but with few services. CMS ran the village and township health centers, in which so-called barefoot doctors, community-based doctors with little health training, provided both Western and traditional Chinese medical care at basic levels.

In the 30 years after 1949 life expectancy increased from 35 to 68 years, infant mortality fell from 200 to 34 per 1,000 live births, and vaccination levels increased, reducing the spread of infectious diseases.

Despite these achievements, the political and economic shifts of the early 1980s initiated the disintegration of most of the health care system. In the 1980s, China began a dramatic shift toward a market-based, privatized economy. For health care this meant that the formerly collectivist structure became more privatized, individually financed, and shifted its orientation from prevention to acute care. In 1978, the central government began to transfer financial responsibility for health care to the regional and local governments. The 1982 constitution made this shift official. Budgetary decisions were delegated to local governing bodies, and much more of the funding came from payments from individuals instead of the national government. These changes reinforced the preexisting disparities between care in the coastal, urban provinces *and* the inland, rural provinces. In addition, power over national health care transferred from the Communist Party (CCP) to the Ministry of Health (MOH). Because fiscal decision making had been decentralized to local and provincial governments, the MOH could not implement nationwide policy changes.

Prior to the early 1980s, the government had tight controls over how much hospitals and clinics could charge for most services. But as part of the 1980s reforms, the government also imposed a new price-regulation system that increased costs and decreased access. It allowed facilities to earn profits on drugs and tests. Physicians also began to receive bonuses for bringing in more revenue in a fee-for-service model. Around the same time, the rural health insurance scheme collapsed as a result of rising premiums and subsequent disenrollment, causing hundreds of millions of rural citizens to lose their coverage. Most of the previously government-sponsored clinics transformed into expensive, fee-for-service health centers. To even make a living, the barefoot doctors, now unemployed, turned to private health care provision— charging high fees, selling drugs, and abandoning their previous emphasis on preventive care.

Health care costs increased dramatically. Between 1980 and 2000 national health expenditures rose by 4,000%. In response, the government reintroduced some price controls, but this gave patients an economic incentive to stay in hospitals longer than medically necessary, thus wasting resources and exacerbating shortages of medical services.

Faced with high operating costs and little government support, hospitals started charging high markups for specialty services, tests, and drugs not covered by price regulations. By 1992, these markups accounted for about three-quarters of hospital funding. Demand for hospital services grew as rural residents with the means to travel began to come to cities seeking care. Focus on public health diminished because physicians had few incentives to emphasize preventive measures. Population health progress slowed, and some infectious diseases began to reemerge.

Since 2000, China has taken major steps to overhaul its health care system. After an outbreak of SARS in 2003, the government reinvigorated its preventive health measures, initiating thousands of local-level projects to prevent and control disease. In 2002, President

Hu Jintao's government began to look at ways to decrease costs and increase access.

Insurance reforms had already begun in 1998 with the creation of the Urban Employee Basic Medical Insurance (UEBMI), which combined and replaced the old GIS and LIS systems. UEBMI put all workers at urban, state-owned enterprises into a citywide risk pool, which stabilized the enterprises' finances. All employers—private and state owned—were required to offer employee coverage with medical savings accounts (MSAs) and catastrophic coverage, funded by payroll taxes. However, the UEBMI pools were largely populated by aging and retiring workers. Consequently, costs began to grow. Although enrollment was mandatory, UEBMI often did not cover younger people because they were migrant workers and not considered urban residents eligible for the insurance. In 2007, the government introduced a 2nd urban insurance scheme called Urban Resident Basic Medical Insurance (URBMI), targeted at unemployed or informally employed urban residents. This plan included students, children, the elderly, poor, and disabled. The central government heavily subsidized it.

Beginning in 2003, rural health care received a similar overhaul. China established the New Cooperative Medical Scheme (NCMS), a re-creation of the old CMS overseen by the MOH. Unlike its predecessor, NCMS was voluntary and focused on acute care. It pooled risk at the county level and was geared toward covering hospital and emergency expenditures. Government subsidies were initially low, which required high out-of-pocket payments. Nevertheless, by 2007, 86% of China's counties enrolled in NCMS, covering 730 million rural residents.

In 2009, following 4 years of internal debate over how to resolve the issues of declining coverage rates, limited rural access to care, increased incidence of public health crises, and rapidly rising out-of-pocket costs, China introduced a comprehensive reform plan. This reform had 5 objectives:

1. Expand insurance coverage.
2. Increase funding of public health.
3. Expand local-level health care infrastructure.
4. Form an Essential Drugs List (EDL).
5. Improve public hospital operations.

This required an enormous investment by the central government, which by 2015 had reached $354 billion USD annually. Unfortunately, the plan fell short of its goals.

Although at the end of 2011, 95% of the population was covered, this was more in name than in reality. About 200 million rural-to-urban migrant workers, who may have been covered by NCMS in their hometowns, lacked coverage in the cities where they actually lived and worked. In addition, most inpatient and outpatient coverage still required high out-of-pocket payments, often totaling more than 50% of the bill. Public health funding increased from $2 to $3.50 USD (15 RMB to 25 RMB) per capita, but it is unclear if this has had a tangible effect on population health.

The central government worked with local governments to create township health centers (THCs) that housed primary care physicians who focused on both acute and preventive care, but rural residents still preferred to use village clinics and county hospitals. The Essential Drugs List (EDL), a list of 520 medications covered by public insurance and required to be sold at cost, was created, and some prices dropped. But many hospitals either did not comply with the law or even induced demand for inpatient services to offset revenue lost through lower drug prices. Even worse: the reforms to the public hospital system, which were supposed to improve the efficiency of care, were slow to materialize.

More recently, reforms have been incremental. In 2015, the government announced that it was removing price controls on most drugs, with new regulations that would rely partly on market pricing. Similarly, in 2015 the government encouraged more private-sector involvement in the health care system, allowing patients with public insurance to receive reimbursement for privately provided services. The government has also begun to investigate—and prosecute—corruption in the health care sector. And it pledged to increase health care spending to 7% of GDP by 2020 in an effort to combat chronic illnesses.

The disparities between URBMI and the NCMS were apparent from the beginning. In the rural areas the NCMS risk pools were province based. Consequently, they were smaller, riskier, and cost more than urban risk pools. In addition, because rural health care was much harder to access—and therefore more expensive than care in urban areas—NCMS enrollees were paying more out of pocket for fewer and lower-quality health care services. Finally, premium contributions in the rural insurance scheme were significantly higher as a percentage of income than in the urban one.

Significant portions of the population who technically had health insurance coverage were in reality unable to receive services. Chinese residents had to register with their local municipality and could only receive benefits from social insurance programs in the locality where they were registered. Thus, migrant workers who leave rural areas for work in the cities are denied social insurance program benefits, including health coverage, because they live outside their registered municipality. Furthermore, each locality is assigned either urban or rural status. Residents in rural localities could only enroll in NCMS, while those assigned urban status could only enroll in URBMI. But as the urban-rural distinction was being phased out throughout the early 2000s and 2010s, provinces began to merge their NCMS and URBMI programs. To mitigate the problems of paying for migrants' health care, in 2017 the Chinese launched a cross-province medical settlement program that benefited a few million workers.

In December 2016, the national government announced that it would formally integrate NCMS and URBMI into one program: the Urban and Rural Resident Basic Medical Insurance (URRBMI). Each province was required to submit a plan to merge the 2 systems at the provincial level by the end of 2019. In 2018, a new government agency, the National Health Commission (NHC), was formed to oversee all state health coverage.

By 2016, many urban provinces had in reality almost no NCMS enrollees, and so this enormous shift in governance was less arduous than it might have seemed. Still, this period of transition will test whether China can truly create a unified system of universal coverage.

As with many aspects of government, the Chinese health care system is centralized in theory but fragmented in fact. This produces significant disparities between cities, provinces, and programs based on wealth and location, and it makes coordination difficult. As these issues emerge, the government must continually grapple with the challenges of insuring the world's largest population through a decentralized and underfunded system.

COVERAGE

China is a country of 1.4 billion people, 60% urban and 40% rural, spread across 22 provinces, 4 municipalities, and 5 autonomous regions (which, for the purposes of health insurance, are considered part of China).

There is no universal legal mandate for health insurance coverage. URRBMI—the new health insurance system introduced in 2016 to cover both urban and rural residents—is voluntary. Nevertheless, China is nearing universal health coverage. Approximately 95% of the population is covered by one of the publicly funded programs.

Public Health Insurance
All publicly funded coverage is person specific. This means that health insurance programs cover individuals, not their family or dependents, and therefore each person must enroll separately.

Two publicly funded health insurance programs cover 85% of China's population. First, the Urban Employee Basic Medical Insurance (UEBMI) provides health insurance to all urban employees of government agencies, state-owned enterprises, and private enterprises. Participation in UEBMI is mandatory for employees *and* employers. In 2017, UEBMI covered 303.2 million people, but it does not include coverage for employees' family members and dependents.

Second, the Urban and Rural Resident Basic Medical Insurance (URRBMI) provides health insurance to other urban residents, including children, the self-employed, students, and elderly adults, as well as to all rural residents regardless of whether they work. Enrollment is also voluntary, and the government pays most of the cost for covered services with low individual premiums. By 2017, URRBMI covered 873.6 million people. URRBMI was supposed to be fully implemented at the end of 2019. It should now cover the entire population formerly covered by the URBMI and the NCMS—or more than a billion people. It remains to be seen whether URRBMI will succeed in providing coverage for all

Figure 1. Health Care Coverage (China)

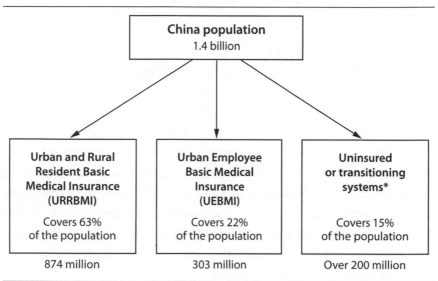

*Government reports 5% uninsurance; remainder still transitioning from the New Cooperative Medical Scheme (NCMS) to URRBMI.

those people and expanding coverage to those who previously struggled to obtain it.

Foreign citizens residing in China are also entitled to coverage under whichever program is applicable to their employment status.

There is no nationally standard basic benefits package. Covered services vary widely between provinces because local health officials can determine some aspects of coverage. In theory both UEBMI and URRBMI cover primary care, specialist care, emergency room visits, hospitalization, and mental health care along with prescription drug expenses. Traditional Chinese Medicine, some dental and optometry services, and sometimes home and hospice care are covered depending upon the province. In most areas, though, only acute inpatient and outpatient care are actually covered, although UEBMI enrollees can use their medical savings accounts to cover other health expenses, such as drugs or dental care. Neither plan covers long-term care.

Preventive health care is covered separately through a public health program funded by the central government and administered by local government health clinics. Every Chinese citizen is entitled to free preventive care, including immunizations and disease screenings. Public health clinics also track and manage infectious diseases in local communities.

Private Health Insurance

Only about 5% of Chinese residents have any form of private insurance. Private health insurance is often sold in combination with life insurance. Most of these policies are critical-illness policies, which apply only to prespecified illnesses—such as cancer—and pay out a lump sum if the policyholder is diagnosed with one of those conditions. Private health insurance is largely supplementary to public insurance and is often offered by large multinational employers, although some higher-income individuals only use private insurance. Private insurance can offer access to better-quality care because some private hospitals, which tend to be less crowded and of higher quality than public ones, do not accept public insurance.

Despite encouragement from the government to expand its reach after the 2009 health reforms, the private health insurance market has remained small. In 2015, the market was about $36.7 billion USD (250 billion RMB) and has grown at about 36% each year since 2010. This market will likely continue to grow as more middle- and upper-middle-class citizens look for a way to cover the superior care they hope to receive at private hospitals.

FINANCING

China spends about $1.33 trillion USD (9.2 trillion RMB)—6.2% of its GDP—on health care annually. This translates to roughly $960 USD per capita. Of this, about 62% is funded by public sources. The rest comes from private spending, including supplemental insurance plans, private care, and, mainly, out-of-pocket payments for various drugs and services that public insurance does not fully cover. Health care expenditures have risen almost 12% annually since 2010.

Public/Statutory Health Insurance

UEBMI, the employment-based public insurance scheme for urban workers, is funded by a payroll tax. Employees pay 2% of their salary

Figure 2. Financing Health Care (China)

A. URBAN EMPLOYEE BASIC MEDICAL INSURANCE (UEBMI)

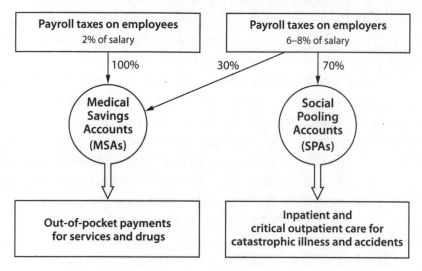

B. URBAN AND RURAL RESIDENT BASIC MEDICAL INSURANCE (URRBMI)

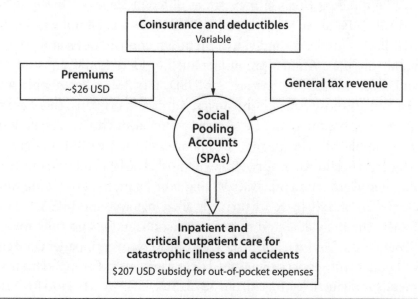

and employers contribute 6% to 8% of the employee's salary. This money is divided into 2 pools. Each individual has a medical savings account (MSA), made up of their contribution plus 30% of the employer's contribution. The other 70% of the employer's contribution goes into a social pooling account (SPA). Retirees are exempted from the employee contribution but are still covered by UEBMI.

Administered by the individual, the MSA is mainly used for out-of-pocket payments for outpatient services and drug purchases. Local governments administer the social pooling account. The SPAs cover in- and outpatient services for acute and catastrophic illnesses or accidents. Before the SPA coverage goes into effect, individuals must pay a deductible, set at about 10% of the average annual wage of a local worker. Individuals are also responsible for a coinsurance of 5% to 20% of the health bill. The SPA will pay health care costs up to 6 times the local employees' average annual wage. At this point, if the MSA is also exhausted, all expenses must be paid out of pocket. Unspent money in MSAs is rolled over to the next year.

The details of each province's exact URRBMI financing structure will be different because they are at different stages of merging the old URBMI and NCMS to create URRBMI. As an example: in Beijing URRBMI is funded by individual premium contributions and government subsidies. Annual premiums for the elderly, children, students, and those of working age are $26 USD (180 RMB). For people with disabilities, those beneath the poverty line, and orphans, there are no premiums, but there may be high individual deductibles. The national government contributes the vast majority of the URRBMI budget out of general tax funds. In 2015, 78.2% of the old URBMI budget came from the central government; URRBMI might be financed in the same way.

Unlike UEBMI, there are no medical savings accounts (MSAs) in URRBMI. The individual and government contributions go only into an SPA. Like the SPA for UEBMI, the URRBMI SPA covers inpatient and critical outpatient services—but much less generously. For inpatient treatment, the deductible ranges from $43 to $188 USD (300 to 1300 RMB) for the first hospitalization (depending on the type of hospital) and half the original deductible for subsequent admissions, with 20% coinsurance. The maximum the SPA will pay for inpatient coverage is $28,969 USD (200,000 RMB). After that, individuals must pay all health expenses out of pocket. For critical outpatient treatment there is a $14 USD (100 RMB) deductible and 45% coinsurance. Each person also gets a $207 USD (1430 RMB) subsidy from the government for out-of-pocket expenses.

Private Health Insurance

Individuals purchase private health insurance policies out of pocket. There is no government subsidization of private health insurance. Some large multinational corporations purchase group reimbursement policies for their employees. These policies cover care at private hospitals, but they are fairly rare.

Long-Term Care

The one-child policy has created a rapidly aging population without sufficient familial and social support for the elderly. Recognizing this, in June 2016, the Ministry of Human Resources and Social Security (MoHRSS) launched an experimental long-term care insurance program. The goal was to create a national long-term care system by 2020. Long-term care insurance is currently only available in the 15 pilot cities designated by the MoHRSS. The MoHRSS provided fairly little guidance to the pilot cities on how to structure their systems, suggesting only that the policy should:

- cover those with long-term disabilities,
- be limited to UEBMI enrollees,
- be funded by alterations to the structure of UEBMI funding,
- pay 70% of the costs that meet reimbursement requirements, and
- gradually expand both the covered population and the benefit package over the course of the pilot.

Few details on individual cities' financing structures are currently available.

Public Health

All Chinese citizens can receive basic public health services, including immunizations and other preventive care, at no upfront cost through a national public health service program. In 2016, this program had a per capita budget of $6.50 USD (45 RMB), funded by the central government. It is under the purview of the National Health Commission (NHC).

PAYMENT

Payments to Hospitals

There are 2 different payment schemes for hospitals.

Small- and medium-sized local (known as Class I and Class II, respectively) hospitals receive annual prospective payments from the National Health Commission (NHC). At the beginning of each year, the NHC will estimate what the hospital's costs will be. Monthly it disburses payments. At the end of the year, there is an adjustment payment if costs were above or below the prospective payment. Hospitals can receive bonuses if their costs were under 80% of the estimation. If costs were above 120% of the estimation, hospitals must share 50% of the excess expense. Patients at local hospitals must only pay the out-of-pocket portion of their bill; the prospective government payment covers the insured portion.

Large cross-district and national hospitals (Class III) are the most prestigious and have the most highly regarded doctors on staff. These hospitals are mostly funded by patients' out-of-pocket payments. Patients at Class III hospitals must pay the full bill at the point of service and then send receipts to the local government to be reimbursed for the insured portion of the bill. However, this practice is beginning to change. In 2018, patients could use their digital social security cards to settle their medical bills at the point of service at most public hospitals.

Private hospitals can receive payments from the government in the same way that Class III hospitals do as long as they have been designated, or appointed, by the government. Local governments can designate hospitals, functionally making them in network for government health insurance payments.

Payments to Ambulatory Care Institutions

Township and community health centers, which provide most of China's primary care, have 3 sources of revenue: fee-for-service (paid by

Figure 3. Payment to Hospitals (China)

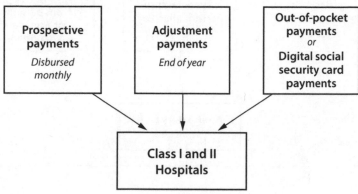

A. CLASS I AND II HOSPITALS

| Prospective payments
Disbursed monthly | Adjustment payments
End of year | Out-of-pocket payments
or
Digital social security card payments |

Class I and II Hospitals

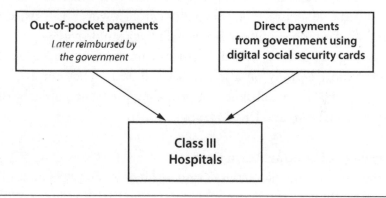

B. CLASS III HOSPITALS

| Out-of-pocket payments
Later reimbursed by the government | Direct payments from government using digital social security cards |

Class III Hospitals

health insurance or patients), drugs (from dispensing medications), and government subsidies. The government subsidizes the gap between clinics' revenue and expenditures. On average, subsidies are about half of total revenue for primary care institutions.

Payments to Physicians

Doctors in outpatient primary care institutions are paid a salary, which is determined by 2 factors: Basic Performance Pay and Encouraging Performance Pay. Basic Performance Pay is a fixed amount that varies from doctor to doctor depending on job title, experience, location, and

Figure 4. Payment to Ambulatory Care Physicians (China)

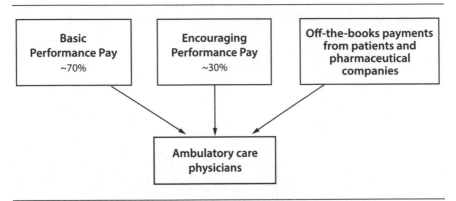

place of practice. It usually makes up about 70% of a physician's wage. The other 30% is Encouraging Performance Pay, which is theoretically intended to encourage better-quality care. However, it is usually paid out based on the volume of services a physician provides.

Village doctors, providing primary care in rural village clinics, are paid almost entirely on a fee-for-service basis. They receive low per capita government subsidies for providing the basic public health services that UEBMI and URRBMI cover.

Payments for Long-Term Care

Other than in the pilot cities designated by the MoHRSS in 2016, long-term health care is paid for by patients and their families entirely out of pocket.

Payments for Complementary and Alternative Medicine

Traditional Chinese Medicine (TCM) is covered by the public health insurance system. Payments for such services are made the same way as payments for Western health care services, whether they are administered in primary care institutions or in hospitals.

Payments for Public Health/Preventive Medicine

There is no upfront payment for basic public health services. The central government distributes low per capita subsidies to clinics and other primary care institutions for providing these services.

DELIVERY OF HEALTH CARE SERVICES

For many reasons, health care delivery in China is extremely hospital centric. The vast majority of physicians are specialists practicing in hospitals. This is in large part because care in physician offices is viewed by both physicians and patients as much lower quality and much less prestigious. Consequently, prominent physicians do not offer nonhospital outpatient care, and new physicians are hesitant to practice in nonhospital settings. Thus, there are few freestanding outpatient physician offices. There is no gatekeeper model. Patients do not need a primary care physician or GP referral to see a specialist.

Reinforcing these cultural practices that emphasize hospital-centric care is the payment system. Because the 2 social insurance schemes do not cover much beyond inpatient and critical outpatient care, patients go to hospitals as the main point of contact for health care services.

Hospital Care

As of 2017, there are 30,000 hospitals in China, with 6.1 million hospital beds. Of these hospitals, 12,000 are public and 18,000 are private.

Hospitals in China are divided into 3 groups, Class I (primary), Class II (secondary), and Class III (tertiary) hospitals. Primary hospitals are typically small, with 100 or fewer beds, providing little specialized care. Secondary hospitals are larger (100 to 500 beds) and usually serve a broader region. They provide comprehensive medical care and also perform medical research and education at the regional level. Tertiary hospitals are national and cross-regional, and they perform both specialized care and specialized research. They usually have more than 500 beds and are the most prestigious.

Hospital care is in high demand, as citizens believe—often correctly—that hospitals are the best place to receive quality care. Rural residents will often travel long distances to urban hospitals. As a result, hospitals tend to have long waits.

Ambulatory (Outpatient) Care

Doctors, village doctors, and nurses provide ambulatory care in health centers and clinics throughout the country. As of 2017, there were

37,000 township health centers, 35,000 community health service centers, 230,000 clinics, and 638,000 village clinics delivering such services.

In most urban areas physicians see their patients at hospital facilities. Except for a small but growing number of private physician offices, the vast majority of ambulatory care is provided in hospital facilities.

Mental Health Care

Mental health care is largely cordoned off from other medical care, although the government is attempting to integrate it more fully into primary care. There are around 30,000 psychiatrists, 60,000 psychiatric nurses, and 450,000 psychiatric beds for a population of 1.4 billion—about the same number of practitioners as the United States for a population 4 times the size. Like most health care in China, mental health care is hospital based.

Around 45% of all mental health resources—institutions and personnel—are located in 11 eastern provinces, indicating an even more unbalanced distribution of resources than is typical in the Chinese health care system. Areas composed mostly of ethnic minorities, such as the Tibet Autonomous Region, have few to no psychiatrists.

Long-Term Care

There is no public structure for long-term care delivery, although the number of nursing homes is rising rapidly and private in-home nursing services are becoming more widely available in cities. In 2017, there were approximately 145,000 nursing homes. Most long-term care is informal and administered by family members. But with a one-child policy, there is only one female caregiver—the married daughter or daughter-in-law in a couple—for 4 parents.

Complementary and Alternative Medicine

There are about 4,000 Traditional Chinese Medicine (TCM) hospitals and 42,528 TCM clinics, with roughly 450,000 TCM practitioners. TCM facilities across the country receive about 910 million annual visits. All TCM practitioners are required to pass exams administered by provincial-level TCM organizations and obtain recommendations from at least 2 previously certified TCM practitioners. Allopathetic physicians may also specialize in TCM.

Preventive Medicine
Local health institutions deliver preventive care services, including disease screening and immunizations.

PHARMACEUTICAL COVERAGE AND
PRICE CONTROLS

Pharmaceutical Market
China's pharmaceutical market is the 2nd largest in the world after the United States. It reached $108 billion USD in 2016 after 5 years of annual growth rates exceeding 25%. Pharmaceutical expenditure comprises 1% of total GDP and 17% of total health care spending. There are 5,000 to 7,000 individual local pharmaceutical manufacturers, with most producing a small slate of generic products. Of total drug sales, just under two-thirds are generic drugs, making the Chinese generic market the largest in the world.

Coverage Determination
After the Chinese Food and Drug Administration grants prescription drugs market authorization, the drugs can be placed on 2 reimbursement lists. The Essential Drugs List (EDL), created in 2009, catalogs medicines that the Chinese government considers essential and that every public primary care clinic must be fully stocked with by 2020. There are around 700 drugs on the EDL, and about one-third are TCMs. Currently the process for selecting EDL drugs is undergoing reform.

The National Reimbursement Drug List (NRDL) was created in 2000. As of 2017, it covers about 1,300 Western drugs and 1,250 TCMs. The National Health Commission (NHC) selects drugs for its formulary in 2 lists, or tracks. List A drugs are completely covered by state health insurance and are given priority use at public hospitals and clinics. Regardless of province, the UEBMI and URRBMI insurance schemes cover these drugs. Most List A drugs are widely used, generic drugs that

Figure 5. Regulation of Pharmaceutical Prices: Competitive Bidding (China)

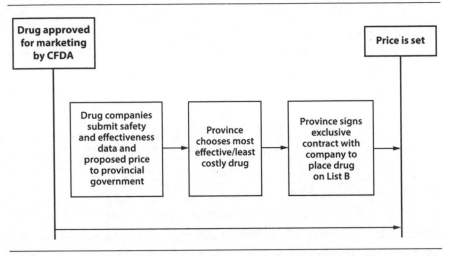

are relatively inexpensive and considered essential. There is substantial overlap between the drugs on List A and the EDL, as the NRDL predates the EDL by almost a decade.

In contrast, List B drugs are not completely covered. Provincial governments may remove up to 15% of the drugs from the national List B, add an equivalent number of different drugs to their provincial List B, and designate those drugs as covered. List B drugs also may require co-pays, which are determined by the provincial governments and can be substantial. Drugs on List B tend to be newer, and many do not yet have generic substitutes.

Drugs that are not included on the EDL or the NRDL must be paid for out of pocket. Drugs are added to the formulary about every 5 years as part of the same process by which their price is determined.

Price Regulation
China currently has 2 different drug pricing systems. It is gradually moving from a negotiating process toward a competitive bidding one.

Under the negotiation system currently being phased out, there are 3 phases of price determination. Negotiations under this system last took place in 2017. In the first phase, expert committees made up of doctors, academics, and government experts selected drugs to participate in price negotiations. In the 2017 round of negotiations, about 4,000 experts participated in the selection process, and 44 drugs were chosen for negotiation.

In the 2nd phase, the government established 2 independent groups of experts to determine a target price at which to begin negotiations. One group evaluates the pharmacoeconomic value of the drug in question, and the other looks at the government's capacity to reimburse the drug. This process is confidential, and manufacturers are not told the target price even once it is reached.

Finally, in the 3rd phase, the manufacturers are given a chance to negotiate the price. If manufacturers offer a price more than 15% higher than the target price, negotiations cannot begin, and the drug will not be admitted to the formulary; if they offer a price less than 15% greater, negotiations can begin. However, the negotiated price cannot exceed the government's target price. This process, although strange, gives manufacturers an incentive to open negotiations with a lower price, thus giving the government a good chance at getting a low price. In the last round of negotiations in 2017, 36 of the 44 drugs were admitted to List B of the formulary, and none had more than a 20% co-pay. On average, the final prices were 44% lower than prices under the previous drug negotiation scheme.

Recently China introduced a competitive bidding process for pharmaceuticals that is being piloted in 4 large cities and 7 provinces. In this process drug companies submit safety and effectiveness data to the provincial or city government along with a proposed price. The provincial government then chooses the drug that is effective and the least costly; it then signs a contract with the producer to place that drug on their province's List B. The company then must sell that drug at the agreed price, completely crowding out competition in the province. The first round of this bidding ended in December 2018, and prices fell an average of 52% from previous negotiated prices.

This pilot process will likely be scaled up to the national level in the next 5 years.

Regulation of Physician Prescriptions

There is little regulation of physician prescriptions. This, in combination with relatively low physician salaries, has led to endemic corruption among doctors. Physicians often take large payouts from pharmaceutical companies in exchange for prescribing their drugs. Although illegal, this practice is pervasive because it allows physicians to substantially increase their income.

Prices Paid by Patients

In theory, patients are well insulated from high drug prices. But, as in many parts of the Chinese health care system, reality is bleaker. Few drugs are fully covered, and those that are covered often come with high co-pays. In addition, many drugs are not included on either List A or List B, so they must be paid for totally out of pocket.

The government claims that individuals pay no more than 30% of their health care spending out of pocket. However, according to one prominent health care researcher, "Many other data indicate that individuals pay more than 30% because there are many drugs not on the formulary, so individuals pay a lot out of pocket."

HUMAN RESOURCES

Physicians

There are 3 kinds of doctors in China: licensed doctors, who must complete medical school; licensed assistant doctors, who need only complete 3 years of junior medical college; and village doctors, who can work in village clinics with only a technical school degree. In 2017, there were 3.4 million licensed doctors and licensed assistant doctors, or about 2.4 doctors per 1,000 people, up from 1.7 per 1,000 people in 2000.

As in most countries, Chinese students who want to become licensed doctors begin training immediately after graduating from high school. Training takes 5 years for a medical bachelor's degree or 3 years in a junior medical college. Students may then choose to continue for 2 or 3 more years to gain a master's or doctorate in medicine, which usually focuses on either experimental medicine or clinical diagnosis. About half of medical students continue on to graduate education. Importantly, an advanced degree is not required to become a practicing physician in hospitals or clinics. The Ministry of Education requires all 5-year programs to provide training in TCM as part of the mandatory curriculum. Doctors may choose to specialize in TCM at the medical bachelor's, master's, and doctoral level.

There are about 180 medical universities, graduating about 600,000 students each year, but only about 100,000 of those go on to become doctors. The rest enter research, biotech, or other higher-paying disciplines. TCM doctors make up about 10% of doctors in China.

Most physicians are public-sector employees, working in strict hierarchies within public hospitals and without much autonomy over their work. The vast majority are specialists. In urban settings, general or family medicine is not as common as in other countries. In 2016, there were only 206,000 primary care physicians in all of China. Lower salaries and lower social standing contribute to the dearth of primary care physicians. The Chinese government is currently encouraging more physicians to become general practitioners, including lowering barriers to enter GP practice and strengthening GP education in public medical schools.

As with many countries, in China there is a substantial urban-rural maldistribution of physicians. In urban areas there are about 4 doctors per 1,000 people, but in rural areas this falls to 1.7 per 1,000 people.

Far more common in rural areas are village doctors, who follow in the midcentury tradition of the barefoot doctors. They are only permitted to practice in village clinics, where they take responsibility for almost all primary and preventive care at the village level. They receive training in basic medical and paramedical treatment. In 2017, there were 968,000 village doctors and assistants working in 632,000 village clinics. About 93% of villages have a clinic, which is often the only accessible health care provider.

Doctor salaries range widely depending on location, experience, place of practice, and specialty. Salaries rarely exceed $30,000 USD (203,000 RMB) a year, and typical salaries are far lower. In reality, however, doctors often take home bonus pay because of kickbacks for prescribing certain drugs, fees from private patients, and even bribes from patients, so called red envelopes. These kickbacks have added to the perception that doctors are corrupt. As a result, violent physical assaults on doctors, usually by patients or their families, oc-cur regularly.

Nurses

The supply of nurses has grown rapidly in the past 2 decades. In 2000, there was only 1 nurse per 1,000 people. By the end of 2017 that number had grown to 2.7 nurses per 1,000 people, or 3.8 million total. How-ever, the supply of nurses is still quite low relative to the size of the population, the number of hospital beds, and international standards. Consequently, there is a high nurse vacancy rate in most hospitals. In addition, nurses are concentrated in urban areas, contributing to the shortage of providers in rural areas. In cities there are 5 nurses per 1,000 people but only 1.6 per 1,000 in rural areas.

Aspiring nurses are required to pass an examination (held once a year) and obtain a professional nursing certificate from the govern-ment. This requirement is waived for those with certain nursing de-grees. Registered nurses are regularly reviewed and required to sit for an examination each year to keep their certificates.

Nurses have somewhat limited roles. Unlike in the Netherlands, for example, they cannot stand in for doctors in simple procedures. They administer tests, shots, and medicines; observe patients and maintain the medical record; and answer questions from patients and their fam-ilies. However, they typically handle large patient loads compared to nurses in other countries. They are also not paid as well as nurses in many other countries. The typical salary for recent nursing graduates is as low as $300 USD (2,032 RMB) per month. As a result, nursing is not a highly regarded profession in China.

CHALLENGES

China has made tremendous leaps in relatively little time toward estab-lishing national access to health insurance for 1.4 billion people through 2 insurance programs. Although gaps in access and out-of-pocket costs relative to income are much larger than in most Western high-income countries, 95% of the population has some form of health insurance.

But, because of its size and political history, the Chinese health care system faces a number of unique and substantial challenges, especially in the delivery of care.

First, the legacy of the one-child policy has broad implications for social policy writ large. Without an adequate number of young workers contributing to the social safety net, health costs will rise as the population ages and fewer workers are contributing to the insurance funds. This problem is exacerbated by the increase in the prevalence of costly chronic illnesses like diabetes and hypertension. The one-child policy also exacerbates the problems of long-term care. Traditionally, adult male children and their wives cared for the husband's parents in their old age. But the one-child policy gives each adult couple 2 sets of parents to care for, which will strain the younger generation's resources. Informal, family-based care is no longer a sustainable solution for this growing elderly population. China urgently needs to address long-term care insurance and infrastructure.

China's large and rapidly growing middle class is beginning to demand better medical care as well. But its health care delivery system is the most hospital centric of all the systems I studied. It is very expensive to build and staff new hospitals to meet the middle class's rising expectations for high-quality care. And it is far more expensive to deliver care in a hospital than in a physician office, clinic, or community health center, which makes combating widespread diseases all the more challenging. Yet China faces serious barriers to moving more care out of hospitals into physician offices and clinics. This would require encouraging more—and more prestigious—physicians to provide clinic- or office-based care. In part, this could be incentivized by raising salaries for nonhospital primary care and specialist physicians. It may also require having physicians who want to practice in hospitals to also practice part of the time in nonhospital office settings. The mismatch between the populations' rising expectations for high-quality health care and providing care predominantly in the hospital will be difficult to resolve given the current system's structure and financing.

A related challenge is how China can introduce more private enterprise into health care. An aging population and the costs of building new hospitals mean that government financing and provision of health care and long-term services will be difficult. One possibility is to introduce more private-sector insurance and delivery of care. Not only might this relieve the government of meeting rising expectations; it might also allow more innovation in the Chinese system. The government, though, seems ambivalent about greater privatization of the health care system. The government's hesitancy of permitting more private health care—and the threat of cutting down whatever emerges—makes it hard to see how a private system can flourish.

The difference in access to care between rural and urban areas also continues to be a challenge. Resources, institutions, and personnel are very unevenly distributed, creating substantial shortages in more rural areas. There are about 4 doctors per 1,000 people in urban areas, but this falls by more than half in rural areas. This maldistribution is even more extreme in the Tibet Autonomous Region and other areas mostly composed of ethnic minorities, like Xinjiang, where quality health care is hard to find. The government needs to incentivize physicians and nurses to move to rural areas as well as to invest more heavily in primary care and GP training, which is more mobile and cheaper to bring to rural areas.

Most troubling, however, is the lack of trust between doctors and patients. Health care—especially public health—requires trust that the system and physicians are acting in patients' best interests and do not need to be bribed to do so. One source of the distrust is both real and perceived corruption in the Chinese health care system. For decades, doctors have been allowed to receive kickbacks from pharmaceutical companies while simultaneously upcharging patients for the very same drugs. Although new laws forbid these practices, both researchers and the public believe that they are still fairly common. Years of corruption have bred mistrust. The ultimate expression is the common violence against doctors and nurses committed by patients or their relatives dissatisfied with their care or its price. In addition, recent rumors that the government is using compulsory health exams to collect DNA to track minority populations further undermines trust. This lack of trust may have the most adverse impact in a public health emergency, as we have seen with the recent coronavirus outbreak. Because of the government's tendency to understate the magnitude of public health crises, patients have not trusted the public health advisories, and the government's suppression of crucial information about the virus's spread has only fostered more distrust. The government needs to build trust in the medical system by making and rigorously enforcing laws to root out corruption. But to have physicians and nurses adhere to these laws and refuse bribes, they will have to be paid much better. This will raise costs.

The Chinese household registration (*hukou*) system in which people are registered in a municipality even if they live and work in far-off urban communities also continues to limit access. Merging URBMI and NCMS will certainly ease some of the issues that rural-to-urban migrants faced in obtaining care, but these issues will not be completely solved until the household registration system is abolished.

Relative to most high-income countries, China lags substantially in mental health care. Like other care in China, mental health care is still hospital based, and resources are unevenly distributed. Mental health disorders are also highly stigmatized in Chinese society; researchers have estimated that fewer than 10% of people with diagnosable mental health disorders seek treatment. As a consequence of the stigma there is a tremendous shortage in mental health personnel. As chronic care becomes an increasingly large portion of health care spending, China will need to address comorbid anxiety and depression, and the government needs to be working harder to create more resources for those in need as well as destigmatize mental illness.

The structural problems in health care are exacerbated by the administrative decentralization. Although from the outside China looks very centralized, with a command-and-control economy, the reality in health care is quite different. Provinces have substantial autonomy over funding, coverage, and prices. This means the central government has difficulty managing costs and transforming practices that inhibit progress. And, because most provinces are either primarily urban or primarily rural, they face fundamentally different structural challenges and funding.

In addition, the last 20 years have brought dozens of different health reforms. In the last 5 years alone, the government has merged 2 major public insurance schemes, overhauled the drug pricing and approval process, moved oversight of health insurance to a new government agency, and abolished the one-child policy. It is hard to evaluate the effects of any one of these changes when they occur in such quick succession. The system needs some stability to allow doctors, patients, and administrators to effectively implement and evaluate the new programs.

The demands on the Chinese system are immense. It needs to serve more than a sixth of the world's population. Although it has achieved an impressive feat by providing health insurance to almost its entire population through 2 health insurance schemes, it also faces unique—and hard-to-change—structural, cultural, and behavioral barriers in delivering high-quality care. The system is excessively focused on hospitals. The population thinks high-quality care can be delivered in Class III national hospitals. The demand for such hospitals will grow as the middle class expands—and it is almost impossible to meet such demand even with big investments. Low trust in the health care system is pervasive because of corruption and other factors. Restoring trust requires increasing physician salaries and changing physician practices. Because of the one-child policy, China has grown old before it has grown rich. The demand for long-term care will put a huge financial burden on families and the government.

To confront these fundamental structural problems, China will need innovation in both the financing and delivery of health care. Yet the system is not structured to foster innovation—or permit more of it in an entrepreneurial private sector. To truly reform and meet growing population demands for better health care services, China will need to change the structure of its health care system. That is no easy task, but the consequences of failing to act could have significant political and social ramifications.

CHAPTER TWELVE

WHO'S THE BEST?

THE LESSONS LEARNED

I began this project with a simple question: Which country has the best health care system?

After studying 11 systems, my answer is: None.

None is a frustrating, annoying, and evasive answer. The reader might feel disappointed—even duped—and tempted to throw this book in the trash. That would be a mistake—or I hope it would be a mistake. Although it is not possible to select the *best* health care system overall, it is possible and reasonable to make judgments about *better* and *worse* systems.

In this book I analyzed each country by considering 7 topics: history, coverage, financing, payment, delivery, pharmaceutical regulation, and workforce. Across these topics I delineated different dimensions of analysis: 3 historical lessons and 22 discrete criteria for evaluating health system performance (see Table 12-1). Countries can—and typically do—perform well on some dimensions and poorly on others. I provided a detailed evaluation based on each criterion. Clearly, just like countries, patients prioritize each dimension differently. That is why it is impossible to claim one system is the "best." It is always important to ask the question: best for whom?

Whereas health policy wonks may care about all 22 evaluative criteria, including effective limits on total spending, alignment of payment incentives, and progressivity of financing, my discussions with patients suggest that they have different priorities. They tend to zero in on health care for themselves and their families. Older patients or

Table 12-1. Performance on 22 Dimensions

Domain	Dimension	Best-Performing Countries	Notably Poor-Performing Countries
Coverage	Universal coverage	Australia Canada France Germany Netherlands Norway Switzerland Taiwan United Kingdom	United States
	Simplicity and ease of obtaining coverage	Australia Canada Norway Taiwan United Kingdom	United States
	Comprehensiveness of benefits	France Germany Netherlands Norway Taiwan United Kingdom United States	Canada China
	Affordability at point of service	Canada Germany Norway United Kingdom	France Switzerland United States
Financing	Progressive financing	Canada United Kingdom	Australia Switzerland United States
	Specially subsidized groups—low income, children, and chronically ill	Canada Germany Netherlands Norway Taiwan	Switzerland United States
	Dedicated mechanism for financing long-term care	Germany Netherlands	China Taiwan

Domain	Dimension	Best-Performing Countries	Notably Poor-Performing Countries
	Effective limits on total health care spending	Netherlands Norway Taiwan United Kingdom	Australia France Switzerland United States
Payment	Alignment of payment incentives	—	China Norway Germany
	Simplicity in paying by patients	Canada Germany Taiwan United Kingdom	United States
	Simplicity in payment to physicians and hospitals	France Taiwan	United States
	Innovation in payment	Netherlands United States	China
Delivery	Choice of physicians and hospitals	France Germany Netherlands Norway Switzerland Taiwan	China United States
	Simplicity of getting services	Canada Germany Norway Taiwan United Kingdom	China United States
	Excellent primary care	Netherlands United Kingdom	China
	Excellent chronic-care coordination	Netherlands United Kingdom United States (all selective areas)	China France Germany Norway Switzerland
	Waiting times	Germany Switzerland Taiwan	Australia Canada Norway United Kingdom

(continues)

Table 12-1 (continued)

Domain	Dimension	Best-Performing Countries	Notably Poor-Performing Countries
	Excellent mental health care	Netherlands United States (all selective areas)	China Switzerland
	Innovation in care delivery	Netherlands United Kingdom United States	China Germany Switzerland
Pharmacy Prices	Low drug prices	Australia Norway Taiwan	Switzerland United States
	Access to innovative drugs	Switzerland United States	
	Rigorous and objective mechanism to price drugs	Australia Norway United Kingdom	United States

those caring for parents put a high priority on long-term care. Conversely, many people emphasize choice of insurer or physician. Today in the United States, many people ask about prescription drug costs. In other countries there tends to be more preoccupation with shorter waiting times for important elective procedures like hip replacement or cataract surgery.

Taking these different dimensions into account, it is clear that although not outstanding in every way, some countries are performing very well. The top tier would include Germany, the Netherlands, Norway, and Taiwan. The top achiever among them would depend upon which set of criteria is being prioritized. For instance, the Netherlands excels at choice of primary care physician and hospital as well as chronic care coordination, and it is one of only 2 countries not muddling through the financing of long-term care—it has explicitly tackled the issue. Importantly, the Netherlands does not perform poorly on any specific dimension. Similarly, Germany offers free choice of sickness fund, any physician, and any hospital in the country; affordable care; no waiting times; and, like the Netherlands, a dedicated funding mechanism for long-term care. Its deficiencies are a significant overuse of hospital care, no system for chronic care coordination, and no real data and incentive to systematically improve the quality of care. In addition, Germany has over 100 sickness funds (insurance companies) that do not seem to really compete and strive to improve quality, thus consuming money with no clear added benefit to patients. Norway is another top-performing country, with good affordability of physicians, hospitals, and pharmaceuticals. It also has a wide choice of physicians and hospitals, although choices narrow for patients once they are admitted to a hospital. The deficits are a heavy financial burden for long-term care on patients and families; suboptimal care coordination, especially for chronic illnesses; and persistent waiting times for certain procedures. Taiwan has excellent choice of physicians and affordability of care, including pharmaceuticals; an outstanding electronic health care system; and nonexistent waiting times. The flip side is that Taiwanese patients have very limited interaction with doctors, who see way too many patients very quickly, Spartan hospitals, no chronic care coordination, and no coherent system for long-term care.

Many countries might be just below the top tier because they do excel at certain metrics but face bigger challenges. For instance, the Swiss are excellent on free choice of physicians and waiting times. The French are excellent on choice of physicians and pharmaceutical costs. The Australians—in the public sector—excel on affordability of services including pharmaceuticals. But each has other deficiencies: The Swiss face high costs, including for pharmaceuticals—2nd only to the United States—and quality is more an article of faith in all things Swiss than an empirical fact. The French have poor care coordination and utilization of preventive services such as vaccines and cancer screening tests. And the Australians have long waiting times (in the public health system) for many procedures.

Finally, there are 2 decidedly poor performers. Maybe not surprisingly, I confirmed the view that the United States underperforms across many dimensions. By far the United States is the most expensive country overall, at the point of care, and on pharmaceuticals. Ironically—and maybe surprisingly to many readers—the choice of physician is much more limited in the United States than in most other countries—not by the government, but by private insurers. (Medicare has excellent choice, but private insurers have constantly changing networks.) And there is no coherent mechanism for financing long-term care. Conversely, probably to the surprise of many readers too, the United States does excel in having many delivery organizations with best-in-class chronic care coordination. It is also the case that although no country has found a "solution" to mental health, the United States—like the Netherlands—has pockets of excellence and promising, innovative initiatives that are worthy of further study and, potentially, emulation.

Even worse than the United States is China. The Chinese system is overly focused on hospitals, with a poorly developed ambulatory care sector and very low patient trust. This is a structural problem built into how doctors are licensed and public perceptions, neither of which are easily altered. There is extensive lack of trust in the system and its physicians, even leading to violent attacks on doctors. There are challenges regarding mental health care and long-term care based on stigma and demography that also seem structural. Maybe most importantly, there is little private-sector experimentation and little sustained drive in the public sector to innovate, especially in trying new mechanisms to improve the delivery of care.

Having tiered the countries, I hope the reader will refrain from chucking the book and read on to my analysis of all 22 dimensions. I begin with 3 key lessons from my historical survey of how the health care systems evolved to where they are today. There are some important surprises in the history worth highlighting.

HISTORY

1. Universal health coverage, even in high-income countries, is relatively recent.

When it comes to health insurance, many people believe that all high-income countries achieved universal coverage long ago and that the United States is a historical outlier. This impression is misleading. Although many countries began extending coverage to portions of their population many decades ago—even in the 19th century—the assurance of *universal* coverage is much more recent.

The earliest truly universal health insurance scheme was established in 1946 when the UK implemented the National Health Service Act. Although many people identify Bismarck's enactment of health insurance in Germany in the 1880s as the beginning of universal coverage, Bismarck's plan only applied to urban industrial workers—10% of the population. The other 90% remained uninsured. Only in 1972, after adding select groups—such as agricultural workers, the self-employed, and the unemployed—in a stepwise fashion over many decades, did all segments of (West) German society achieve truly universal coverage.

Most other countries have had similar paths of slowly expanding coverage. France introduced national insurance in 1945 for commercial and industrial workers, but it was not until 2000 that coverage became truly universal. In 1912, Switzerland began regulating and subsidizing health insurance funds. In 1914, Basel became the first Swiss municipality to mandate health insurance coverage. Other municipalities and cantons followed suit, and by 1959 80% of the Swiss population had health insurance. However, Switzerland did not achieve universal coverage until 1994, with the passage of the Federal Health Insurance Law, which legally mandated that individuals purchase health insurance or face severe penalties. Australia uniquely achieved universal coverage, repealed it, and then reinstituted it. In 1972, the Labor Party passed Medibank, a compulsory universal health insurance system. The Liberal coalition repealed Medibank in 1981, but the Labor Party returned to power in 1983 and passed Medicare, the current compulsory universal health insurance system.

China's first universal health plan began in 1949 when Mao Zedong came to power, but it only theoretically covered the entire population. Much of rural China lacked access to basic medical services. Over the next 30 years barefoot doctors helped expand care, mostly rudimentary and preventive services throughout the country, but true universality for all 1.4 billion Chinese to modern medicine remains elusive.

Universal coverage came to Taiwan in 1995—in a single burst. Taiwan had relied on independent insurance funds, which served different parts of the labor market, leaving 40% of the population with no coverage. Then, in the 1990s, the economy was growing at breakneck speed and the political system was liberalizing rapidly. The public demanded health insurance coverage, and political leaders wanted to "catch up" with other developed countries.

Although other countries may have achieved universal coverage much later than is commonly assumed, they have insured over 99% of the population. The United States has not, making it an outlier among developed countries. The Affordable Care Act created a framework for universal coverage, but about 10% of the US population remains uncovered. However, that some states, such as Massachusetts, have achieved nearly 98% coverage suggests the framework can get universal coverage. Unfortunately, due to ideology, inadequate subsidies, and complexity, universal coverage remains elusive for the United States.

2. Paths to universal health coverage have varied, but universality has never been fully reversed.

Different countries have come to universal coverage in different ways.

Conventional wisdom suggests that countries enact sweeping legislation only during crises: wars, economic depressions, or both. Germany enacted its first health reform in 1883 in response to major labor unrest and threats of revolution during industrialization. During World War II the United States incentivized expansion of private employer-based health insurance to keep the labor market afloat, and Nazi occupation brought to the Netherlands mandatory health insurance for low- and middle-income people. World War II catalyzed the establishment of the British NHS and France's expansion of health insurance coverage to all workers. Even the Affordable Care Act coincided with the Great Recession.

However, in many other countries neither military nor economic crisis precipitated universal coverage. The Dutch began considering a system of managed competition among private insurance companies with an individual mandate in the late 1980s and finally enacted the system in 2006, an otherwise quiet period in Dutch history. The current managed competition system in Switzerland was legislated in 1994—not a time of military or economic crisis. In the mid-1960s, Norway made health coverage one of the tax-financed benefits as part of an integration of its welfare state programs; no war or major economic crisis prompted this legislation. In Australia, health care was the focus of political conflict between the Liberal and Labor parties for decades.

A sweeping Labor Party electoral victory—in a campaign focused on health care—was the pivotal event. The impetus for universal coverage in Taiwan was when its political system opened up. The nationalist party that had run the country since the 1940s began to allow real democracy and competition among parties, unleashing public demands for better health care that officials felt compelled to answer.

There is no consistent path to universal coverage. Sometimes a crisis catalyzes a leap to universality. Sometimes the path is more gradual or piecemeal. Importantly, except for a brief, 2-year moment in Australia, there is no case in which universal coverage, once achieved, has been undone. And even in Australia, when the Liberal (conservative) government repealed universal coverage, they were devastated at the polls.

3. Health care systems are path dependent.

The global story of universal coverage vividly illustrates how path dependence works, both within countries and across them. The German health and pension systems, instituted in the 1880s, had significant influence on subsequent policies adopted in Europe and the United States. Germany institutionalized 65 as the age of eligibility of government-funded pensions, used payroll taxes with employer and employee contributions, and cultivated a central role for employer-based private insurance—that is, sickness funds. Other countries subsequently adopted many of these structures. The United States, France, and the Netherlands all use payroll taxes to finance government-supported health coverage. Similarly, private insurance plays a major role—with government sanction and/or financial support—in France, the Netherlands, Switzerland, Australia, and the United States.

On the national level certain structural decisions are hard to undo. Subsequent reforms almost always work within the constraints of existing institutions. Even Taiwan's single-payer system, which represented a relatively clean break with its past, adapted elements of its earlier sickness fund system. Officials deliberately created a benefits package that would resemble—but exceed—what prior sickness funds offered.

When financing models do shift, the most typical change is gradual: from exclusively single payer to a greater role for private health insurance. This is usually intended to lower health care costs and restrain government spending by shifting costs to the private sector and attempting to inject more competition into the system. In the mid-1990s and 2000s, both Switzerland and the Netherlands introduced a kind of managed competition with an individual mandate to purchase coverage from competing private health insurance companies. Similarly, Australia, France, and the UK have encouraged private insurance so as to restrain government health care spending.

I found no system that transitioned from well-developed private financing to single payer. Two factors probably explain this single direction of evolution. Shifting toward government financing requires higher taxes, which is politically difficult in any country, especially ones with aging populations and increasing demands for pensions and long-term care. Moreover, once insurance companies become entrenched, their economic power, political influence, and central administrative role stymie efforts to dislodge them. If the United States successfully shifts to single payer, that would be a historic moment, unique among the countries I examined.

COVERAGE

An overriding goal of every health care system, regardless of the country, is to provide health *care* to *all* its citizens. Universal coverage is necessary, but it is not sufficient. The simplicity of obtaining coverage, comprehensiveness of benefits, and affordability to individuals are also of fundamental importance. This yields 4 dimensions for evaluating countries' performance coverage: (1) universality, (2) simplicity and ease of getting care, (3) comprehensiveness of benefits, and (4) affordability at the point of service (see Table 12-1).

All countries make trade-offs between universality, comprehensiveness of benefits, and affordability. When the US National Academy of Medicine made recommendations regarding essential benefits in the ACA, it noted that universality and affordability should take priority over comprehensiveness of benefits. This is a common—and correct—view.

Gro Brundtland, former prime minister of Norway and former director general of the WHO, said that the goal is for a system to achieve universality and retain affordability before covering every possible benefit. It is widely accepted that some health care services provide less benefit than others and can ethically be left to individual discretion without a major impact on health. But it is important that those trade-offs not exclude benefits that are truly indispensable, such as cancer care or vaccinations. Consequently, many countries have excluded coverage of dental and vision care from their health care benefits, leaving it to supplemental insurance or out-of-pocket costs. Other countries exclude these services for adults but cover them for children. These decisions may be controversial, especially with our growing knowledge about the link between oral and more general physical health, but it is the norm rather than the exception.

Norway may have the best performance on all 4 dimensions. Coverage is universal: fully 99.6% of Norwegian residents have health insurance. Getting coverage is simple: all residents—not just citizens—are automatically enrolled when they pay taxes. The tax-financed benefits are comprehensive, with the major exception being long-term care, which has high out-of-pocket costs. Similarly, Taiwan's National Health Insurance (NHI) is also truly universal, simple, comprehensive, and affordable. The benefit package includes just about everything—inpatient and outpatient services, Western medicine, traditional Chinese treatments, and dental and vision care for both children and adults. The excluded benefits in Taiwan are idiosyncratic, including birth control, abortion, smoking cessation therapy, and drug addiction therapy. Although there is significant cost sharing for some, Taiwan, like many countries, reduces or eliminates out-of-pocket spending for people with certain serious conditions or low incomes. Similarly, the UK's National Health Service is universal, simple, comprehensive, and affordable at the point of care. Just showing up to get care ensures enrollment. NHS benefits are also relatively comprehensive—dental care is covered with a co-pay—and there are no costs at the point of service.

France has achieved universal coverage with a broad benefits package, but the financial protection is shallow. The French benefits package, though comprehensive, requires significant cost sharing. Consequently, about 95% of the population has supplementary private insurance to address cost-sharing burdens.

As France opted for comprehensive benefits with significant co-pays, Canada went in the opposite direction. Canada has no cost sharing for any service deemed medically necessary, although "medically necessary" is more narrowly construed: it does not cover dental and vision care nor long-term care. And, perhaps most surprisingly, most provinces do not cover prescription drugs. Consequently, nearly 67% of Canadian residents purchase supplemental insurance for drugs, dental care, and vision care.

In Germany, the Netherlands, and Switzerland, coverage is universal, but the process of getting it is more complex. Individuals must select a plan and pay premiums to private insurance companies or sickness funds.

Clearly the United States performs poorly on universality, simplicity, and affordability. About 10% of the population still has no health insurance, and getting coverage is complex and cumbersome. It is estimated that most of the uninsured actually are eligible for some sort of coverage at a reasonable price, but the processes of establishing Medicaid eligibility or buying insurance on the exchanges are complex, time consuming, and confusing.

However, the 10 essential benefits that US health insurers are required to cover are comprehensive, including the usual care categories as well as services for mental health and substance abuse, drug coverage, and dental and vision care for children. In addition, some crucial services, including an annual wellness visit and a host of preventive services, are free at the point of care. As with many countries, a big deficiency for an aging population in the United States is the absence of long-term care insurance except if a person becomes impoverished and is eligible for Medicaid. And affordability for individuals is increasingly problematic: high-deductible plans have become more pervasive and drug costs increasingly burdensome, especially for individuals with chronic illnesses—only Switzerland imposes higher out-of-pocket costs than the United States.

FINANCING

Health care in any developed country is expensive, and financing it requires substantial, value-laden decisions. I identified 4 dimensions to assess health care financing across the countries: (1) progressivity of financing, (2) financial protections for vulnerable populations, (3) sustainable long-term care financing, and (4) mechanisms to control health care spending growth.

The American debate over health care financing is often between advocates of single payer versus those of private insurance. As I learned, this is too simplistic—and, in some countries, just inaccurate. There are at least 5 different ways of financing health care (see Table 12-2). How the financing measures up against the 4 dimensions is more important than whether it is structured more as single payer or private insurance.

The UK is at one end of the spectrum, with a socialized system funded through taxes and with government ownership of most of the delivery system. A private health insurance system parallels the NHS, but it is not integral to the function of the NHS. There is no dedicated NHS tax, so the financing is as progressive as the underlying tax system—which by OECD measures is the 4th most progressive, after the United States, Italy, and Ireland.

Many countries have eschewed fully socialized medicine, opting for single-payer systems, with the government financing almost all health care, while leaving some insurance and much of the delivery system private. In Canada and Norway, over 90% of financing is public, but there are tiny private insurance sectors and predominantly private physicians, and some hospitals are private.

In France and Australia, a single-payer system is the foundation of the coverage model. But unlike Canada and Norway, there is a substantial and structural role for the private health insurance system. Put another way, the public system heavily relies on—and encourages—a functioning private insurance market.

Germany and the Netherlands have a single payer but rely on multiple private insurers to actually pay for care. In Germany, the public statutory health system covers nearly 90% of the population and is financed by payroll taxes that are distributed to private sickness funds. In addition, about 11% of the population, based on income and type of job, have private health insurance totally separate from the statutory health system. In the Netherlands, the government requires that all people have health insurance, collects payroll taxes to distribute to private insurers, and uses general revenues to subsidize the purchase of private insurance.

Table 12-2. Different Mechanisms of Financing Health Care

Country	Socialized Medicine	Single Payer with Very Limited Private Insurance	Single Payer with Substantial Private Insurance	Single Payer Channeled Through Private Insurance	Individuals Purchase Private Insurance with Government Subsidies
Australia			X		
Canada		X			
China		X			
France			X		
Germany				X	
Netherlands				X	
Norway		X			
Switzerland					X
Taiwan		X			
United Kingdom	X				
United States	VA	Traditional Medicare parts A and B, some state Medicaid	Traditional Medicare and Medigap	Medicare Advantage and Managed Medicaid	Exchanges and employer-sponsored insurance

Switzerland is not a single-payer system at all. It mandates that individuals purchase private health insurance. It provides government subsidies to help low- and middle-income families pay the private insurance premiums.

The complex US system has every kind of financing arrangement. Like the UK, the Department of Veterans Affairs is a socialized system. Like Canada and Norway, traditional Medicare payment for hospitals (Part A), physician services (Part B), and some state Medicaid programs are true single-payer systems. Like France, Medicare patients are able but not required to buy supplemental private insurance—Medigap plans—to help cover co-pays and additional services in traditional Medicare. The German model is analogous to Medicare Advantage (Part C) and states with managed Medicaid plans. In these cases, the federal and state governments collect money and then allocate it to private insurers who organize and pay for the actual care. Like Switzerland, the health insurance exchanges and employer-sponsored insurance allow individual Americans to buy insurance with government assistance. In the insurance exchanges the subsidies are income based, and in the employer-sponsored part of the American system, subsidies flow through the tax exclusion. One way of describing this complexity in the US financing of health care is an incomprehensible mess that has grown up over time devoid of design and rationality—and now justification. Doubtless, that fuels part of the appeal of Medicare for All.

The first financing dimension is how progressive or regressive the system is. Ultimately, because health costs are so large, few citizens can afford to pay for health insurance on their own. Every system relies heavily on government financing, either directly or through subsidies for private insurance. Thus, how progressive a system is depends on how much it relies on premiums and which taxes are used for financing. In general, relying heavily on a flat premium—that is, the same across income levels—is regressive because it is more financially burdensome to low- and middle-income individuals even if there are some subsidies. Similarly, heavily relying on premiums and some taxes, such as value-added taxes (VAT), means the system will be regressive.

Switzerland may be the most regressive country in this regard because it heavily relies on individuals paying premiums that are not income linked, with modest government subsidies for low- and middle-income individuals. The United States heavily relies on private insurance premiums, and the tax exclusion for employer-sponsored insurance that disproportionately benefits high-income citizens further exacerbates the system's regressivity. A surcharge on the wealthy, implemented by the ACA, to finance expansion of coverage has slightly ameliorated the regressive payroll tax that funds part of traditional Medicare.

In primarily publicly financed systems—such as Australia, Canada, China, France, the Netherlands, Norway, and the UK—the progressivity of financing health care is a function of the underlying tax system. For instance, the relatively high Norwegian VAT used to finance much of the government is regressive. Germany largely uses more regressive payroll taxes for the statutory health system. Conversely, in Canada payment comes from general tax revenue, which is mostly generated by progressive income taxes. Overall, the UK and Canada, with their relatively progressive tax systems, probably have the most progressive health care financing arrangements.

The 2nd dimension of financing is how well vulnerable populations are protected from excess health care costs. There are 3 specific financially vulnerable groups who typically receive special financial protection: low-income individuals, those with chronic conditions that require significant amounts of health care, and children.

All systems have some way of subsidizing low-income individuals, with varying degrees of effectiveness. In some cases—such as Canada and the UK—low-income individuals pay little to no taxes but get the same health benefits as everyone else in the public system, often with no co-payments at the point of service.

Australians earning under about US$16,000 are exempt from the 2% Medicare tax, and those earning under US$20,000 pay only a portion of it. Despite the fixed income payroll tax in the Netherlands, the government subsidizes the additional premiums paid to insurers for all families with incomes under US$41,000. Taiwan subsidizes low-income residents and has some other plans to help them, including interest-free loans for people who have outstanding medical debt.

Similarly, Americans who earn below 138% of the poverty line (approximately $34,000 for a family of 4) are eligible to receive premium-free health coverage through Medicaid, but only in the 37 states and Washington, DC, that have expanded Medicaid. In Medicare, the premiums assessed for physician services and drugs are income-linked and subsidized at about 75% of the cost. In addition, the exchanges have income-linked subsidies for the purchase of private insurance for households earning up to 400% of the poverty line ($100,000 for a family of 4).

Switzerland may have the worst subsidization of low-income individuals. Although the government requires that all cantons subsidize low-income individuals and provides funds for those subsidies, the number of subsidies, income level for eligibility for subsidies, and how individuals apply for relief varies by canton.

Low-income populations also receive special treatment with regards to co-pays and other out-of-pocket payments. The UK and Canada have no payment at the point of service, automatically making it friendlier to people with low incomes. In Germany, low-income individuals are exempt from all co-pays. Taiwan waives out-of-pocket expenses for its poorest residents, veterans, children under 3, and patients with catastrophic illnesses like cancer. Additionally, Taiwan's NHI waives prescription co-pays for roughly 100 chronic conditions— including diabetes and high blood pressure—as well as co-pays for certain intense physical therapies; it also reduces co-pays for people living in remote areas. In Norway, the government handles all co-pays once they exceed about $250 per year for an individual, regardless of income. The Australian government sets an annual out-of-pocket limit of $330 on payments for all nonhospital care.

In the United States, the states set the co-pays on Medicaid, although the federal government establishes a low out-of-pocket maximum for those co-pays. For instance, co-pays cannot exceed $4 for physician office visits and $75 for hospitalizations. In the insurance exchanges cost-sharing subsidies are applied for all individuals earning under $30,000 per year and families earning under $60,000. (Previously the federal government compensated insurance companies for these subsidies, but now they are built into the premiums because President Trump canceled the payments.) Many people in the employer-based market have out-of-pocket limits as well, but they are set too high to offer relief for many middle-class Americans.

Many countries also protect patients with specific expensive conditions. In France the government pays 100% of health care costs for people with a chronic illness. In the Netherlands and Switzerland community rating subsidizes the premiums for sicker-than-average patients. In many countries patients with chronic illnesses are often not required to pay co-pays or they pay much lower rates. For instance, in Norway, patients with HIV/AIDS—but not other chronic diseases—have no co-pays for primary care physician visits. In Germany, patients with chronic illnesses are exempt from co-pays once they pay 1% of gross income in co-pays. The UK waives prescription co-pays for people with some chronic illnesses, including diabetes and cancer, and Taiwan does the same.

Most countries insulate families with children from pediatric health care costs. In the Netherlands, the government pays premiums for all children under 18. Similarly, in Germany the payroll taxes used to finance the statutory health system are the same for single individuals and those who are married or have children, and there are no co-pays for children. Norway covers all dental and vision care for children at no cost to parents. Switzerland subsidizes 50% of insurance premiums for children and young adults aged 18 to 25 in low- and middle-income households. The UK waives all co-pays for prescription drugs for children.

The United States has the least financial protection for families with children. Private health insurance premiums for such families are not subsidized, placing a huge burden on families. Frequently, families face high deductibles and co-pays for pediatric care. The difference between individual and family premiums in employer-sponsored insurance is about $14,000.

A 3rd dimension is the financing of long-term care. Every developed country is facing both increases in the absolute number of elderly people and a relative rise in the proportion of nonworking elderly compared to workers who finance their care.

The Netherlands and Germany stand out because both have dedicated taxes to finance long-term care. In the Netherlands payroll taxes, patient co-pays for services, and government subsidies from income taxes finance long-term care. Coverage historically focused on institutional care, but it has since evolved to include care at home. Germany's long-term care insurance parallels its health insurance, functioning partly through statutory sickness funds and partly through private health insurance. Most of the 3.3 million beneficiaries receive cash payments for care at home. The payments can compensate family caregivers or be used for the hiring of professional care providers.

In Norway, municipalities are responsible for funding long-term care through the single-payer social and health insurance system. This creates a trade-off between funding primary health care services and long-term care. Norway prioritizes younger people, subsidizing primary care, especially for children, and imposing high out-of-pocket costs on the elderly for long-term care.

In recognizing its oncoming demographic crisis, China is beginning to experiment with long-term care insurance at the provincial level. A pilot program is focused on those with disabilities and aims to cover 70% of the costs of care. Long-term care is the biggest gap in Taiwan's coverage scheme. Paying for it remains a challenge and, since 2000, has been the subject of 2 major legislative efforts. An attempt to integrate long-term care into national health insurance fell apart when the party that favored it lost control of the government. Taiwan presently handles long-term care through a separate program that operates more like welfare than social insurance, leaving many residents paying large out-of-pocket costs.

In the United States Medicaid covers long-term care for low-income elderly people, but qualifying is complex and requires impoverishment. For the vast majority of elderly, there is no mandatory long-term care coverage. Indeed, an attempt to include voluntary long-term care insurance in the ACA was repealed because of insufficient and unstable financing. In addition, private, long-term care insurance is disappearing. Where it continues, it is limited to short, usually 3-year terms.

THE FINAL DIMENSION of financing relates to whether a country has effective limits on total health care spending. Many countries have a fixed health care budget that imposes discipline on spending and spending growth. The UK, with its socialized system, and other countries with predominantly single-payer financing and limited private insurance have governmental budget limits on total health care spending. Norway's Ministry of Health sets the budget for the 4 regional health associations that, in turn, set total hospital spending. The

Dutch minister of health sets a total health budget and, if it is exceeded, is empowered to recoup money from insurers. Initially, Taiwan did not have a national health budget, but shortly after introducing the national health insurance scheme it added one to control spending. Taiwan adjusts payment levels to physicians quarterly to remain within its budget.

Conversely, countries such as Switzerland and the United States, which rely on private insurance for a substantial portion of the financing, have no mechanism to establish a total health care budget and cannot impose limits on spending growth. In the United States, Medicare and Medicaid comprise over $1.3 trillion in spending, and while they are government programs, they do not have fixed budgets; they are open-ended entitlements. Although the government sets prices, total expenditures fluctuate based on use, which is determined largely by physicians—and often the severity of an influenza season. However, to limit health care cost increases, several US states, such as Massachusetts, have begun linking permissible increases in spending to a combination of the aging of the population and growth in the state GDP.

Because many factors affect per capita health care expenditures, a budget alone does not correlate with low spending. For instance, we know that the higher a country's per capita income, the higher its per capita health care spending. Norway is the best example of this. Nevertheless, countries without budgets, such as Switzerland and the United States, tend to have higher per capita health care spending. Conversely, countries with strict government budgets and effective enforcement mechanisms—such as Canada, Germany, Taiwan, and the UK—have lower per capita health care spending (see Table 12-3). France, which depends heavily on private insurance to supplement the public sector, has a moderately high per capita spending. Thus, it appears that having a global, government-established budget restrains health care costs and cost growth effectively.

PAYMENT

There are 4 key dimensions of payment: (1) alignment between different providers to optimize care and care coordination, (2) simplicity

Table 12-3. Health Care Spending

Country	Health Care Spending as Percentage of GDP (2017 or most recent available)	Health Care Spending per Capita in USD (2017 or most recent available)
Australia	10.3[1]	$5,200[1]
Canada	11.3[2]	$4,800[2]
China	6.2[3]	$960[3]
France	11.5[4]	$4,600[5]
Germany	11.5[6]	$6,200[6]
The Netherlands	10.1[7]	$5,000[7]
Norway	10.4[8]	$7,400[8]
Switzerland	12.2[9]	$9,700[9]
Taiwan	6.3[10]	$1,500[10]
United Kingdom	9.6[11]	$3,900[11]
United States	17.9[12]	$10,700[12]

1. Australian Institute for Health and Welfare, "Reports & Data," Australian Institute of Health and Welfare, www.aihw.gov.au/reports-data.

2. Data for 2018. Canadian Institute for Health Information, *National Health Expenditure Trends, 1975 to 2018* (Ottawa, ON: CIHI, 2019), www.cihi.ca/en/health-spending/2018/national-health-expenditure-trends.

3. Data for 2016. National Bureau of Statistics of China, *China Statistical Yearbook 2017*. China Statistics Press; 2017. http://www.stats.gov.cn/tjsj/ndsj/2017/indexeh.htm.

4. Data for 2016. Santé MdSedlm Les dépenses de santé en 2017—Résultats des comptes de la santé—édition 2018, 2018, http://drees.solidarites-sante.gouv.fr/IMG/pdf/cns_2017.pdf.

5. Data for 2016. OECD, *Health at a Glance 2017—OECD Indicators* (Paris: Organisation for Economic Co-operation and Development, 2017), www.oecd.org/health/health-systems/health-at-a-glance-19991312.htm.

6. Statistisches Bundesamt, "Health Expenditure," Destatis, 2019, www.destatis.de/EN/Themes/Society-Environment/Health/Health-Expenditure/_node.html.

7. CBS Netherlands, "Health Expenditure: Functions and Financing for International Comparisons, June 21, 2019, https://opendata.cbs.nl/statline/#/CBS/en/dataset/84043ENG/table?ts=1548188388918.

8. Organisation for Economic Co-operation and Development, "Health Expenditure and Financing," OECD.Stat, 2019, https://stats.oecd.org/.

9. Data for 2016. Swiss Confederation, *Statistical Data on Health and Accident Insurance* (Federal Office of Public Health FOPH, 2018), www.bag.admin.ch/bag/en/home/zahlen-und-statistiken/statistiken-zur-krankenversicherung/weitere-statistiken-zur-krankenversicherung.html.

10. Data for 2016. Ministry of Health and Welfare, *2018 Taiwan Health and Welfare Report* (Taipei, Taiwan: Ministry of Health and Welfare, 2018), www.cdway.com.tw/gov/mhw2/book107/book1e/#p=22.

11. Office for National Statistics, *Healthcare Expenditure, UK Health Accounts: 2017* (Office for National Statistics, 2019), www.ons.gov.uk/peoplepopulationandcommunity/healthandsocialcare/healthcaresystem/bulletins/ukhealthaccounts/2017.

12. Centers for Medicare & Medicaid Services, *National Health Expenditures 2017 Highlights* (Department of Health and Human Services, 2018), www.cms.gov/Research-Statistics-Data-and-Systems/Statistics-Trends-and-Reports/NationalHealthExpendData/Downloads/highlights.pdf.

for patients, (3) simplicity for physicians and hospitals, and (4) introduction of innovative mechanisms to achieve higher quality and lower costs.

No country had optimal alignment of payment incentives. Many systems have legacy payment mechanisms that rigidly segregate ambulatory care from hospital care and hospital-based specialty care. This is a cautionary lesson. Segregating payments inhibits—if not totally precludes—alignment in care delivery, especially between hospitals and primary care. It impedes the shift of medical services out of expensive hospital facilities and into lower-cost ambulatory care settings and even patients' homes. This frustrates the coordination of care, which is especially important for chronically ill patients. Typically, the party financially responsible for ambulatory and home care resists shifting care out of hospitals.

In Norway, municipalities pay for primary care, home care, and long-term care, whereas the national government pays for hospital services. In Australia, it is the reverse: the national government pays for physician services, whereas the state and territory governments have the largest financial liability for hospital care. In Germany, sickness funds pay hospitals for services, state governments pay hospital capital costs, and sickness funds pay the state physician associations, which then pay physicians based on a risk-adjusted fee-for-service basis.

These types of divided payments create misaligned incentives. In Norway deinstitutionalization lowers costs for the regional health authorities that cover hospital costs while also increasing costs for the municipalities, thus disincentivizing municipalities from expanding ambulatory care services, home care, and long-term care. Germany's divided payments lead to over-hospitalization. For political reasons, German states are loath to close hospitals, so they spend on hospitals' capital and building costs, generating an oversupply of hospital beds and increasing costs for sickness funds.

Alignment is more likely when the same organization pays for both ambulatory care and hospital care. This typically occurs when insurance companies or one governmental body is responsible for the full payment. Therefore, in addition to having one party be financially responsible for both settings, the mechanism of payment matters too. Fee-for-service tends to inhibit alignment, whereas capitation and bundles improve it. No country excelled at aligning payment to incentivize coordinated care. More work needs to be done in this area.

Simplicity in payment is a virtue. There are 2 main perspectives on simplicity—the patient's, and the physician and hospital's. A simple, successful payment system should be easily navigable for patients and should minimize administrative hassles for hospitals and physicians. The UK excels at such simplicity. Patients have no deductibles and co-pays for primary care; co-pays are restricted to a limited range of services, such as examinations for life and disability insurance. Primary care providers are paid risk-adjusted capitation, with bonuses for quality performance and some fee-for-service payments for providing "enhanced services." Hospitals are paid DRG and receive additional add-on payments for research, training, and services not in the DRG, such as mental health. In the world of health care financing, this qualifies as simple.

In Canada, payment is also simple for patients: most physician office visits and hospitalizations have no co-pay and no coinsurance. In Germany, there is a low, flat, daily co-pay for hospitalizations and no co-pay for physician visits. However, payment from sickness funds to physicians is more complex: physicians receive only a percentage of their total billings; the amount depends upon total billings of all primary care or specialist physicians in the state. Hence, their exact payment for services is known only after they have delivered the services—a point they sorely complain about.

In Switzerland, primary care physicians and specialists are paid fee-for-service, based on a uniform, national fee schedule (tariff). Billing patients above the set fee is illegal. In managed care some primary care physicians are paid capitation. Swiss patients choose their insurance option and know what they are paying in advance, and physicians know the fee schedule for each visit and procedure.

The French payment system is also laudably simple. Physicians are paid fee-for-service, based on rates set in a national contract between the Ministry of Health and the National Union of Health Insurance Funds (UNCAM). Less than 10% of physician payment comes from incentive payments. Physicians who do not balance bill receive the fixed rate per patient as well as certain financial benefits, including a 2% reduction in the rate for social security payments.

In Australia, payment is simple for patients with Medicare at a publicly financed hospital: free—no deductible, no co-pay, no coinsurance. Patient payment to physicians is a bit more complicated, though. For primary care, Medicare pays 100% of the Medicare schedule fee, but if the physician's charge is higher than the Medicare schedule fee, the patient is responsible for the difference (gap fees). Typically, the patient pays the physician the full amount, and Medicare electronically reimburses the patients' bank account within a few days for the Medicare schedule fee amount.

Taiwan's system is relatively simple. Patients face modest out-of-pocket expenses at the point of service, with certain vulnerable populations facing no out-of-pocket payments. However, the back-end system—the payment to physicians and hospitals—is more complex. The primary method of reimbursement is fee-for-service, with payments that the government adjusts each quarter based on use patterns to stay within the national budget. But there is also a DRG system that covers about one-quarter of inpatient care.

Finally, because fee-for-service and DRG payments do not reward higher quality or more efficient care, some countries are innovating and experimenting with new payment models, with the United States and the Netherlands leading the way. Ironically, the complexity and high cost of the US health care system incentivizes innovation. Under the label of value-based payments, for the last decade the United States has been actively experimenting with alternatives that incentivize greater attention to restraining total cost of health care while also improving quality. For primary care, this typically means some kind of risk-adjusted capitation that includes financial risk for total cost of care and/or quality. In addition, there are experiments with bundling, which are lump-sum payments mainly to surgeons and specialists to reimburse for all costs associated with an episode of care. Bundles usually include hospital care, all physician visits, and posthospital care for a period of time, typically 90 days. The payment innovations are moving toward 2-*sided* risk: financially rewarding higher-quality and lower-cost care and penalizing lower quality and higher costs. Increasingly, the emphasis has been on total cost of care, which incentivizes shifting care to lower-cost settings such as the home. Similarly, the Dutch have experimented with bundled payments for certain chronic conditions, such as diabetes and COPD.

Other countries are tracking these innovations in the hopes of implementing the most successful policies. For example, several of the French health policy experts I met with were interested in the design and results of bundled payment experiments in the United States.

DELIVERY SYSTEM

I have identified 7 important dimensions of health care delivery systems: (1) choice of physicians and hospitals, (2) simplicity of navigating the system to get appropriate care, (3) quality of primary care services, (4) good coordination of care for chronically ill patients, (5) waiting times, (6) mental health care, and (7) innovation in care delivery methods.

When it comes to choice, Germany, Switzerland, and Taiwan seem close to ideal. German patients can see any primary care or specialist physician they want anywhere in the country, and they can see as many of them as they want without restriction. German patients also have free choice of any hospital in the country. And there are no complaints of waiting lists.

Swiss patients with the regular, basic insurance can go to any doctor (insurers are required to cover any willing provider) and can go to any hospital in any canton. Similarly, the Taiwanese have unlimited choice of both physician and hospital without a referral; the only incentive for obtaining a primary care referral is a relatively modest discount in out-of-pocket costs. Patients can even show up at ambulatory centers and hospitals and ask for tests on their own, without physician orders.

Other countries have free choice of primary care providers, but there are restrictions on access to specialists. In Norway, patients have the right to choose any primary care provider and can switch twice a year. Similarly, in the Netherlands, France, and Australia, patients have free choice of primary care provider and can switch at any time. But the primary care gatekeeper model may restrict choice of specialists and hospitals. France has a relatively weak primary care gatekeeper model, and patients can easily go to any specialist. In Australia, Norway, and the Netherlands, access to specialists and other parts of the system requires a referral from a primary care provider to a specific specialist or clinic. This is typically enforced by limiting or prohibiting payment when there is no referral.

Simplicity for patients is a crucial dimension of delivery. It should be easy for patients to navigate the health care system and get care without barriers. The Norwegian, Canadian, German, and UK systems shine here. Although there may be wait times and primary care referrals are necessary, there are no prior authorizations from insurers, no out-of-network providers with higher co-pays, and no or few costs at the point of service.

On the dimensions of patient choice and simplicity in use, the United States fails miserably. Many patients are subject to opaque and constantly shifting networks that limit their choice of physicians and hospitals. In addition, many patients need navigators to help them figure out who to get care from. With ever-shifting networks of physicians and hospitals and physicians at in-network hospitals who themselves might be out of network, the need for prior authorization, along with many other barriers, it is hard to figure out who and what is actually covered by insurance.

Outstanding primary care services are critical for a successful delivery system. In this regard, the Netherlands stands out. Dutch primary care providers are the first and principal line of care for all patients. Primary care physicians ensure that patients receive necessary preventive services, are promptly cared for by someone who has access to their medical history, have access to competent after-hours urgent—but not emergency—care, and get quick referrals to competent specialists. In addition, most primary care physicians have nurses dedicated to providing first-line mental health care. To retain their medical registration, Dutch primary care physicians must participate in after-hours cooperatives for at least 50 hours a year. These cooperatives efficiently provide after-hours care and are open daily until at least 8:00 p.m., including weekends and holidays, providing prompt primary care and emergency referrals. Dutch primary care physicians act as strong gatekeepers. Their professional societies have robust care guidelines, which promote an ethos of not overtesting or overtreating. Providing this level of primary care requires systematic recordkeeping as well as outreach for cancer screenings and immunizations, same-day appointments for urgent problems, and a good call system with shared electronic records.

Other countries, such as France, also have good primary care physicians but may make it easy for patients to go directly to specialists without referrals or fail to disincentivize the use of specialists when primary care physicians might be just as good. Not incentivizing the use of primary care physicians or allowing patients to go to specialists without referrals can inhibit care coordination.

THE 4TH DIMENSION is coordination of care for chronically ill patients—an issue of growing importance as chronic conditions become a greater disease burden. All countries are transitioning from a 20th-century acute and reactive health system, designed around hospital-based interventions, to the 21st-century "chronic, connected, and proactive" health system, designed around frequent and proactive engagement with patients in outpatient settings. Chronic care coordination means not waiting for patients to present with problems but instead having frequent interactions initiated by the medical team to identify problems early and forestall exacerbations that can require expensive hospital care.

Many countries have poor coordination across provider groups—primary care physicians, specialists, and hospitals. As noted, much of this is rooted in the health care system's structure and financing. In many countries, such as Norway, specialists are frequently restricted to hospital service, and communication with primary care physicians is often haphazard. In many systems these structural barriers are reinforced by anachronistic payment systems that do not incentivize the use of primary care physicians or the coordination of care. For instance, German health policy experts bemoan the rigid divide in payment and administration between ambulatory and hospital-based care that inhibits coordination of care.

No country has systematically and effectively deployed chronic care coordination throughout its health care system. Yet there are 2 bright spots of innovation and achievement in chronic care coordination. The highly regarded Diabeter model for diabetes care in the Netherlands creates a care team, including care coordinators, and uses a data platform that collects and presents to providers physiological, quality-of-life, and other data on patients. Bundled payments facilitate this model of comprehensive diabetes care, and it has achieved high quality of care and low hospitalization rates.

Although far from perfect, the United States has some excellent models of chronic care coordination as well. Interestingly, even though they evolved independently, these models are often similar to Diabeter. They identify patients at risk for high cost exacerbations or hospitalizations. A care coordinator is then embedded in the primary care physician's or specialist's office and takes responsibility for monitoring and managing a small group of high-risk patients. The chronic care coordinators ensure that patients are taking their medications and getting the right tests. They reach out to patients if there are medical, family, social, or other problems that could exacerbate symptoms. If so, care coordinators intervene by sending a home care team or bringing the patient to the office for a visit. Many provider groups throughout the United States have implemented this model to improve care and reduce costs, but the model is not yet widespread.

When a patient has a clear medical problem, they should not need to wait for care. In many countries I studied, waiting times are present and problematic, especially for imaging services and elective surgical procedures. The biggest problems are often for hip replacements, cataract surgery, and CT and MRI imaging, but they can sometimes include services that might not qualify as elective, such as cardiac surgery. The public is attuned to long waiting times, and in many countries they have become major electoral issues.

Australia, Canada, Norway, and the UK have highly visible and public waiting time problems. In Australia, it appears physicians manipulate waiting times in the public insurance sector in order to shift patients to the private sector, where physician fees are higher. In Norway one response has been to put waiting times for various procedures online, and patients can use that information to choose the hospital with shorter waits. In Canada supplemental insurance can reduce waiting times.

Waiting times seem to be less salient—but not necessarily less prevalent—in the countries where private financing predominates: the United States, Switzerland, and the Netherlands. This is not because there is hard evidence that waiting times are nonexistent or shorter; rather, it may be because there is no single entity, such as Britain's National Health Service or Australian Medicare, on which patients can focus their anger and complaints.

On waiting times, Taiwan is an outlier. It is a single-payer system with relatively low spending, free choice of provider, and not a particularly high number of physicians. In short, it is the type of system that would seem prone to long queues. Yet waiting times appear nonexistent, even for specialty care. The dominant explanation is that physicians churn through patients quickly so that the Taiwanese see the doctor frequently and easily, but they do not get a lot of time or attention when they do. So although patients may have high access to physicians and no waiting times, the burden is loaded on overworked physicians. This has Taiwanese officials concerned about burnout and quality.

For more than a century, mental health care has been clinically, financially, administratively, and geographically isolated from "regular" health care. Historically, mental health has been stigmatized as not "real" medicine. The result was poor care, both for patients with severe psychiatric disorders, such a bipolar disorder and schizophrenia, and "normal" patients with comorbid depression and/or anxiety. Increasingly, medical experts and health care systems appreciate that mental health conditions are widespread and both complicate and increase the cost of providing regular care.

Over the last half century most countries have gone through a process of deinstitutionalization, shifting care from sequestered asylums to outpatient settings in communities. But, like chronic care coordination, no country I studied has "solved" mental health challenges, either for patients with comorbid conditions or those with serious disorders. And most countries have poor mental health care.

However, there are some initiatives that were encouraging. In many countries, such as Norway and the Netherlands, treatment for mild or moderate mental health problems has been to entrust primary care physicians with referrals if patients' conditions require more special-ized practitioners. Typically these systems added training and financial incentives for the primary care physicians. In the Netherlands, about 88% of primary care physicians have hired nurses to provide first-line mental health care. It is unclear whether these approaches have signifi-cantly improved the identification and treatment of mental health is-sues, especially for those with comorbid depression and anxiety.

Some health practices in the United States have instituted a process of systematic screening for depression and anxiety and then, like the Dutch, offering care through mental health providers embedded in primary care and specialist physicians' offices. The embedded provid-ers are usually psychiatric social workers, health psychologists, or spe-cialized nurse practitioners. As providers have increasingly assumed financial risk for the total cost of care, these embedded mental health provider models are spreading. Preliminary data suggest that the model may work well for patients with depression and anxiety. But both rigor-ous evaluation and refinement as well as scaling throughout the system are needed.

Finally, all delivery systems I studied need improvements to reduce unnecessary and wasteful care, increase the consistency of care, reduce costs, and improve the coordination of chronic and mental health care. Innovation means having a system that offers and encourages oppor-tunities to try new approaches to delivering care, systematically evalu-ates new interventions, and scales the successful ones.

The Dutch, American, and UK systems excel at innovation in the delivery of care. In part, this may be cultural. Historically, these soci-eties have more open cultures that value innovation and reward en-trepreneurs. Whereas the NHS is underfinanced and under pressure to deliver better care within a limited budget, the Dutch and American systems have private payers that are under pressure to lower costs and can align financial incentives across different parts of the delivery sys-tem. These systems have experimented with imposing financial risk on physicians and hospitals, which encourages experimentation in new ways of delivering care.

Taiwan's major innovation is a well-functioning, advanced elec-tronic medical record—something many other health systems have failed to accomplish. Taiwanese patients' records are available to any practitioner in any part of the health care system. This successful innovation may have something to do with Taiwan's booming tech sector and how it created a universal coverage system—virtually from scratch—relatively recently. There were no legacy electronic health records or payment systems to eliminate, as is the case in other countries.

PHARMACEUTICAL COVERAGE AND PRICE CONTROLS

Drug prices are a significant issue in every country. Even those countries that regulate prices and have comparatively low drug spending struggle with rising drug costs. But countries deal with the pharmaceutical market in different ways, revealing 3 important dimensions of pharmaceutical coverage and pricing: (1) low prices, (2) access to innovative drugs, and (3) using a rigorous and objective mechanism to price them.

The first dimension is consistently low drug prices. Norway has, if not the lowest, then nearly the lowest drug prices among high-income countries. It uses strict external reference pricing for outpatient drugs. Norway will not pay more than the average price in the countries with the 3 lowest drug prices. Hence, although no single drug may be the absolute cheapest in Norway, across the board Norway has low drug prices. Clearly the United States is an outlier at the other end, with consistently high prices.

Low drug prices are of little value if patients don't have access to new, innovative drugs. Ultimately, patients in all these countries have access to all safe and effective drugs. Controversy centers on how quickly access is granted once regulatory agencies certify a drug as safe and effective. For a variety of reasons this focus on speed of approval tends to focus on patient access to high-cost cancer drugs. Some have claimed that price regulation can delay introduction of cancer drugs. The truth—and the impact on actual health—of this claim is hotly debated. At worst, introducing drugs in these different countries varies by a small number of months.

The US FDA approves new cancer drugs more rapidly than the European Medicines Agency, which evaluates medicinal products' safety and effectiveness for EU countries. A recent assessment of one type of drug used to treat many different cancers suggests that drugs are approved and on the market about 6 months earlier in the United States. Importantly, this difference is not related to the drug price regulation process, but it seems to be linked to *when* drug companies submitted their drug dossiers for approval. Drug companies decide when they will ask for approval to market a drug in a country, and they do not submit to all countries at the same time. They often determine how such approvals might impact pricing and delay introducing drugs to ensure higher prices in countries that use external reference pricing. In addition, the US FDA employs accelerated drug approval pathways more frequently. Put another way, the FDA is willing to tolerate lower evidence of safety and effectiveness. However, this has resulted in high rates of safety recalls or warnings in the United States. Thus, the difference in timing for access seems to have less to do with price regulation than with drug company behaviors and regulatory approvals based on safety and efficacy.

Indeed, in many countries there are strict timelines for establishing drug prices that prevent or limit delays in access to drugs. For instance, German drug price regulation does not prolong time to market, as companies can market the drug while the ultimate price is being established over a legally determined 12-month period. In the Netherlands, the Ministry of Health, Welfare, and Sport has 90 days after receiving the dossier from the company to establish both the wholesale price to distributors based on the drug price in other countries (reference pricing) *and* whether it will be included in the basic insurance package.

In some countries, especially those using cost-effectiveness analyses, there is controversy over access to certain drugs that are expensive but either might extend life only a few months or minimally improve quality of life. These controversies are politically charged. In the UK they have led to special approval processes and cost thresholds. Ultimately this is a small number of drugs affecting a relatively small number of patients and providing, by definition, minimal impacts on health.

How countries regulate prices should be evidence driven, objective, and sufficiently transparent to avoid arbitrary decisions. Countries adopt 2 broad approaches to setting prices: (1) reference pricing and (2) rigorous value-based pricing and cost-effectiveness analysis (CEA), or what some countries term health technology assessments.

In reference pricing, a country assesses prices by looking at costs for the same or similar drugs. In external reference pricing, the country assesses the prices charged for the same drug in other countries (external) and uses the median, average, or average of the lowest prices to establish its price. The Netherlands, Canada, France, Norway, and Taiwan use international reference pricing in setting prices, with the exact process varying among countries. Whereas Norway indexes to the 3 *least* expensive countries, Canada indexes to 7 expensive countries, which has led Canada to pay significantly more for drugs than Norway. One consequence is that Canada is currently changing how it sets drug prices.

Internal reference pricing is when a country takes a newly approved drug and establishes the price based on what is charged in the country for other drugs in the same class. Many countries—such as Australia, Canada, China, and Germany—use internal reference pricing for many drugs, such as statins for cholesterol.

The other main way of establishing drug prices is through rigorous value-based pricing and cost-effectiveness analysis (CEA). Australia, Canada, France, Taiwan, Norway (predominantly for hospital-based drugs), and the UK use CEA. Typically these countries use a sliding scale threshold, usually close to about US$30,000 to US$40,000 per QALY, for noncancer or non-life-saving medications, with higher thresholds for cancer and life-saving medications. CEA analysis is often not used to set a price but instead to inform price negotiations between a governmental agency and the pharmaceutical companies.

I am agnostic about how best to regulate drug prices through price comparisons or value-based pricing. However, it is clear that having *some* objective and rigorous system for setting prices is definitely better than leaving it to drug companies with monopoly pricing power. Nevertheless, the Australian and UK systems impressed me. They do not rely on the prices charged in other countries, which is probably one reason they are often among the basket of countries used for reference pricing. Among countries using reference pricing, the way Norway pegs its prices to the lowest charged in other countries seems most rational.

THROUGHOUT THIS STUDY it became clear that the United States is a relatively poor performer. Along almost all criteria, the American system is more complex and costlier than any other system. And despite placing a high premium on patient choice, American patients actually have less choice than patients many other countries. In large measure because of the health system's complexity and high cost, the United States excels at innovation in payment, the delivery of care for the chronically ill, and providing mental health care in some areas. Complex, privatized, and diffuse systems will always be more flexible and innovative but less equitable. Every country will need to determine what kind of trade-offs it will accept between those goals. Hopefully, some successful innovations in payment and delivery of care will eventually permeate across all delivery organizations in the American system and make their way abroad, just as DRG payment did for hospital payment over the last 30 years.

But because the US system is doing poorly overall, it behooves us to return to the motivation behind the question that audiences have persistently asked me:

Based on other countries' experiences and successes, what changes can the United States adopt to improve its health care?

CHAPTER THIRTEEN

CONCLUSION

Six Lessons for Improving the US Health Care System

This comparison of the US health care system and 10 other countries' offers at least 4 clear conclusions for those curious and persistent Americans who kept asking me: Which country has the best health care?

First—and most clearly—the US health care system is not the best, 2nd best, or even 3rd best in the world. It significantly underperforms on numerous dimensions.

Once, maybe in the 1950s and 1960s, the United States had the best health care in the world. At some facilities and for some conditions, the United States currently offers fantastic care. Cancer care may be such a condition. But overall today the United States is way behind many other countries. Only 90% of the US population has coverage, while almost every other country manages to get over 99% coverage. On cost, the United States spends 27% more per person than the next most expensive country and 50% more than most countries.

For all that money, the US health care system performs poorly on many dimensions, including ones that Americans prize highly, such as patient choice of hospitals and physicians, with Canada, France,

Germany, the Netherlands, Switzerland, Taiwan, and other countries exceling and outperforming the United States on this very dimension. And there is ample data that quality in the United States is—to put it charitably—inconsistent; the United States ranks poorly in many areas amenable to health care interventions, such as infant and maternal mortality. On many dimensions, US health care is not in the top 10 globally.

Second, although not the best, the United States also does not have the worst health care system in the world. As I said, the Chinese system seems to be both poorer performing for today and less innovative for the future.

The 3rd conclusion is that the United States does excel on some dimensions, particularly innovation and experimentation in payment models and care delivery (especially for chronic conditions). These innovations are a work in progress, but the United States—along with the Netherlands and perhaps the UK—is far more invested in these experiments and demonstration projects. Ironically, the system's underperformance spurred this drive for innovation. For instance, because US hospitals are so expensive and have high rates of infections and complications, there are strenuous efforts to avoid hospitalizations and deliver what hitherto was hospital-level care in the outpatient setting and patients' homes. Similarly, because the fee-for-service payment model incentivizes overuse of high-margin tests, treatments, and unnecessary care, the United States leads in the development of alternative payment models. This innovation is one reason I am optimistic about the US system's long-term performance. In the next decade or 2, the United States will again become one of the best systems in the world.

Considering the US system's underperformance and innovativeness, it is appropriate to ask what this study of other countries can teach us about what changes would improve the US system. In other words: Where should we focus that innovative energy?

As one expert wrote, "It is not desirable [or even possible] to 'lift and shift' health system parts from one country to another." Nevertheless, what my audiences have asked for is possible. We can learn specific lessons from other countries that can be implemented in the United States to significantly improve the system.

This evaluation of 10 other systems reveals 6 feasible and beneficial changes to the American system: (1) ensuring universal coverage, (2) enhancing financial protection for children, (3) mandating simplification across all forms of health insurance, (4) emphasizing primary care, (5) accelerating the innovation and dissemination of best practices in chronic care coordination and mental health, and (6) regulating drug prices.

Lesson #1: Ensuring universal coverage with auto-enrollment and larger subsidies

Fully 10 years after the Affordable Care Act the United States has seen great improvement in coverage, but still we can barely get to 90% coverage. Even worse, the last few years of Republican attacks on the ACA's coverage mechanisms—such as repealing the mandate, reducing funding for advertising and navigators, and weakening the insurance exchanges—have caused the uninsured rate to rise—the opposite of what we expect with falling unemployment and a growing economy. A high uninsured rate is not a law of nature, and the United States can achieve near-universal coverage without massive, systemic change.

Most people who are uninsured today are eligible for highly subsidized, relatively affordable health insurance through Medicaid or the exchanges. Over 6 million uninsured Americans are eligible for Medicaid. Even states that have expanded the program have hundreds of thousands of residents who are eligible but have not signed up. Similarly, the health insurance exchanges are designed to help people with incomes above 100% of the poverty level but no affordable employer-based insurance—think independent contractors and Uber drivers in the new gig economy. The exchange plans cover all preventive services and annual checkups without a deductible or co-pay. With the subsidies, plans for some people have almost no premium and often cost low-income individuals less than US$100 per month. But many independent contractors or people working in small businesses that do not offer health insurance are unaware of the subsidies and/or do not have the time to shop during a limited enrollment window. As a result, millions of low-income Americans are uninsured despite the existence of programs to cover them.

What can we learn from other countries about getting to true universal coverage? Automatic enrollment with substantial subsidies has enormous power.

In Norway and the UK everyone has health coverage by virtue of being a resident. That's all it takes. Furthermore, Norway has a simple form of auto-enrollment: all residents pay taxes to fund the National Insurance Scheme, which insures all residents. Any resident can show up, get care, and have it paid for from the system. Amazingly, the United States has a nearly identical system in Medicare Part A, which pays for hospital care for seniors.

Although auto-enrollment is a bit more complex in systems based on private health insurance, it is still achievable. In the Netherlands and Switzerland, the government automatically enrolls people who do not obtain health insurance themselves. In Switzerland every person needs to register with a canton (state) as a resident and then has 90 days to buy health insurance. After 90 days the government can randomly select a plan for new residents and require them to pay both a premium and a penalty. The Netherlands operates a similar system at the national level, and the penalty is stiff. Importantly, both the Netherlands and Switzerland provide generous subsidies to between 33% and 60% of the population to purchase the mandatory private insurance. (On subsidies, the Netherlands is much more generous than Switzerland.) Hence, despite having coverage through competing private insurance plans, the Netherlands and Switzerland have over 99% coverage through a combination of strong financial penalties, substantial subsidies for low- and middle-income families, and auto-enrollment if individuals do not initiate enrollment themselves.

Behavioral economics suggests that automatic enrollment would dramatically reduce the uninsured rate in the United States. When programs automatically enroll people, who can also opt out if they wish, participation goes way, way up. For instance, in countries that have automatic enrollment in organ donation (organ donation is assumed at the time of death unless a person has explicitly refused for religious or other reasons) more than 90% of the population agrees—or at least does not object—to organ donation. Conversely, in opt-in countries, where people need to explicitly agree to organ donation when they get their driver's license, such as the United States, only about 15% of the population volunteers as donors.

The complex patchwork of insurance programs in the United States makes it harder to design an auto-enrollment program. Americans are eligible for different programs based on employment status, age, income, and geography. Often they need to select an insurance company and pay a premium—more burdensome choices. However, even with these complications, it is possible to have a modified version of auto-enrollment. It is not even partisan or fantastical—analysts from both the left-leaning Brookings Institution and right-leaning American Enterprise Institute have written extensively about how to leverage automatic enrollment. This could slash the uninsured rate to under 5%. Indeed, there are 6 states and the District of Columbia that have achieved over 95% coverage under the ACA, showing that small changes can significantly improve coverage.

One approach is to auto-enroll people without insurance into Medicaid. If people show up at a physician's office, urgent care center, emergency room, or hospital without any insurance, the provider would be legally required to bill Medicaid. Medicaid would keep that person enrolled unless it determines the person is eligible for some other coverage—say, in the exchanges or through Medicare. It would then enroll them in that alternative coverage. Another possibility is to auto-enroll uninsured people into the lowest- or 2nd-lowest-cost silver plan on the insurance exchanges and add an assessment for the premium—after subsidies—to their taxes at the end of the year. Switzerland does this.

These auto-enrollment mechanisms would require changes in laws and regulations. For instance, the income eligibility determination mechanisms in Medicaid and the insurance exchanges are not aligned. For most individuals Medicaid uses a person's previous month's pay, while exchange subsidies are based on the previous year's income. Using Medicaid's income determination process in the exchanges—and eliminating the claw-back of subsidies should a person's income be higher than expected—would greatly facilitate auto-enrollment. These legal and regulatory changes to facilitate auto-enrollment are hardly brain surgery and should not be the excuses to do nothing.

In addition to auto-enrollment, 2 key issues seem to be the premium charged and, relatedly, the level of subsidies in the insurance exchanges. Two easy ways for the United States to drive down premiums in the exchanges are to make reinsurance permanent and to pay for the cost-sharing subsidies. Reinsurance reduces the risk of super-expensive patients for insurance companies, and this, in turn, reduces premiums. Another way to reduce premiums would be to reinstate the federal government's payment for the cost-sharing subsidies. Estimates are that this would reduce premiums about 10% to 15%. Research has shown that low-income individuals are extremely price sensitive when it comes to buying health insurance, and reducing premium sticker prices dramatically increases enrollment.

Similarly, the United States could increase subsidies for the purchase of health insurance in the exchanges. While the United States is generous up to about US$62,000 for a family of 4—the median household income—with substantial help for families buying insurance and with deductibles and co-pays, it becomes much less generous for slightly-better-off families. There has been much discussion about increasing subsidies for insurance premiums and out-of-pocket expenses and extending them to families with incomes over US$100,000. The lessons—particularly from the Netherlands—suggest this: higher subsidies than those currently in the ACA would help induce people who qualify for the exchanges to buy private insurance.

Other countries' experiences suggest that auto-enrollment with reinsurance and more generous subsidies would be effective and important policy mechanisms to get to universal coverage—more important than public versus private financing, the role of insurance companies, a public option, and so on. The United States needs to adopt some form of auto-enrollment and improve the generosity of subsidies for middle-income families.

Lesson #2: Cover children at no additional cost to their parents and families

"Our children are our most valuable asset."

How often do we hear politicians, business executives, and civic leaders utter this phrase? When it comes to health care in the United States, however, this seems mostly to be an empty phrase, not a living reality. This comparative study of health care reveals that in most countries children are viewed as both a treasure and an investment in the future. Consequently, society collectively pays for children's health insurance and provides them services with no deductible or co-pay. But in the United States, the financial burden for children's health care falls on each individual family through higher premiums, deductibles, and co-pays.

The United States has made important progress in covering children at low or no cost to their parents. In the 1990s, a bipartisan coalition led by Senator Ted Kennedy (D-MA) and Senator Orrin Hatch (R-UT) enacted the Children's Health Insurance Program (CHIP), which covered children whose parents earned too much money to be eligible for Medicaid but who did not have private health insurance. It now provides health coverage to about 9 million children, and the uninsured rate for children has fallen about 65% since CHIP's enactment. Not only has the United States expanded coverage for children, we also have made the benefits more comprehensive. In 2010, the ACA mandated that all insurance companies include pediatric dental and vision care as one of the 10 essential health benefits.

Although these are important improvements, they remain inadequate. About 4 million American children—or 5%—are uninsured. Outrageously, almost a third of these uninsured children live in just 2 states: Texas and Florida. In Texas alone 11% of children lack health insurance. Nearly 60% of all uninsured children are eligible for Medicaid and/or CHIP but are not enrolled, and these states create barriers to enrolling children.

Another problem is that even insured children can be a significant financial burden on their parents. On average, family premiums for employer-sponsored insurance are nearly 3 times those for individuals—US$7,188 for individuals versus US$20,576 for families in 2019. Indeed, an average worker's contribution to an individual, employer-sponsored health insurance plan was US$1,242 in 2019 but US$6,015 for family coverage—nearly 5 times more. After paying higher premiums, families must then pay deductibles and co-pays for their children as well.

My comparative study reveals that almost all other countries liberate families from the financial burden of paying for their children's health care. Some countries do this by directly subsidizing premiums for children's health insurance and eliminating deductibles and co-pays for pediatric services. In the Netherlands, all children under 18 *need* to have health insurance, but families do not pay any additional premiums to cover children with the standard package. In Germany, all workers at a company earning similar salaries pay the same in payroll taxes for their health insurance regardless of whether they have a family or not. And workers' family members—nonearning spouses and children—get health coverage without any additional payments from the employer or employee.

Countries without typical insurance premiums also strive to make children free to parents. In Australia, the tax (levy) for the mandatory government Medicare program does not change based on family size. In addition, Australian children are typically added to private health insurance plans at no additional cost to the family. In Norway, there is no co-pay when children under 16 go to the primary care physician to receive health services, and pediatric dental care is free. Rather than loading the premiums (or taxes) and out-of-pocket costs for a child's health coverage on individual families, these countries see children as an investment and spread the cost across all of society.

Such policies strongly communicate family values—the valuing of families and their children. Having society pay the full cost of children's health care also helps to fulfill the ideal of equality of opportunity by ensuring that all children will get access to the same set of essential health services regardless of their parents' income and social status. It also serves a coldly self-interested purpose: How much future economic productivity is lost by denying children access to needed care today?

The United States—all Americans, together—should assume the financial liability for children's health insurance. There are several policy changes that would accomplish this.

First, the United States could require employers to charge the same health insurance premiums to workers, whether they are individuals or have dependent children. This would distribute the cost of family health coverage among all workers—not just adults with families. Second, the United States could emulate almost all other countries and require private insurers to eliminate all deductibles and co-pays when children under 18 receive medical services, including visits to the pediatrician, the urgent care clinic, the dentist, or the hospital and for prescription drugs.

When it comes to public health coverage, another policy would be to ensure that 100% of children receive health coverage by enacting auto-enrollment into Medicaid and CHIP without requiring any verification of family income or other requirements. There should be no co-payments for pediatric care in Medicaid and CHIP.

Finally, because of low reimbursement rates, many physicians refuse to take Medicaid or CHIP patients or limit the number of patients with these types of coverage they are willing to treat. For 2 years, in 2013 and 2014, the ACA increased payment to physicians caring for Medicaid patients. The result was a significant improvement in both the number of physicians taking Medicaid patients and the promptness of the services the patients received. And today 19 states have voluntarily continued the policy of higher Medicaid reimbursement for physicians. To ensure that all children with Medicaid or CHIP coverage have access to pediatricians and specialists *and* receive timely care, the US government could permanently increase Medicaid's reimbursement rates for pediatric services.

Enacting these policies would ensure 100% of American children receive health coverage and that this coverage is not a substantial financial burden to their families.

Lesson #3: Simplify the American health care system

Every health care system in every high-income country is complex. That does appear to be a law of nature. But this study of 10 other health systems reveals that the American system is unique in that it is significantly more complex than the system of any other country. It needs simplification—urgently.

Complexity is burdensome. Patients spend too much time trying to figure out which type of coverage they are eligible for, which specific plan to sign up for, which physicians and hospitals are in network, how much they owe in deductibles and co-pays, how to dispute inaccurate bills, and so on. There is woefully little time left for patients to ensure they are getting optimal, evidence-based care. Purchasing insurance is so complex that employers hire consultants to design their employees' health benefits. The multitude of insurance products—usually dictated by employers—and complex insurance billing processes mean that US physician practices spend 4 times more on administration compared to their Canadian counterparts.

Complexity is also financially costly, and these costs are ultimately borne by all Americans. In 2012, the National Academy of Medicine (NAM) estimated that the United States has disproportionately high administrative costs. In 2019, the Center for American Progress updated NAM's estimate, showing that the United States spends nearly US$500 billion on billing and insurance-related costs. Nearly half of that, over US$240 billion, is classified as "excess"—read, waste—that could be eliminated with a simpler system.

American policymakers, insurers, and others did not intend to design a mind-bogglingly complex system. It is path dependence at work. Nobody considers simplicity an imperative in developing new laws, regulations, or policies. Rather than trying to simplify existing systems, lawmakers layer programs onto each other to address problems and deficiencies—and to satisfy hospitals, insurance companies, drug and device companies, and scores of other interest groups. Most importantly, they add various provisions to secure enough votes for legislation to be passed—with little attention to how the added provision will affect administration. Here is a simple example I recently witnessed. A well-intentioned congresswoman wanted to reduce patients' burgeoning out-of-pocket costs, so she suggested eliminating deductibles and co-pays for 5 primary care visits and 3 specialist visits for established chronic conditions each year. Just imagine the complexity of keeping track of the number of visits as well as identifying which visits are to primary care doctors versus specialists treating a specific, qualifying condition.

A key lesson from studying other countries is that there is much that can be done to simplify the US health care system in 3 important areas: (1) the differing ways Americans get insurance, (2) the complexity of insurance benefits design, and (3) the relationships among insurers, hospitals, and physicians.

First, the United States needs to simplify the process of buying health insurance. The United States basically has every type of health financing ever invented—socialized medicine (the VA), single payer (traditional Medicare and Medicaid), single payer managed by private insurance (Medicare Advantage and managed Medicaid), private employer-based insurance, and individual purchase (see Table 12-2). This is preposterous.

HERE IS HOW we could simplify getting coverage: reduce the insurance options to either employer-sponsored insurance or Medicare. Within Medicare offer a choice between traditional fee-for-service or a managed care plan. This would require combining Medicare, Medicaid, and the insurance exchanges into one program that allows all people who do not receive employer-sponsored insurance to choose between traditional Medicare or a Medicare Advantage plan operated by a private insurance company. This is essentially the plan proposed by the Center for American Progress and introduced into Congress by Representatives Rosa DeLauro (D-CT) and Jan Schakowsky (D-IL).

Obviously, many details would need to be worked out—how much states would contribute when Medicaid is merged with Medicare, what businesses should contribute if they do not provide health insurance and want their employees to be in Medicare, and how much to charge individuals under 65 who enroll in Medicare. But at the core this change would make it much easier on Americans to navigate health insurance options and would simplify billing by physicians and hospitals. It may be a substantial change given the current political realities, but it is a meaningful step in the right direction that other countries have already taken.

Another simplification is to reduce the myriad health insurance benefit designs. Most countries have significant limitations on the range of services covered, co-pays, balance billing, out-of-pocket expenses, network formation, which services supplemental insurance can offer, and so on. By law, the 22 Dutch insurance companies must cover the same basic benefits and have the same minimum deductible with the same exemptions for primary care physician visits. The ability to accept higher deductibles in exchange for lower premiums is the same across companies. The only thing that really varies is the level of premiums, supplemental coverage, and the physician and hospital networks. Because important factors cannot vary between insurance companies, patient choices are focused on just a few key factors, and this also helps providers know for certain which services are covered.

Such simplification was successfully achieved in the United States within the Medigap program, in which seniors can buy private, supplemental insurance to pay for services and out-of-pocket expenses not covered by traditional Medicare. Through legislation, Congress reduced the number of benefit designs to 10 paradigmatic types. Each type had standardized benefits, limited the duration of exclusions for preexisting conditions, and required minimum medical-loss ratios. Thus, seniors' choices were reduced to selecting among the 10 insurance designs.

The government could do the same for employer-sponsored insurance and drug benefits. Today, it is largely employers and their benefit design consultants that require variations in the design of their insurance benefit. There is woefully little evidence that these benefit designs help with improving quality, reducing costs, or improving employee health. But we are sure they are a main reason administrative costs are so high. Needing to determine what patients are covered for, their deductibles, the network, and all the other variables is administratively costly. The federal government already took a step in the direction of simplification with the passage of the ACA, which delineates 10 essential benefits that all plans must cover. The government should further reduce plan variability and define up to 10 prototypical plans with standardized benefits, co-pay and deductible levels, drug benefits, and other consumer-facing parameters. This would reduce employers' *and* employees' costs and would also allow patients to more easily compare insurance options.

Finally, simplification needs to occur at doctors' offices, hospitals, and other facilities. There are endless paper registration forms filled out by hand, recording and rerecording addresses, past medical problems, allergies, medications, and emergency contacts. In the digital era, this is completely wasteful, and health care providers are only slowly switching to digital registration voluntarily.

In contrast, the Taiwanese system has developed a useful digital medical card that makes registration analogous to the swipe of a credit card. We should not reinvent the wheel. The federal government should mandate that within 3 years all physicians, urgent care centers, hospitals, and other providers have digital registration either by electronic card or a biomarker (fingerprint or eye scan). This would link to verifying insurance eligibility and benefits as well as past registration that could be corrected. It would also allow patients to have a reasonable upfront estimate of what their physician visits cost.

Another level of complexity relates to physician and hospital billing. Reducing the different types of health offerings to 10 should reduce the complexity of billing, but more importantly, there should be administrative simplification of bills. The United States needs a single clearinghouse for medical bills, with a standardized form that prevents each insurer from using its own mechanisms to request additional information.

Finally, prior authorization requirements, despised by doctors but required by insurers for many high-cost tests and treatments, need reform. They take time, and they are costly. Although physicians and patients hate prior authorization, the tools are effective because physicians frequently do not practice evidence-based medicine. Physicians often order unnecessary—even harmful—tests, treatments, and excessively priced medications. The only way to get rid of prior authorization is for physicians to adhere to proven care pathways.

Until that day comes, prior authorization can be simplified in 2 ways. First, it can be put in the flow of physician ordering. This will take technical improvements and upgrades in EHRs, but it is coming. Insurers could also more widely institute "gold carding," which would allow physicians who consistently (over 95% of the time) adhere to treatment guidelines to be exempt from prior authorization. Second, rapidly shifting to alternative payment models in which physicians are held accountable for the total cost of care should, over time, reduce unnecessary and inefficient tests and treatments because such models align the physicians' interests with adhering to evidence-based care.

Simplification has a cost, though.

It applies a handful of rules to everyone, treating all people the same. It reduces exceptions and taking account of unique circumstances. But having exceptions for each person, group, or employer—which is the current system—creates substantial and costly complexity. The US health care system has gone way too far in the direction of complexity, which imposes substantial burdens on all of us. We need to bring the pendulum back toward simplicity. And to this end, every organization

and person in the health care system should evaluate what they are doing by the simplicity standard: How can I make this simpler and less
time intensive?

Lesson #4: Emphasize and increase the reimbursement for primary care

The United States has too many adult-focused specialists, who are paid
more to perform procedures and provide consultations than primary
care physicians and pediatric specialists. The United States needs to
prioritize primary care.

Medicare pays a primary care physician about US$160 for a 45-min-
ute discussion of advance care planning, but cardiologists receive
about US$620 for single-vessel stent placement. Does placing a stent in
a heart blood vessel really require nearly 4 times more skill and brain
power than a compassionate 45-minute end-of-life care discussion
with a patient and their family? If so, why do most cardiologists—and
other American physicians—do almost everything they can to avoid
such discussions? Furthermore, specialists in the United States expend
significantly more resources than primary care physicians when they
manage patients with similar conditions. Like many countries, the
United States has too few pediatric specialists and pays them too little.
But unlike many countries, the United States systematically underval-
ues primary care.

My comparative study reveals that a strong primary care system enhances performance. Countries like the Netherlands, Norway, and the
UK have strong primary care models. Primary care physicians manage most patients. Specialists work as consultants to the primary care
physicians and only manage the most complex patients. Conversely,
in Germany patients have wide choice and do not need to get a primary care referral in order to access specialists or surgeons. France has
a system that is in between: primary care referrals are often necessary
to access a specialist, but patients can access any specialist they want
with a referral, and the specialist is not a consultant to the primary care
physician.

The Dutch system has significant advantages, and it is worth shifting the US system more in that direction, even if we are unlikely to go
as far as the Dutch in creating a strong gatekeeper model. First, Dutch

GPs tend to assume responsibility for many more services than US primary care physicians. For example, almost all of them employ nurse practitioners who are allowed to prescribe medications. They often employ mental health nurses for behavioral health conditions, such as comorbid depression and anxiety. Primary care cooperatives provide extensive after-hours telephone triage and even in-person after-hours care so patients do not go to the emergency room in the middle of the night. In addition, patients are financially penalized for going directly to specialists, and specialists have additional administrative burdens if they see a patient without a referral. This also ensures coordination of care through the Dutch primary care physicians.

Changing Americans' behavior regarding primary care and specialist care is not going to be easy. But one thing can be done: change out-of-pocket payments for patients. The United States could make primary care visits free to patients—no deductibles and no co-pays. This could be linked to increasing the co-pay to see specialists without a primary care physician referral.

For this to work effectively, insurers would need to change payments to primary care physicians to incentivize them to assume more responsibility for managing and coordinating patient care. This could be achieved by shifting primary care payments to capitation with financial responsibility for a patient's total cost of care. Primary care physicians could thus realize substantial financial benefits by managing more of their patients' care, ensuring their patients are going to physicians who follow guidelines, and avoiding unnecessary or inefficient tests and treatments.

Lesson #5: Adopt and implement best practices for the care of patients with chronic and mental health conditions

More than 80 cents of every health care dollar in the United States goes toward patients with chronic illnesses: diabetes, asthma, hypertension, congestive heart failure, emphysema, cancer, and other conditions. To lower health care costs and improve quality, care improvement needs to focus on these patients with chronic conditions, especially patients who are at high risk of exacerbation of their illnesses.

No country has universally implemented innovative approaches to chronic care management. But I did find many bright spots and excellent models of chronic care coordination, especially in the Netherlands and in the United States. One of the lessons I learned from this study is that physician groups that perform well in managing patients with chronic illnesses all seem to adopt a similar model of care. The key ingredients are:

- Creating multidisciplinary teams around a care coordinator embedded in the physician practices to manage high-risk patients
- Identifying high-risk, high-cost patients—patients who are likely to have exacerbations—who need added attention and services
- Educating patients and their families about how their condition is treated and teaching patients self-management techniques
- Instituting frequent, proactive outreach to patients not only to ensure compliance with testing, medication adherence, and lifestyle changes but also to address stressors that might lead to exacerbations
- Implementing same-day appointments and home visits for rapid responses to preempt and address potential disease exacerbations
- Using data on patient outcomes and practice performance to iterate and improve processes of care

In the Netherlands and the United States these models are facilitated by alternative payment methods such as capitation or bundling—so that physician practices earn more money when they do a good job of coordination that results in patients' reduced use of hospitals.

These practices work to both improve the quality of care for patients and reduce costs. For instance, the Dutch Diabeter model has a comparatively high percentage of pediatric diabetics with hemoglobin A1c under 7.5% and a very low rate of hospitalization. Many physician practices in the United States have similarly achieved significant savings with embedded, proactive chronic care coordinators as part of multidisciplinary teams. For instance, in 2018 CareMore—a Medicare Advantage plan primarily focused in the Western United States and targeting the frail elderly—had 20% fewer hospital admissions and 23% fewer bed days (a measure of admissions and length of stay) than traditional Medicare patients. Compared to traditional Medicare, it also had a lower hospital readmission rate.

Obviously Diabeter and CareMore programs could be further improved. But they are well above average. And such excellent care for patients with chronic illnesses is less a matter of invention than one of dissemination. The challenge is to scale proven models throughout the health care system. This requires changing physician payment, helping physician practices consistently implement these 6 steps in the way they care for patients, and providing physicians frequent performance assessments so they know whether and how much they are improving. In the United States insurance companies, Medicare, and Medicaid need to continue to expand alternative payment models. This scaling will require the use of performance data, learning collaboratives, and technical assistance to enable physician practices to adopt the right approach.

We have a similar need to address mental health issues. There is a high burden of mental health conditions, which raise costs substantially. About 5% of the general public have depression, and 7% have anxiety. Among cancer patients, 20% have co-occurring depression and 10% have anxiety. Among patients with coronary artery disease, 15% live with depression and 23% have anxiety.

Mental health problems translate into high costs that are not for mental health services; instead, they are for "regular" medical services because of the challenges of managing these diseases that are then complicated by mental health issues. It is hard to get depressed diabetes patients to manage their diet and take their insulin appropriately, and this drives up the costs associated with diabetes. One report showed that symptomatic depression increased costs of caring for adults with diabetes by over US$5,000 compared to diabetic patients with no depression. The same pattern is found for patients with cancer, asthma, and congestive heart failure.

Two of the biggest deficiencies in health care systems have been the lack of diagnosis of mental health conditions and the slowness of providing care once a behavioral health problem is identified. No country has systematic mental health screening of either hospitalized patients or patients with chronic illnesses. In addition, many patients with mental health issues often have difficulty getting an appointment with a psychiatrist or other mental health provider. In the United States it is not unusual for patients to wait 2 or 3 months for an initial appointment with a psychiatrist.

Although no country I looked at excelled system-wide at mental health care, both the Netherlands and the United States had some impressive models. Dutch primary care physicians are responsible for treating mild mental health conditions, and 88% employ mental health nurses to treat patients. In the United States I found a number of groups—from small practices to larger providers, such as Advocate Health Care—doing a good job. Advocate screens all hospitalized seniors for comorbid mental health problems and intervenes within 48 hours. And at some of their larger primary care practices they have embedded psychiatric social workers to care for patients with mental health conditions. These interventions have improved care and lowered costs.

Much of the success of effective programs seems to inhere in consistently implementing a few critical steps:

- Embedding mental health providers—nurses specialized in mental health care, psychologists, or psychiatric social workers—in physician practices or linking to online providers
- Routinely screening patients for depression, anxiety disorders, and substance abuse and having them be rapidly—within 24 to 48 hours—seen by the in-house or online mental health providers
- Using targeted pharmacologic and behavioral interventions with the aim of addressing the mental health problem and returning patients to functionality
- Routinely assessing patients for improvement and giving this feedback to mental health providers

These mental health interventions are not yet as firmly tested and established as the ones for the care of high-risk, high-cost chronically ill patients. They need additional evaluation and refinement. But this process needs to be accelerated. Many small changes could facilitate this process, such as having EHRs seamlessly able to record patients' mental health screening tests and mandating reporting on mental health outcomes for practices. Payers could also assess whether incentives for physician groups that embed mental health providers in the practice lead to effectively intervening to treat mental health problems and reducing medical costs. Once successful programs have been identified, they need to be scaled.

Lesson #6: The United States needs to join the rest of the world in regulating drug prices

When it comes to both drug prices and drug price regulations, the United States is an *extreme* outlier. With less than 4.5% of the world's population, the United States accounts for over 40% of all drug expenditures. It is the only country that grants drug companies monopolies through patents and marketing exclusivity and then allows them to freely set prices. All of the countries I studied explicitly regulate drug prices. Consequently, there are stark differences in drug prices that are not attributable to the number of drugs Americans consume. This study revealed that it is possible to regulate drug prices without stifling innovation or reducing access for patients.

Studying other countries gives insight into an effective approach to instituting drug price regulation. First, all other countries have one price for drugs for the entire population. They may adjust co-payments, but there is one price. Thus, in the United States drug prices should apply nationally, not just to one market segment, such as Medicare or the employer-based market. Second, drug price regulation needs to be informed by independent standards—not just what the drug companies want to charge. Some countries, such as Australia, Norway, and the UK, use a rigorous cost-effectiveness analysis to establish drug prices. Other countries, such as the Netherlands, Canada, France, and Taiwan, largely rely on external reference pricing. These 2 methods place independent benchmarks for acceptable prices. Benchmarks could be used in one of 2 ways. In one approach, the highest price—whether the cost-effectiveness price or the price in other countries—could establish a maximal price for drugs, allowing companies to set their own price below that maximum. Alternatively, these pricing methods could inform negotiations with the drug companies on the final price.

Another important lesson is that the government need not conduct these negotiations. In Germany the government empowers a nongovernmental entity to negotiate the prices with drug companies under legal constraints, with arbitration if they cannot come to an agreement.

This review of practices in other countries suggests that drug price regulation did not lead to significant delays in access to newly approved drugs. The differences in time to market seemed to come more from when drug companies submit applications for drug marketing to countries and the regulatory bodies' time for safety and efficacy assessments. In almost all countries there was a strict timeline to establish drug prices that ranged from a few months to one year. Although drug price regulation might have added a few months to the time to market, it often was because of company resistance to lower prices, and no delay was excessive. What's more, the savings were substantial—the equivalent of US$100 billion in drug spending.

Regardless, one key improvement the United States could make to lower costs for patients and the entire system is to actively regulate drug prices.

How challenging is it to implement these 6 reforms? None of this is going to be easy. Many clearly require federal legislation. For instance, changing the way income is determined for Medicaid and the insurance exchanges, requiring that employers assess families the same insurance contributions as individuals, constraining employers to offer only one of 10 different insurance products, and regulating drug prices all require federal legislation. Given the current partisanship at the federal level, legislating on health care is hard. We cannot seem to get a law passed on surprise medical billing or drug prices, despite large public majorities supporting laws on these issues. I do think some of these proposals can be enacted, especially around shifting more toward auto-enrollment and drug price regulation. But it will take years.

Some of these suggestions could be done, at least in part, by regulation or corporate initiatives and some by greater coordination between Medicare and private insurers. They should be easier to implement. Although administrative simplification was included in the ACA, it has floundered. It could be achieved if the federal government more vigorously pursued it in collaboration with private insurance. Creating a clearinghouse for claims and a standardized claims form used by all payers would be a step in the right direction.

The federal government needs to regularly reevaluate its fee schedule—how much it pays for different physician activities. For a long time it has been urged to increase the value of primary care and lower the value paid for surgical and other procedures. Recent evidence suggests that, at least for some procedures, such as hip and knee replacements, the government overpays. Paying based on the time spent, using empirical data from EHRs, is one way to rebalance the amount spent on surgical procedures. Reevaluating the difficulty of cognitive activities versus procedures is another thing that can be initiated without legislation. But more importantly, the government could work with private insurance companies to more aggressively—and, even more importantly, rapidly—shift toward alternative payment models. For the past 5 to 10 years there have been multiple demonstration projects testing these payment mechanisms. In general, they have modestly improved quality and lowered cost. None has made quality worse or systematically increased costs. There needs to be a coordinated effort between the government and private payers to expand and make permanent these models that would convince health systems and physician practices to invest more in changing their processes of care. And at the top of the list of those changes would be giving more focus to high-risk, high-cost patients who have either chronic conditions and/or mental health issues. These changes are occurring, but they could be significantly accelerated without the need for legislation.

CODA

Coronavirus and the Performance of Health Care Systems

Just as this book was going off to the printer, the coronavirus pandemic arrived. The publisher stopped the presses, ripped up the previous version of the coda, and asked that I take a few moments to consider if there was anything this examination of health care systems could illuminate about coronavirus and what coronavirus might tell us about health care systems. This new coda, written one week after New York City had begun its "pause" and the same weekend as Louisiana had declared its lockdown, is necessarily *very* preliminary. But here are 7 tentative thoughts that quickly emerged from the evidence around the world.

First, coronavirus is not a one-off or a black swan event. We should expect more emergency infectious disease outbreaks. Over the last 2 decades, the world has witnessed an outbreak almost every 3 years: SARS in 2003–2004, H1N1 swine flu in 2009–2010, MERS in 2014, Ebola in West Africa in 2014, Zika in 2016, Lassa fever in 2018, Ebola in the Congo in 2019, and now in 2020 COVID-19. Because of reasons including climate change, the progressive encroachment of humans into animal habitats, greater travel, and more mass displacements, these outbreaks are likely to occur regularly. Thus, health systems will need to be resilient and develop disaster plans that confront the possibility of overwhelming, if limited-term, demand—something they have typically not been prepared to do.

Second, and relatedly, as has become clear with COVID-19, competently and effectively addressing the widespread outbreak of a novel virus for which there is no established herd immunity in the general population is not fundamentally a test of the health care system. It is true that an outbreak can overwhelm the health care system and cause it to fail to adequately care for all patients. But fundamentally, the adequacy of the response depends upon political judgment and leadership to rapidly institute public health measures and the competence of public health infrastructure to implement them effectively and swiftly. The countries that have responded best to COVID-19 and were able to avoid massive outbreaks, high population mortality, and overloading the health care system were those that were able to (1) engender public trust with frequent and accurate pronouncements about the number of COVID-19 cases and other relevant matters, (2) implement physical distancing, (3) deploy extensive population-wide testing, (4) implement rigorous and extensive contact tracing, and (5) isolate and quarantine positive cases. These are not responses of any one health system but of governments and the public health system. While they are related, they are often separate governmental agencies and have very different purposes. Health care agencies typically address the financing of personal health care, while the public health agencies are supposed to focus on population-level problems.

Third, a standout response to COVID-19 was in Taiwan. In 2003 and 2004, SARS was a wake-up call. Health care officials there recognized that with incredibly tight trade and travel connections with China, they had a very high risk of exposure to any novel virus that might arise there. After SARS, the Taiwanese government prepared itself for an outbreak by putting in place the capacity to proactively identify people at risk of carrying the virus and by preparing a stockpile of personal protective equipment. With the novel coronavirus, the government immediately—in a single day—integrated patients' National Health Insurance identification cards with data from its immigration and customs database. This allowed them to identify patients who had traveled recently to China and use that information to alert clinicians of patients with high infectious risk, who were then identified and quarantined. Having an excellent electronic health insurance card system with the ability to not only collect information but also to transmit information back to physicians greatly facilitated Taiwan's response, which led to just 252 COVID-19 cases and 2 deaths at the end of March—far fewer than originally projected.

Fourth, COVID-19 exposed the serious flaws of both the Chinese and American health systems, but for different reasons. China deserves the widespread general criticism it received for its initial suppression of information about the novel disease and the way this endangered the entire planet. More relevant to this book is that China's health care is hospital focused. Fundamentally, there are few other health care facilities. There are vanishingly few physician offices or other ambulatory centers to deliver care. Thus, mild, moderately, and severely ill patients with COVID-19 flooded into the hospitals, crowding together with infected and other noninfected patients, and overwhelmed the entire system. In Hubei province this required the emergency construction of 16 new hospitals, the influx of 30,000 health care workers, and the assembly of equipment and supplies from all over the country to tackle the torrent. While such construction and mobilization of material was nothing short of miraculous, the inevitable delay in getting these resources ready dramatically increased the mortality rate and was hugely inefficient and wasteful. A hospital-centric delivery system is poor at addressing emergent and widespread health needs.

COVID-19 also exposed multiple failings of the US system. The absence of universal coverage and the high-deductible health insurance of many Americans made it hard to convince people with suspect COVID-19 cases to seek medical attention, endangering the wider population—even those with good health insurance. This required emergency action to make COVID-19 testing and other interventions related to the disease free. This emergency response was reminiscent of the decision in the early 1970s to nationalize the payment for dialysis for all patients with chronic renal failure. The policy zigzag plugged one hole rather than comprehensively addressing the entire faulty health insurance system. This patchwork approach is both inequitable and inefficient—inequitable because it favors patients with one condition while ignoring equally worthy patients with other medical needs, and inefficient because it requires legislation, regulation, or other special actions that add ever more complexity to the system and is slow to be delivered.

Fifth, some US physicians were able to adapt their investment in chronic care coordination to facilitate their response to COVID-19. Many primary care physicians in the United States were overwhelmed and uncertain how to proceed—order tests, manage COVID-19 patients, and change their practices. However, there were others who quickly determined that the patients at highest risk from COVID-19 were the elderly with multiple chronic conditions. For practices that had instituted innovative chronic care coordination, these were precisely the kind of patients being followed by coordinators. One primary care practice organization I know of (because the venture firm I work with invested in it), Village MD, was able to identify all high-risk patients and immediately, proactively reach out to them. This allowed coordinators and other staff to inform patients about their risks and the symptoms of COVID-19, advise them to self-quarantine, encourage them to limit visitors, and educate them about how to safely use the health care system, such as calling ahead if they needed emergency services. Village MD was also able to work with their patients to provide telemedicine services instead of in-person visits. Practices that quickly implemented advanced chronic care coordination had an advantage in responding to the outbreak and protecting high-risk patients.

Sixth, the COVID-19 pandemic has changed medical delivery in many countries. Many of these changes need to become permanent. Because of the virus's infectiousness, many routine clinical activities have moved to text, phone calls, video calls, and other modes of virtual medicine. They will be done just as well as when performed face-to-face. In addition, new phone apps or "add-on" technologies will be developed. These virtual medicine interventions should be viewed not as improvised adaptations to COVID-19 but as improvements that become integrated into routine care. A permanent expansion in virtual medicine should allow more time to be devoted to face-to-face interaction for the chronically ill who need more extensive management.

Similarly, because of the threat of overwhelming the system, criteria for hospital admission, performing procedures, and other clinical services have become more stringent. It is important that the medical systems do not revert to practice B.C.—Before COVID-19. In a *Washington Post* op-ed, one physician, Dr. Jeremy Faust, described how, in the B.C. system, physicians would admit patients to the hospital with "small, but non-trivial chances of having a serious medical problem that further testing and observation may reveal." All the hospital demands imposed by COVID-19 have changed this calculation. Faust used the case of a stroke patient to illustrate the kinds of changes in clinical decision making:

> If a physician is evaluating a patient who may have had a stroke, but who did not go to an emergency room until a few days later, we would normally perform a "stroke work-up" to gather more information. We get a CT scan of the brain in the ER, and in some cases, a second more detailed one with dye. We check some bloodwork and make sure that the symptoms aren't being caused by a "stroke mimic," such as an infection that can temporarily worsen the symptoms of a previous stroke, for instance. This all takes a few hours.
>
> However, even in a patient whose symptoms have disappeared and who is "back to baseline," we often admit them to an observation unit or to the hospital to complete the work-up. That usually includes an MRI and other tests, which can take up to a day or more.
>
> But, if we are being honest, we all have come to learn that the "yield" of investigations such as the one described here is pretty low. These patients are not eligible for urgent treatments. About the best that neurologists can do is offer medications that might prevent a future stroke.

The new, much higher threshold for hospital admission needs to become permanent to avoid unnecessary and inefficient care.

Similarly, to conserve personal protective equipment and redirect health care personnel, elective surgery and other procedures have been discontinued at many hospitals and ambulatory surgical centers. When the COVID-19 threat abates, physicians should reassess how many of those procedures were really necessary or whether they were done more for hard-to-justify reasons such as convenience, financial remuneration, and the like. When elective procedures can resume, there should be a higher threshold for performing them too.

These COVID-19-induced changes in physician practices could significantly improve medical care, convenience, and safety as well as reduce costs.

The final observation from the COVID-19 pandemic returns to the main purpose of this book: the importance of other countries. Clearly, COVID-19 reminds us all that the nearly 200 countries of the world are deeply interlinked. Not just in the usual economic, travel, resource ways but also in terms of health. Health outbreaks that happen in one country have an effect on all countries. It is truly impossible to isolate different countries. Countries must work together.

More importantly, the pandemic emphasizes to everyone that studying other countries is very valuable. That question my audiences kept asking me—Which country has the best health care?—is fundamentally right. COVID-19 has made abundantly clear that we can and must learn from how different countries responded and how the viral outbreak affected different countries' health systems. Every country can learn from Taiwan's felicitous use of its health insurance card system to address the urgent public health and health care situation. Other countries might learn from medical practices that were able to adapt a system built for chronic care to handle an acute infectious illness. And we can learn from countries that had poor responses to COVID-19 about the dangers of not sharing information and not implementing public health measures rapidly. If countries truly seek out the lessons from each other about what finance, delivery, and other health system arrangements enhanced the COVID-19 response, then patients everywhere will greatly benefit in ways that go beyond the immediate crisis. That seems like a worthwhile objective from the fight against a frightening new disease.

ACKNOWLEDGMENTS

This book has been a full team effort. First, thanks go to the person I fondly refer to as "the Amtrak guy." Ken Gray happened to see me on Chris Wallace's show. He called my office, saying he wanted to meet and support my work. We did not meet at a fancy foundation or investment office but rather in the lounge at the 30th Street Amtrak train station. And being the kind of person he is, Ken was perfectly comfortable with that. I delineated my various research projects, and on the spot Ken literally gambled on my idea to conduct an international comparison of different countries' health systems. Ken is one of the rarest people in this world: unassuming but brilliant, data-driven, no-nonsense, and thoughtful. His serious commitment to help solve the health care problems of this country and his generosity were both inspirational and indispensable to sustain this project.

Ken Gray's funding made this book possible. But it became a reality with months of research, interviewing, writing, fact checking, editing, and many other activities. This book's existence is a testament to the inexhaustible efforts by my crack research team of Aaron Glickman, Emily Gudbranson, John Urwin, Sarah DiMagno, and Cathy Zhang in performing all these activities. They are as much the authors of this work as I am.

Jonathan Cohn visited Taiwan and reported on that country's health care system for the *Huffington Post*. We were able to expand and transform his reporting and articles into a chapter for this book.

Joseph Fruscione provided invaluable help in reading the entire book, editing it, and making the chapter structure consistent.

Teasel Muir-Harmony read many chapters, and her insightful suggestions and edits made it more "me" and relevant to contemporary debates.

Clive Priddle at Public Affairs has been my publisher and editor for more than a decade. He is a pleasure to work with. His faith in what I have to say, the way he pushes me to be clearer in how I say it, and how he reminds me of the big picture that I want to convey always greatly improves my work. And this book is no exception.

My agent, Suzanne Gluck, has been my advocate and advisor for many, many years. Thanks go to her for taking this harebrained idea of looking at different countries' health care systems and focusing it into a lucid book.

Finally, this book exists because of myriad people in all 11 countries whom my team and I interviewed and harassed for ever more details and insights about their health care system. Of course they bear no responsibility for the content of the chapters, but they did add great illumination and insight that I hope enhances the substance of this book.

US
Stuart Altman

Canada
David Rudoler, PhD
Sara Allin, PhD
Gregory P. Marchildon
John Lavis
Paul Grootendorst
Allan Detsky

UK
Dido Harding
Donald Berwick
Bob Wachter
Malcolm Grant
Richard Murray
Ninjeri Pandit
Simon Stevens

Norway
Reidun Førde
Tor Iversen
Trygve Ottersen
Ole Nordheim
Magne Nylenna
Olaf Aasland
Berit Bringedal
Karin Rø
Fredrik Bååthe

France
Jean de Kervasdoue
Paul Dourgnon
Zeynep Or
Antoine Malone
Michel Naiditch
Fabien Calvo
Laurent Degos
Agnes Couffinhal
Isabelle Durand-Zaleski
Pierre-Yves Geoffard

Germany
George Baum
Stephan Hofmeister
Andreas Gassen
Reinhard Busse
Thomas Renner

Netherlands
Roland Bal
Peter Groenewegen
Danielle Timmermans
Niek Klazinga
Patrick Jeurissen
Wouter Bos
Martine de Bruijne
Jeroen Struijs

Switzerland
Samia Hurst
Rebecca Ruiz
Claudine Burton-Jeangros
Jacques de Haller
Jacques-Andres Romand
Paolo Ferrari
Giorgio Merlani
Omar Kherad

Australia
Andrew Wilson
Paul Dugdale
Gary Freed
Adam Elshaug

Taiwan
Sam Radwan, Enhance
   International LLC
May Wang
May Tsung-Mei Cheng
Phoebe Chi
Shou-Hsia Cheng
Ming-Jui Yeh
Yun Yen

China
Sam Radwan, Enhance
   International LLC
Gordon G. Liu
Elizabeth Zhao
Beth Zhang, Enhance
   International LLC
Roger Xu, Enhance International
   LLC

GLOSSARY OF ACRONYMS

APMs—alternative payment models
CEA—cost-effectiveness analysis
COPD—chronic obstructive pulmonary disease
DRG—Diagnosis Related Group
EHR—electronic health record
EMA—European Medicines Agency
GP—general practitioner
LPN—licensed practical nurse
MSA—medical savings account
MEA—managed entry agreement
NICU—neonatal intensive care unit
NP—nurse practitioner
OECD—Organisation for Economic Co-operation and Development
PCP—primary care physician
QALY—quality-adjusted life year
RN—registered nurse
RVU—relative value unit
SHI—statutory health insurance
VAT—value-added tax
VHI—voluntary health insurance
WHO—World Health Organization

UNITED STATES

ACA—Affordable Care Act (2010)
ACO—Accountable Care Organization
AMA—American Medical Association
CDC—Centers for Disease Control and Prevention
CHIP—Children's Health Insurance Program

CLASS Act—Community Living Assistance Services and Supports
    Act (2010)
CMMI—Center for Medicare and Medicaid Innovation
CMS—Centers for Medicare and Medicaid Services
CPT code—Current Procedural Terminology code
DSH—Disproportionate Share Hospital
FDA—Food and Drug Administration
FMAP—Federal Medicaid Assistance Percentage
FQHC—Federally Qualified Health Clinic
GME—graduate medical education
HMO—health maintenance organization
IHS—Indian Health Service
IME—indirect medical education
MS-DRG—Medicare Severity Diagnosis Related Groups System
NAM—National Academy of Medicine
PBM—pharmacy benefit management companies
PMPM—per-member-per-month
PPO—preferred provider organization
VA—Department of Veterans Affairs

CANADA

CADTH—Canadian Agency for Drugs and Technologies in Health
CDR—Common Drug Review
CHA—Canada Health Act (1984)
DIN—Drug Identification Number
HIDS Act—Hospital Insurance and Diagnostic Services Act (1957)
HPFB—Health Products and Food Branch
LHIN—Local Health Integration Network
MAPP—maximum average potential price
MCA—Medical Care Act (1966)
NAFTA—North American Free Trade Agreement (1993)
NDS—New Drug Submission
NOC—Notification of Compliance
ODB—Ontario Drug Benefit
OHIP—Ontario Health Insurance Program

OHIP+—Ontario Health Insurance Program Plus
pCPA—pan-Canadian Pharmaceutical Alliance
PDIP—Public Drug Insurance Plan
PMPRB—Patented Medicines Prices Review Board
TDP—Trillium Drug Program

UNITED KINGDOM

ABPI—Association of the British Pharmaceutical Industry
ADLs—activities of daily living
APMS—Alternative Provider Medical Services
BMA—British Medical Association
BPT—Best Practice Tariff
CCG—clinical commissioning group
CHAI—Commission for Healthcare Audit and Inspection
CQC—Care Quality Commission
CQUIN—Commissioning for Quality and Innovation
GMC—General Medical Council
GMS—General Medical Services
HRG—Healthcare Resource Group
ICER—incremental cost effectiveness ratio
ICS—integrated care systems
MFF—market forces factor
MHIS—Mental Health Investment Standard
MHRA—Medicines and Healthcare products Regulatory Agency
NHS—National Health Service
NICE—National Institute for Health and Care Excellence
NI—National Insurance
NMC—Nursing and Midwifery Council
NPfIT—National Programme for IT
PBR—Payment by Results
PCN—Primary Care Network
PCT—primary care trust
PMS—Personal Medical Services
PPRS—Pharmaceutical Price Regulation Scheme
QOF—Quality and Outcomes Framework

SHA—strategic health authority
STPs—Sustainability and Transformation Partnerships
TAC—Technology Appraisal Committee
VPAS—Voluntary Scheme for Branded Medicines Pricing and Access

NORWAY

DPOS—District Psychiatric Outpatient Service
HELFO—Norwegian Health Economics Administration
    (Helseøkonomiforvaltningen)
HTA—health technology assessment
NIS—National Insurance Scheme (Folketrygden)
NoMA—Norwegian Medicines Agency (Statens legemiddelverk)
RHA—Regional Health Authority

FRANCE

ALD—Chronic Disease (Affection de Longue Durée)
APA—Personalized Allowance for Autonomy
CEESP—Economic and Public Health Assessment Committee
CEPS—Economic Committee for Health Products
CMU—Universal Health Coverage Act (1999)
CNAMTS—National Health Insurance Fund for Salaried Workers, or
    the General Fund
CNSA—National Solidarity Fund for Autonomy
CSG—General Social Contribution
DMP—Personal Medical Record (Dossier Médical Personnel)
ENCC—National Cost Studies with Common Methodology
GHM—Homogeneous Group of the Sick (Groupe Homogène des
    Malades)
HAS—High Authority on Health
IAB—improvement in additional benefit
PUMA—Universal Disease Protection Act (2016)
SMR—medical service rendered (service médical rendu)
UNCAM—National Union of Health Insurance Funds

GERMANY

DMP—disease management program

GBA—Federal Joint Commission (Gemeinsamer Bundesausschuss)

INEK—Institute for Reimbursement in the Hospital (Institute fur das Entgeltsystem im Krankenhaus)

IQWiG—Institute for Quality and Efficiency in Health Care (Institut für Qualität und Wirtschaftlichkeit im Gesundheitswesen)

KBV—National Association of Statutory Health Insurance Physicians (Kassenärztliche Bundesvereinigung)

NUB—new diagnostic and treatment methods (Neue Untersuchungs- und Behandlungsmethoden)

NETHERLANDS

AWBZ—Exceptional Medical Expenses Act (1967)

BKZ—Health Care Budget

CAK—Central Administration Office

CBS—Statistics Netherlands

CGS—College of Medical Specialists

CIZ—Care Assessment Agency

DBC—Diagnosis Treatment Combination

DFHCS—Diabetes Federation Health Care Standard

GVS—Pharmaceutical Reimbursement System

MSB—specialist-owned partnership

NMG—Netherlands Medical Association

NZA—Dutch Healthcare Authority

SVB—Social Insurance Bank

ZBCs—independent treatment centers

ZIN—National Health Care Institute

ZVW—Health Insurance Act (2006)

SWITZERLAND

AI—Disability Insurance

ANQ—National Association for Quality Improvement in Hospitals and Clinics

AVS—Old Age and Survivors Insurance

FDC—Federal Drug Commission

FDHA—Federal Department of Home Affairs

FOPH—Federal Office of Public Health

GDK/CDS—Conference of the Cantonal Ministers of Public Health

HMG/LPTh—Federal Law on Therapeutic Products (Heilmittelgesetz/Loi sur les produits thérapeutiques) (2000)

KUVG/LAMA—Federal Law on Sickness and Accident Insurance (1911)

KVAG/LSAMal—Federal Law on the Supervision of Mandatory Health Insurance (2014)

KVG/LAMal—Federal Health Insurance Law (1994)

LAA—Federal Law on Accident Insurance (1981)

LAI—Law on Disability Insurance (1959)

TARMED—Tarif Médical

AUSTRALIA

ARTG—Australian Register of Therapeutic Goods

BDF—basic daily fee

CDL—Combination Drug List

CHSP—Commonwealth Home Supports Program

DUSC—Drug Utilization Subcommittee

EMSN—Extended Medicare Safety Net

ESC—Economics Subcommittee

GPG—Greatest Permissible Gap

IHPA—Independent Hospital Pricing Authority

LHC—Lifetime Health Cover

MBS—Medicare Benefits Schedule

MSAC—Medical Services Advisory Committee

NDIA—National Disability Insurance Agency

NDIS—National Disability Insurance Scheme

NEP—National Efficient Price

NWAU—National Weighted Activity Unit

OMSN—Original Medicare Safety Net
PBAC—Pharmaceutical Benefits Advisory Committee
PBS—Pharmaceutical Benefits Scheme
PHIAC—Private Health Insurance Administration Council
PHNs—Primary Health Networks
TGA—Therapeutic Goods Administration
VMO—Visiting Medical Officer

TAIWAN

CDE—Center for Drug Evaluation
FPICP—Family Physician Integrated Care Project
LTC 2.0—Long Term Care 2.0
NHIA—National Health Insurance Administration
NHI—National Health Insurance
PBR—Pharmaceutical Benefit Review
TCM—Traditional Chinese Medicine

CHINA

CMS—Cooperative Medical Scheme
EDL—Essential Drugs List
LIS—Labor Insurance Scheme
MOH—Ministry of Health
MoHRSS—Ministry of Human Resources and Social Security
NCMS—New Cooperative Medical Scheme
NHC—National Health Commission
NRDL—National Reimbursement Drug List
SPA—social pooling account
THC—township health center
UEBMI—Urban Employee Basic Medical Insurance
URBMI—Urban Resident Basic Medical Insurance
URRBMI—Urban and Rural Resident Basic Medical Insurance

RECOMMENDED READING

CHAPTER ONE. UNITED STATES

Blumenthal, D. "Employer-Sponsored Health Insurance in the United States—Origins and Implications." *New England Journal of Medicine* 35, no. 1 (2006): 82–88. doi: 10.1056/NEJMhpro60703.

Centers for Medicare & Medicaid Services. *National Health Expenditures 2017 Highlights.* Department of Health and Human Services, 2018. www.cms.gov/Research-Statistics-Data-and-Systems/Statistics-Trends-and-Reports/National HealthExpendData/Downloads/highlights.pdf.

Emanuel, Ezekiel J. *Prescription for the Future: The Twelve Transformational Practices of Highly Effective Medical Organizations.* New York: PublicAffairs, 2017.

Rice, T., P. Rosenau, L. Y. Unruh, A. J. Barnes, R. B. Saltman, and E. van Ginneken. "United States of America: Health System Review." *Health Systems in Transition* 15, no. 3 (2013): 1–431.

Starr, P. *The Social Transformation of American Medicine: The Rise of a Sovereign Profession and the Making of a Vast Industry.* New York: Basic Books, 2017.

The Commonwealth Fund. "The U.S. Health Care System." In *International Profiles of Health Care Systems,* edited by E. Mossialos, A. Djordjevic, R. Osborn, and D. Sarnak, 173–181. The Commonwealth Fund, 2017.

Vignette Adapted From

Hearing on "No More Surprises: Protecting Patients from Surprise Medical Bills." 2123 Rayburn House Office Building: House Committee on Energy and Commerce, 2019. https://energycommerce.house.gov/committee-activity/hearings/hearing-on-no-more-surprises-protecting-patients-from-surprise-medical.

CHAPTER TWO. CANADA

Brandt, J., B. Shearer, and S. G. Morgan. "Prescription Drug Coverage in Canada: A Review of the Economic, Policy and Political Considerations for Universal Pharmacare." *Journal of Pharmaceutical Policy and Practice* 11, no. 1 (2018): 1–13. doi: 10.1186/s40545-018-0154-x.

Canadian Institute for Health Information. *National Health Expenditure Trends, 1975 to 2018*. Ottawa, ON: CIHI, 2019. www.cihi.ca/en/health-spending/2018/ national-health-expenditure-trends.

Canadian Institute for Health Information. *Physicians in Canada, 2016: Summary Report*. Ottawa, ON: CIHI, 2017. https://secure.cihi.ca/free_products/Physicians _in_Canada_2016.pdf.

Allin, S. and D. Rudoler. "The Canadian Health Care System." In *International Profiles of Health Care Systems*, edited by E. Mossialos, A. Djordjevic, R. Osborn, and D. Sarnak, 21–30. The Commonwealth Fund, 2017.

Marchildon, G. P. "Canada: Health System Review." *Health Systems in Transition* 15, no. 1 (2013): 1–79.

Morgan, S. G. and K. Boothe. "Universal Prescription Drug Coverage in Canada: Long-Promised yet Undelivered." *Health Management Forum* 29, no. 6 (2016): 247–254.

Santé, MdSedl. "Les dépenses de santé en 2016—Résultats des comptes de la santé—édition 2017." 2017. http://drees.solidarites-sante.gouv.fr/IMG/pdf/cns _2017.pdf.

Seroussi, B. and J. Bouaud. "Adoption of a Nationwide Shared Medical Record in France: Lessons Learnt After 5 Years of Deployment." *AMIA Annual Symposium Proceedings* (2016): 1100–1109.

Stone, C. P. "A Glimpse at EHR Implementation Around the World: The Lessons the US Can Learn." The Health Institute for E-Health Policy, 2014. www .e-healthpolicy.org/docs/A_Glimpse_at_EHR_Implementation_Around_ the_World1_ChrisStone.pdf.

Vignette Adapted and Quoted From

Kassam A. "The Serious Flaw in Canada's Healthcare System: Prescription Drugs Aren't Free." *The Guardian*, October 20, 2017. www.theguardian.com/ world/2017/oct/20/canada-national-pharmacare-prescription-drugs.

CHAPTER THREE. UNITED KINGDOM

British Medical Association. "General Practice in the UK—Background Briefing." April 2017.

Cylus, J., E. Richardson, L. Findley, M. Longley, C. O'Neill, and D. Steel. "United Kingdom: Health System Review." *Health Systems in Transition* 17, no. 5 (2015): 1–125.

Department of Health and Social Care. *The 2019 Voluntary Scheme for Branded Medicines Pricing and Access: Chapters and Glossary*. GOV.UK, 2018. https://assets .publishing.service.gov.uk/government/uploads/system/uploads/attachment

_data/file/761834/voluntary-scheme-for-branded-medicines-pricing-and
-access-chapters-and-glossary.pdf.

Gershlick, B. *Best Practice Tariffs: United Kingdom (England)*. The Health Foundation, 2016. www.oecd.org/els/health-systems/Better-Ways-to-Pay-for-Health-Care -Background-Note-England-Best-practice-tariffs.pdf.

Milne, C. "Mental Health Spending in the English NHS: Full Fact." May 17, 2019. https://fullfact.org/health/mental-health-spending-england/.

Office for National Statistics. *Healthcare Expenditure, UK Health Accounts: 2017.* Office for National Statistics, 2019. www.ons.gov.uk/peoplepopulationand community/healthandsocialcare/healthcaresystem/bulletins/ukhealth accounts/2017.

Robertson, R., J. Appleby, H. Evans, and N. Hemmings. *Public Satisfaction with the NHS and Social Care in 2018*, 2019. www.kingsfund.org.uk/publications/public -satisfaction-nhs-social-care-2018.

Thorlby, R. and S. Arora. "The English Health Care System." In *International Profiles of Health Care Systems*, edited by E. Mossialos, A. Djordjevic, R. Osborn, D. Sarnak, 49–58. The Commonwealth Fund, 2017.

Vignette Adapted and Quoted From

Central Office of Information for the Ministry of Health. *The New National Health Service*, February 1948.

CHAPTER FOUR. NORWAY

Apotekforeningen. "Key Figures 2017: Pharmacies and Pharmaceuticals in Norway." 2018. www.apotek.no/Files/Filer_2014/Engelske_sider/Pharmacies%20 and%20prescriptions%20-%20%20Key%20Figures%202017.pdf.

Brekke, K. R., T. H. Holmås, and O. R. Straume. *Are Pharmaceuticals Still Inexpensive in Norway?: A Comparison of Prescription Drug Prices in Ten European Countries.* Bergen: SNF, 2010. https://openaccess.nhh.no/nhh-xmlui/handle/11250/ 165071.

Ernst & Young Global Limited. *The Norwegian Processes for Implementation of Medicinal Products and the Associated Tenders: Specialist Health Services.* EYGM Limited. 2019. www.ey.com/Publication/vwLUAssets/Er_anbud_alltid_losningen_for_ legemidler/$FILE/B18022no-Implementation-Medical%20products_07LR_ final.pdf.

European Monitoring Centre for Drugs and Drug Addiction. "Norway, Country Drug Report 2019." www.emcdda.europa.eu/publications/country-drug -reports/2019/norway_en. Published June 2019.

Johansen, I. H., T. Morken, and S. Hunskaar. "How Norwegian Casualty Clinics Handle Contacts Related to Mental Illness: A Prospective Observational

Study." *International Journal of Mental Health Systems* 6, no. 1 (2012): 3. doi: 10.1186/1752-4458-6-3.

Lindahl, A. K. "The Norwegian Health Care System." In *International Profiles of Health Care Systems*, edited by E. Mossialos, A. Djordjevic, R. Osborn, and D. Sarnak, 129–138. The Commonwealth Fund, 2017.

Ministry of Health and Care Services. *The Primary Health and Care Services of Tomorrow—Localised and Integrated*. Norwegian Ministry of Health and Care Services, 2015. www.regjeringen.no/en/dokumenter/meld.-st.-26-20142015/ id2409890/.

Ringard, Å., A. Sagan, I. Sperre Saunes, and A. K. Lindahl. "Norway: Health System Review." *Health Systems in Transition* 15, no. 8 (2013): 1–162.

Statistics Norway. "Earnings." Statbank, 2019. www.ssb.no/en/arbeid-og-lonn/ statistikker/lonnansatt.

Steihaug, S., B. Paulsen, and L. Melby. "Norwegian General Practitioners' Collaboration with Municipal Care Providers—A Qualitative Study of Structural Conditions." *Scandinavian Journal of Primary Health Care* 35, no. 4 (2017): 344–351. doi: 10.1080/02813432.2017.1397264.

Vignette Adapted and Quoted From

Brune, V. "What Happens When You Get Sick in Norway // My Story & All You Need to Know." *Nordic Wanders*, May 9, 2018. https://nordicwanders.com/ blog/2018/05/experience-norwegian-healthcare-system.

CHAPTER FIVE. FRANCE

Chevreul, K., K. B. Brigham, I. Durand-Zaleski, and C. Hernández-Quevedo. "France: Health System Review." *Health Systems in Transition*, 2015. www.euro .who.int/__data/assets/pdf_file/0011/297938/France-HiT.pdf.

Durand-Zaleski, I. "The French Health Care System." In *International Profiles of Health Care Systems*, edited by E. Mossialos, A. Djordjevic, R. Osborn, and D. Sarnak, 59–68. The Commonwealth Fund, 2017.

Dutton, P. *Differential Diagnoses: A Comparative History of Health Care Problems and Solutions in the United States and France*. Ithaca, NY: ILR Press, 2007.

Rodwin, V. G. "The Health Care System Under French National Health Insurance: Lessons for Health Reform in the United States." *American Journal of Public Health* 93, no. 1 (2003): 31–37.

Seroussi, B. and J. Bouaud. "Adoption of a Nationwide Shared Medical Record in France: Lessons Learnt after 5 Years of Deployment." *AMIA Annual Symposium Proceedings*, 2016: 1100–1109.

Stone, C. P. "A Glimpse at EHR Implementation Around the World: The Lessons the US Can Learn." *The Health Institute for E-Health Policy*, 2014. www.e-health

policy.org/docs/A_Glimpse_at_EHR_Implementation_Around_the_World1
_ChrisStone.pdf.

Vignette Adapted From
The World Health Report 2000: Health Systems: Improving Performance. Geneva: WHO,
2000. www.who.int/whr/2000/en/whr00_en.pdf?ua=1.

CHAPTER SIX. GERMANY

Blümel, M. and R. Busse. "The German Health Care System." In *International Profiles
of Health Care Systems,* edited by E. Mossialos, A. Djordjevic, R. Osborn, and D.
Sarnak, 69–76. The Commonwealth Fund, 2017.

Busse, R. and M. Blümel. "Germany: Health System Review." *Health Systems in Transition* 16, no. 2 (2014): 1–296.

Busse, R., M. Blümel, F. Knieps, and T. Bärnighausen. "Statutory Health Insurance
in Germany: A Health System Shaped by 135 Years of Solidarity, Self-Gov-
ernance, and Competition." *The Lancet* 390, no. 10097 (2017): 882–897. doi:
10.1016/S0140-6736(17)31280-1.

European Commission. *Germany: Country Health Profile 2017.* OECD, 2017. www.oecd
.org/publications/germany-country-health-profile-2017-9789264283398-en
.htm.

Statistisches Bundesamt. "Health Expenditure." Destatis, 2019. www.destatis.de/
EN/Themes/Society-Environment/Health/Health-Expenditure/_node.html.

CHAPTER SEVEN. NETHERLANDS

Alders, P. and F. T. Schut. "The 2015 Long-Term Care Reform in the Netherlands:
Getting the Financial Incentives Right?" *Health Policy* 123, no. 3 (2019): 312–316.
doi: 10.1016/j.healthpol.2018.10.010.

CBS Netherlands. "Health Expenditure: Functions and Financing for International
Comparisons." June 21, 2019. https://opendata.cbs.nl/statline/#/CBS/en/data
set/84043ENG/table?ts=1548188388918.

de Graaff, R. and I. Spee. *Current Developments in the Dutch Healthcare Market: 2018.*
Seijgraaf Consultancy B.V., 2018. www.welfaretech.dk/media/6800/current
-developments-in-the-dutch-healthcare-market.pdf.

Government of the Netherlands. Ministry of Health, Welfare, and Sport, 2019.
www.government.nl/ministries/ministry-of-health-welfare-and-sport.

Government of the Netherlands. Zorginstituut Nederland, 2019. www.zorg
instituutnederland.nl/.

Hendriks, R. H. M., K. F. E. Veraghtert, B. E. M. Widdershoven, and K. P. Companje. *Two Centuries of Solidarity: German, Belgian and Dutch Social Health Insurance 1770–2008*. Amsterdam: Aksant Academic Publishers, 2009. doi: 10.26530/OAPEN_353800.

Kroneman, M., W. Boerma, M. van den Berg, P. Groenewegen, J. de Jong, and E. van Ginneken. "The Netherlands: Health System Review." *Health Systems in Transition* 1, no. 2 (2016): 1–239.

Organisation for Economic Co-operation and Development. "Health Expenditure and Financing." OECD.Stat, 2019. https://stats.oecd.org.

Smits, M., M. Rutten, E. Keizer, M. Wensing, G. Westert, and P. Giesen. "The Development and Performance of After-Hours Primary Care in the Netherlands: A Narrative Review." *Annals of Internal Medicine* 166, no. 10 (2017): 737–742. doi: 10.7326/M16-2776.

van Loenen, T., M. J. van den Berg, S. Heinemann, R. Baker, M. J. Faber, and G. P. Westert. "Trends Towards Stronger Primary Care in Three Western European Countries: 2006–2012." *BMC Family Practice* 17, no. 1 (2016): 59. doi: 10.1186/s12875-016-0458-3.

Wammes, J., P. Jeurissen, G. Westert, and M. Tanke. "The Dutch Health Care System." In *International Profiles of Health Care Systems*, edited by E. Mossialos, A. Djordjevic, R. Osborn, and D. Sarnak, 113–120. The Commonwealth Fund, 2017.

Vignette Adapted and Quoted From

Avery, L. "Healthcare in the Netherlands: Is It Really That Good?" *DutchReview*, November 2016. https://dutchreview.com/expat/health/healthcare-in-the-netherlands-2/.

CHAPTER EIGHT. SWITZERLAND

Commonwealth Fund. "Generic Drugs Often Cost Double in Switzerland." *Commonwealth Fund International Health News Brief*, April 19, 2018. www.commonwealthfund.org/publications/newsletter-article/2018/apr/generic-drugs-often-cost-double-switzerland.

De Pietro, C., P. Camenzind, I. SturnyI, L. Crivelli, S. Edwards-Garavoglia, A. Spranger, F. Wittenbecher, and W. Quentin. "Switzerland: Health System Review." *Health Systems in Transition* 17, no. 4 (2015): 1–288.

Interpharma. "Swiss Healthcare and Pharmaceutical Market: Pharmacies Remain the Most Important Sales Outlet." Interpharma. www.interpharma.ch/fakten-statistiken/4460-pharmacies-remain-most-important-sales-outlet.

Sturny, I. "The Swiss Health Care System." In *International Profiles of Health Care Systems*, edited by E. Mossialos, A. Djordjevic, R. Osborn, and D. Sarnak, 155–162. The Commonwealth Fund, 2017.

Swiss Confederation. *Health Equity: Facts and Figures for Switzerland.* Federal Office of Public Health, 2018. www.bag.admin.ch/bag/en/home/zahlen-und-statistiken /zahlen-fakten-zu-chancengleichheit.html.

Swiss Confederation. *Statistics of Medical Professions 2017.* Federal Office of Public Health, 2018. www.bag.admin.ch/bag/en/home/zahlen-und-statistiken/ statistiken-berufe-im-gesundheitswesen.html.

CHAPTER NINE. AUSTRALIA

Aged Care Financing Authority. "Aged Care Financing Authority Annual Reports." Australian Government Department of Health, August 10, 2019. https://aged care.health.gov.au/reform/aged-care-financing-authority/aged-care-financing -authority-annual-reports.

Australian Institute for Health and Welfare. "Reports & Data." Australian Institute of Health and Welfare. www.aihw.gov.au/reports-data.

Boxall, A.-M. and J. A. Gillespie. *Making Medicare: The Politics of Universal Health Care in Australia.* Sydney: NewSouth Publishing, 2013.

Duckett, S. J. and S. Wilcox. *The Australian Health Care System.* 5th ed. South Melbourne, Victoria, Australia: Oxford University Press, 2015.

GlaxoSmithKline Australia Pty Ltd and ViiV Healthcare Pty Ltd. *The Pharmaceutical Benefits Scheme in Australia: An Explainer on System Components,* 2018. https:// au.gsk.com/media/421635/gsk-viiv-the-pbs-in-australia-feb-2018.pdf.

Glover, L. "The Australian Health Care System." In *International Profiles of Health Care Systems,* edited by E. Mossialos, A. Djordjevic, R. Osborn, and D. Sarnak, 11–20. The Commonwealth Fund, 2017.

Goddard, M. S. "How the Pharmaceutical Benefits Scheme Began." *Medical Journal of Australia* 201, no. 1 (2014): S23–S25. doi: 10.5694/mja14.00124.

Healy, J., E. Sharman, and B. Lokuge. "Australia: Health System Review." *Health Systems in Transition* 8, no. 5 (2006): 1–158.

Vignette Adapted and Quoted From
Aubusson, K. "AMA Name-Dropped on 'Egregious' $18,000 Sydney Surgeon Bill." *Sydney Morning Herald,* June 3, 2018. www.smh.com.au/healthcare/ama -name-dropped-on-egregious-18-000-sydney-surgeon-bill-20180601-p4ziy8 .html.

Duckett, S. "Australia's Health System Is Enviable, but There's Room for Improvement." *The Conversation,* September 21, 2017. http://theconversation.com/ australias-health-system-is-enviable-but-theres-room-for-improvement -81332.

Victoria State Government Department of Health and Human Services. "Hospital Costs and Payments." Better Health Channel, September 2015. www

.betterhealth.vic.gov.au:443/health/servicesandsupport/hospital-costs-and
-payments.

CHAPTER TEN. TAIWAN

Cohn, J. "If You Don't Believe Single Payer Can Work, See How They Do It in Taiwan." *HuffPost*, September 8, 2018. www.huffpost.com/entry/single-payer
-medicare-taiwan_n_5b9295ede4b0511db3e1d45a.

Cheng, T.-M. "The Taiwanese Health Care System." In *International Profiles of Health
Care Systems*, edited by E. Mossialos, A. Djordjevic, R. Osborn, and D. Sarnak,
163–172. The Commonwealth Fund, 2017.

Hsiao, W. C., S.-H. Cheng, and W. Yip. "What Can Be Achieved with a Single-Payer
NHI System: The Case of Taiwan." *Social Science & Medicine* 233 (2019): 265–271.
doi: 10.1016/j.socscimed.2016.12.006.

Reinhardt, U. E. "Humbled in Taiwan." *BMJ* 336, no. 7635 (2008): 72. doi: 10.1136/
bmj.39450.473380.0F.

Palfreman, J. *Sick Around the World*. Frontline, 2008. www.pbs.org/wgbh/pages/
frontline/sickaroundtheworld.

Ministry of Health and Welfare. *2018 Taiwan Health and Welfare Report*. Taipei, Taiwan: Ministry of Health and Welfare, 2018. www.cdway.com.tw/gov/mhw2/
book107/book1e/#p=22.

National Health Insurance Administration. "2017–2018 National Health Insurance Annual Report." Taiwan Ministry of Health and Welfare, 2018. www
.nhi.gov.tw/english/Content_List.aspx?n=8FC0974BBFEFA56D&topn=ED
4A30E51A609E49.

Price Waterhouse Cooper. "Taiwan Health Industries: An Introductory Market Over-
view." 2018. www.pwc.tw/en/publications/assets/taiwan-health-industries.pdf.

Yeh, M.-J. "Long-Term Care System in Taiwan: The 2017 Major Reform and Its Challenges." *Ageing & Society* (January 2019): 1–18. doi: 10.1017/S0144686X18001745.

Vignette Adapted and Quoted From

Cohn, J. "If You Don't Believe Single Payer Can Work, See How They Do It in Taiwan." *HuffPost*, September 8, 2018. www.huffpost.com/entry/single-payer
-medicare-taiwan_n_5b9295ede4b0511db3e1d45a.

CHAPTER ELEVEN. CHINA

Blumenthal, D. and W. Hsiao. "Privatization and Its Discontents—The Evolving
Chinese Health Care System." *New England Journal of Medicine* 353, no. 11 (2015).
doi: 10.1056/NEJMhpro51133.

Burns, L. R. and G. G. Liu. *China's Healthcare System and Reform* (Cambridge: Cambridge University Press, 2017).

Fang, H. "The Chinese Health Care System." In *International Profiles of Health Care Systems*, edited by E. Mossialos, A. Djordjevic, R. Osborn, D. Sarnak, 31–38. The Commonwealth Fund, 2017.

Hu, D., W. Zhu, Y. Fu, M. Zhang, Y. Zhao, K. Hanson, M. Martinez-Alvarez, and X. Liu. "Development of Village Doctors in China: Financial Compensation and Health System Support." *International Journal of Equity Health* 16 (2017). doi: 10.1186/s12939-016-0505-7.

Huang, F. and L. Gan. "The Impacts of China's Urban Employee Basic Medical Insurance on Healthcare Expenditures and Health Outcomes." *Health Economics* 26, no. 2 (2017): 149–163. doi: 10.1002/hec.3281.

Li, X., J. Lu, S. Hu, K. K. Cheng, J. De Maeseneer, E. Mossialos, D. R. Xu, et al. "The Primary Health-Care System in China." *The Lancet* 390, no. 10112 (2017): 2584–2594. doi: 10.1016/S0140-6736(17)33109-4.

Liu, X. and H. Cao. "China's Cooperative Medical System: Its Historical Transformations and the Trend of Development." *Journal of Public Health Policy* 13, no. 4 (1992): 501–511.

Luo, Y., W. Bossany, J. Wong, and C. Chen. "Opportunities Open Up in Chinese Private Health Insurance." Boston Consulting Group, August 24, 2016. www.bcg.com/publications/2016/insurance-health-care-payers-providers-opportunities-open-up-in-chinese-private-health-insurance.aspx.

Ma, J., M. Lu, and H. Quan. "From a National, Centrally Planned Health System to a System Based on the Market: Lessons from China." *Health Affairs* 27, no. 4 (2018): 937–948. doi: 10.1377/hlthaff.27.4.937.

Mossialos, E., Y. Ge, J. Hu, and W. Liejun. *Pharmaceutical Policy in China: Challenges and Opportunities for Reform.* Copenhagen, Denmark: WHO Regional Office for Europe, 2016. www.euro.who.int/__data/assets/pdf_file/0020/320465/Pharmaceutical-policy-China-challenges-opportunities-reform.pdf?ua=1.

National Bureau of Statistics of China. *China Statistical Yearbook 2017.* China Statistics Press, 2017. www.stats.gov.cn/tjsj/ndsj/2017/indexeh.htm.

National Bureau of Statistics of China. *China Statistical Yearbook 2018.* China Statistics Press, 2018. www.stats.gov.cn/tjsj/ndsj/2018/indexeh.htm.

OECD. "OECD Health Statistics 2014: How Does China Compare?" 2014. www.oecd.org/els/health-systems/Briefing-Note-CHINA-2014.pdf.

Pu, X., Y. Gu, and X. Wang. "Provider Payment to Primary Care Physicians in China: Background, Challenges, and a Reform Framework." *Primary Health Care Research and Development* 20 (2018). doi: 10.1017/S146342361800021X.

Que, J., L. Lu, and L. Shi. "Development and Challenges of Mental Health in China." *General Psychology* 32, no. 1 (2019): e100053. doi: 10.1136/gpsych-2019-100053.

Ren, X., J. Yin, B. Wang, and M. R. Schwarz. "A Descriptive Analysis of Medical Education in China." *Medical Teacher* 30, no. 7 (2008): 667–672. doi: 10.1080/01421590802155100.

Wang, Q., Y. Zhou, X. Ding, and X. Ying. "Demand for Long-Term Care Insurance in China." *International Journal of Environmental Research and Public Health* 15, no. 1 (2018). doi: 10.3390/ijerph15010006.

Yang, L., L. Sun, L. Wen, H. Zhang, C. Li, K. Hanson, and H. Fang. "Financing Strategies to Improve Essential Public Health Equalization and Its Effects in China." *International Journal of Equity in Health* 15 (2016). doi: 10.1186/s12939-016-0482-x.

Zhu, K., L. Zhang, S. Yuan, X. Zhang, and Z. Zhang. "Health Financing and Integration of Urban and Rural Residents' Basic Medical Insurance Systems in China." *International Journal for Equity in Health* 16, no. 1 (2017).

Vignette Adapted and Quoted From

Nie, J.-B., Y. Cheng, X. Zou, N. Gong, J. D. Tucker, B. Wong, and A. Kleinman. "The Vicious Circle of Patient-Physician Mistrust in China: Health Professionals' Perspectives, Institutional Conflict of Interest, and Building Trust Through Medical Professionalism." *Developing World Bioethics* 18, no. 1 (2018): 26–36. doi: 10.1111/dewb.12170.

INDEX

Act on Specialized Clinical Services
    (Netherlands), 208
Act to Strengthen Competition in
    Statutory Health Insurance, 2007
    (Germany), 172
Affordable Care Act (ACA/United
    States), 21–22
  children, 391
  and churn, 25
  costs/reducing costs, 36, 50
  exchange plans coverage, 22, 25, 28,
    387
  health care delivery, 36
  hospital penalties, 38
  hospital readmissions, 38–39
  improving quality, 36
  innovation, 34, 36
  nursing shortages, 50
  passage, 21
  payments, 34
  policy changes, 22
  preventive medicine, 36
  simplification, 396, 404
  subsidies, 28, 387, 388, 390
  Trump/Republican attacks on, 22,
    28, 52, 367, 387
  uninsured, 52, 387
Aged Care Act, 1997 (Australia), 268–269
Aged Care Assessment Team
    (Australia), 280
Alberta Health Services, 66
alternative medicine. See
    complementary/alternative
    medicine
alternative payment models (APMs)
  bundled payments, 34, 35, 67,

69, 167, 208–209, 211, 372–373,
    374–375, 400
  Canada, 65, 67, 68–69, 68 (fig.), 82
  capitation, 34–35, 68 (fig.), 69,
    96, 124 (fig.), 125, 140, 142, 154,
    372–373, 374, 400
  fee-for-service problems, 32, 34, 35,
    51–52, 96, 405
  France, 151, 154, 167
  Netherlands, 208–209, 211, 400
  Norway, 124 (fig.), 125, 140, 142
  pay for performance, 99, 112, 151, 154
  United Kingdom, 96, 97 (fig.), 99, 112
  United States, 8, 32, 34, 386, 400
Alternative Provider Medical Services
    (APMS/United Kingdom)
    contracts, 98, 98 (fig.)
American Enterprise Institute, 389
American Hospital Association, 37–38
American Medical Association (AMA),
    16, 20, 34
Appraisal Committee (Netherlands),
    220
Association of the British
    Pharmaceutical Industry (ABPI),
    107
Australia, health care, 261–262, 296
  challenges, 296–299
  coverage, 265–269, 266 (fig.)
  delivery, 281–288
  financing, 269–275, 270 (fig.)
  history, 262–265
  human resources, 294–296
  payment, 275–281, 276 (fig.), 278
    (fig.), 279 (fig.)
  pharmaceuticals, 288–293, 289 (fig.)

population size, 266 (fig.)
surprise bills/example, 261–262
Australian Institute for Health and
Welfare, 269, 283, 286
Australian Medical Association, 264
Australian Prudential Regulation
Authority, 273
Australian Register of Therapeutic
Goods (ARTG), 289

BAGSAN (Switzerland), 249
"balance billing" (France), 147, 148, 154,
373
Baylor University Hospital, 19
Berwick, Donald, 99
Best Practice Tariffs (BPTs/United
Kingdom), 99
Better Access initiative (Australia), 287
Bevan, Aneurin, 85
Beveridge Report (1942/United
Kingdom), 84–85
Biologics and Genetic Therapies
(Canada), 74
Bismarck, Otto von, 170, 172
Blair, Tony, 87
Board of Control for Lunacy and
Mental Deficiency (United
Kingdom), 86
Bonded Medical Place Scheme
(Australia), 295
British Institute of Public Opinion, 85
British Medical Association (BMA), 85,
89, 98, 110
Brookings Institution, 389
Brundtland, Gro, 360–361
Burton-Jeangros, Claudine, 235, 248,
256
Busse, Reinhard, 173

California Medical Association, 20
Calvo, Fabian, 159
Canada Health Act, 1984 (CHA), 57
absences, 57
long-term care, 73

Canada, health care
challenges, 81–82
coverage, 58–61, 59 (fig.)
delivery, 70–73
financing, 61–65, 62 (fig.)
history, 56–58
human resources, 79–81
payment, 65–70, 66 (fig.), 68 (fig.)
pharmaceuticals, 74–79, 75 (fig.)
population size, 59 (fig.)
Canada Health Transfer (CHT), 62–63
Canadian Agency for Drugs and
Technologies in Health (CADTH),
75–76
Cancer Core Europe, 159
Care Assessment Agency (CIZ/
Netherlands), 217
Care Quality Commission (CQC/
United Kingdom), 87, 96–97, 103,
104, 104–105
CareMore (United States), 400–401
Catalogue of Tariffs for Physicians
(Germany), 178, 184
Center for American Progress, 394, 395
Center for Drug Evaluation (CDE/
Taiwan), 317 (fig.), 318, 319
Center for Medicare and Medicaid
Innovation (CMMI/United States),
34
Centers for Medicare and Medicaid
Services (CMS/United States), 22
Central Administration Office (CAK/
Netherlands), 206
Central Health Services Council/
councils (United Kingdom),
85–86
Central Reallocation Pool (Germany),
175, 177
Chaoulli v. Quebec (2005), 60–61
Cheng, Tsung-Mei, 301
Chi, Phoebe, 300
Children's Health Insurance Program
(CHIP/United States), 23 (fig.), 24
(fig.), 25, 28, 324, 391

China, health care
  challenges, 346–350
  corruption/distrust, 324, 328, 343–
    344, 345–346, 348–349, 350, 356
  coverage, 330–332, 331 (fig.)
  delivery, 338–341
  financing, 332–336, 333 (fig.)
  history, 325–330
  human resources, 344–346
  payment, 336–339, 337 (fig.), 338 (fig.)
  pharmaceuticals, 341–344, 342 (fig.)
  population size, 331 (fig.)
cholera pandemic (mid-19th century),
  230
Choosing Wisely campaign (United
  States), 249
chronic conditions care/coordination
  Australia, 267, 285
  Canada, 82
  as challenge, 11–12
  China, 347, 349
  comparisons, 366, 367–368, 377–378
  France, 143, 148, 167
  Germany, 172, 177, 185, 186–187, 194
  Netherlands, 208–209, 215–216, 354
  Norway, 139–140
  Switzerland, 258
  Taiwan, 312, 322, 355
  United States, 40–41, 378, 386
Chronic Disease program (France),
  148
clinical commissioning groups (CCGs/
  United Kingdom), 88, 89–90,
  92–93, 92 (fig.), 95, 96, 97 (fig.),
  100, 104
Clinton, William Jefferson, 3, 21
Commission for Healthcare Audit
  and Inspection (CHAI/United
  Kingdom), 87
Commission for Social Care
  Inspection (United Kingdom), 87
Commissioner Forum of New
  Methods (Norway), 134
Commissioning for Quality and
  Innovation (CQUIN/United
  Kingdom), 99

Common Drug Review (CDR/Canada),
  75, 76, 77, 81
Commonwealth Fund, 13
Commonwealth Home Supports
  Program (CHSP/Australia), 280,
  287
Communist Party (CCP), 326
Compassionate Care Benefit (Canada),
  70
complementary/alternative medicine
  China, 338, 340–341
  France, 156
  Norway, 125–126
  Switzerland, 235
  Taiwan, 312, 316
Compulsory Sickness Insurance Act,
  1909 (Norway), 116
Conference of the Cantonal Ministers
  of Public Health (GDK/
  Switzerland), 240, 246–247,
  259
Cooperative Medical Scheme (CMS/
  China), 325, 327
Couffinhal, Agnes, 165
coverage comparisons, 352 (table),
  360–362
  universality/affordability over
    benefits comprehensiveness,
    360–361
coverage/health insurance (Australia),
  265
  chronic conditions, 267
  disabled, 269, 273
  indigenous populations, 266,
    266 (fig.)
  long-term care, 268–269
  Medicare, 266–267, 266 (fig.)
  penalties and, 268
  private supplemental health
    insurance, 266 (fig.), 267–268
coverage/health insurance (Canada),
  58–61, 59 (fig.)
coverage/health insurance (China)
  preventive care, 331
  private health insurance, 332
  public care, 331–332

public health insurance, 330–332, 331 (fig.)

coverage/health insurance (France), 145–148, 145 (fig.)
chronic conditions, 148
employment status, 145–146
out-of-pocket patient costs, 146
private supplemental insurance (voluntary health insurance/VHI), 145 (fig.), 147–148, 156, 159
public/statutory insurance (SHI), 145–147, 145 (fig.), 156, 159

coverage/health insurance (Germany), 145, 173–174, 174 (fig.)

coverage/health insurance (Netherlands)
long-term care, 202
statutory health insurance, 201–202, 201 (fig.)
voluntary, private supplemental insurance, 202

coverage/health insurance (Norway), 118, 118 (fig.)

coverage/health insurance (Switzerland)
alternative medicine, 235
insurers, 235–236
mandatory basic health insurance, 232–235, 233 (fig.)
voluntary private supplemental insurance, 235

coverage/health insurance (Taiwan)
long-term care, 304 (fig.), 305–306, 355, 369
private coverage, 304–305, 304 (fig.)
public insurance/NHI, 303–304, 304 (fig.)

coverage/health insurance (United Kingdom), 89–91, 90 (fig.), 91 (fig.)
mandatory insurance, 89–90, 90 (fig.), 92–93
"postcode lotteries," 90
private insurers, 91
voluntary private insurance, 90 (fig.), 91, 93

coverage/health insurance (United States), 22–26, 23 (fig.), 47 (table)
Blue Cross and Blue Shield/plans history, 20
and "churn," 25
dental/vision care, 26
employer-sponsored insurance, 19, 20–21, 22
history (through 1900s), 19–21
insurance types/uninsured, 23 (fig.)
physicians/AMA early views on, 20
private insurance, 23 (fig.)
surprise bills, 18, 404
tax exemptions (employer-sponsored insurance), 21, 27
uninsured, 23 (fig.), 52
See also specific components/types

CPT code (United States), 33
Curafutura (Switzerland), 236

de Gaulle, Charles, 144
Degos, Laurent, 143
Dekker Committee (Netherlands), 199–200
DeLauro, Rosa, 395
delivery of health care comparisons
choice of physicians/hospitals, 375–376
chronic care/coordination, 377–378
innovations, 380–381
mental health care, 379–380
quality of care, 376–377
simplicity of use, 376
wait times, 378–379
delivery of health care (Australia), 281–288
chronic conditions, 285
hospitals, 282–284
long-term care, 287
mental health care, 283, 286–287
physicians/outpatient care, 284–286
public health/preventive medicine, 288
wait times, 284, 298–299

delivery of health care (Canada)
  ambulatory care, 71–72
  hospitals, 70–71
  long-term care, 73
  mental health care, 72–73
  preventive medicine, 73
delivery of health care (China)
  ambulatory care, 339–340
  chronic conditions care, 347, 349
  complementary/alternative
    medicine, 340–341
  hospitals, 339
  long-term care, 340, 347, 348, 350
  mental health, 340, 349
  preventive medicine, 341
delivery of health care (France),
    156–159
  ambulatory care, 158
  EHRs, 157–158
  hospitals, 157
  long-term care, 159
  mental health care, 158–159
  preventive care, 159, 167–168
delivery of health care (Germany), 157,
    185–188
  ambulatory care, 186–187
  hospitals, 185–186
  long-term care, 187, 195
  mental health care, 187
  preventive medicine, 188
delivery of health care (Netherlands)
  chronic conditions/care groups,
    215–216
  hospitals, 211–213
  long-term care, 216–217
  mental health, 216, 402
  outpatient primary care, 213–214
  public health/preventive medicine,
    217
  specialist care, 214–215
delivery of health care (Norway),
    126–130
  hospital care, 127–128
  long-term care, 130
  mental health care, 129–130
  preventive care, 130

  primary care, 128–129
  specialist care, 128
  Vanessa's story, 115–116
  wait times, 115–116, 140–141
delivery of health care (Switzerland)
  ambulatory care, 247
  EHRs, 249, 256
  home health care, 248
  hospitals, 246–247, 255
  long-term care, 247–248
  mental health, 247
  patient satisfaction, 249
  preventive care, 248
  quality/controls, 248–249,
    255–256
delivery of health care (Taiwan),
    313–316
  ambulatory care, 314–315
  chronic care, 322
  complementary/alternative
    medicine, 316
  EHRs, 300, 308, 316, 380–381,
    396
  hospitals, 313–314
  long-term care, 302–303, 315–316,
    323
  mental health, 315, 322
  preventive medicine, 316
delivery of health care (United
    Kingdom), 101–106
  ambulatory care, 102
  EHRs, 102–103, 113
  hospitals, 101–102
  long-term care, 104
  mental health, 86, 87, 95, 103–104
  patient satisfaction, 105–106
  preventive care, 95, 104
  quality controls, 104–105
delivery of health care (United States),
    36–43, 37 (fig.)
  ambulatory care, 39–41
  hospitals, 37–39, 37 (fig.), 157
  long-term care, 42
  mental health care, 41–42
  preventive medicine, 36, 43
Deming, W. Edwards, 14

dental care, 361
  ACA (United States), 391
  Australia, 265, 266, 274, 279, 296
  Canada, 58, 60, 61, 64, 262
  China, 331
  France, 146, 147, 168
  Germany, 172, 173–174
  Netherlands, 198, 201 (fig.), 202, 224
  Norway, 117, 120, 138, 142, 392
  Switzerland, 234, 235, 239, 241, 244
  Taiwan, 303–304, 307 (fig.), 309, 311,
    314, 361
  United Kingdom, 90
  United States, 26, 391
Department of Health and Social Care
  (DHSC/United Kingdom), 90, 92,
  96, 101, 104, 106
Department of Health and Social
  Security (United Kingdom), 86
Department of Health (Australia), 266,
  267, 289–290
Department of Veterans' Affairs
  (Australia), 266
Department of Veterans Affairs (VA/
  United States), 23 (fig.), 25, 36, 45
Detsky, Allan, 67, 69
Diabeter (Netherlands), 215–216,
  377–378, 400, 401
Diagnosis Treatment Combinations
  (DBCs/Netherlands), 208, 209,
  211
DisabilityCare Australia Fund, 273
disease management programs
  (DMPs/Germany), 186–187, 195
District Psychiatric Outpatient
  Services (DPOS/Norway),
  129–130
Drug Identification Number (DIN/
  Canada), 74
Drug Tariff (United Kingdom), 107
drugs, medicinal. See pharmaceuticals
Durand-Zaleski, Isabelle, 143, 158, 167
Dutch Diabetes Federation Health
  Care Standard (DFHCS), 211
Dutch Healthcare Authority (NZA),
  205, 207, 208, 215

Economic and Public Health
  Assessment Committee (CEESP/
  France), 162
Economic Committee for Health
  Products (CEPS/France),
  161–163
Economist Intelligence Unit of
  Quality of Death (world-wide
  survey), 323
electronic health records (EHRs)
  France, 157–158
  Germany, 195
  importance/advantages, 53, 396–
  397, 402–403, 405
  Switzerland, 249, 256
  Taiwan, 300, 308, 316, 380–381, 396
  United Kingdom, 102–103, 113
  United States, 49, 53
Emergency Hospital Service (United
  Kingdom), 84
Essential Drugs List (EDL/China), 328,
  341–342
European Medicines Agency (EMA),
  160, 161 (fig.), 188, 218
European Observatory on Health
  Systems and Policies, 13, 17
Exceptional Medical Expenses Act,
  1967 (AWBZ/Netherlands), 199
Executive Yuan (Taiwan), 309
Extended Medicare Safety Net (EMSN/
  Australia), 274–275

Family Health Groups (Ontario), 71
Family Health Networks (Ontario), 71
Family Health Organizations
  (Ontario), 73
Family Medicine Groups (Quebec), 71
Family Physician Integrated Care
  Project (FPICP/Taiwan), 314–315
Federal Association of SHI Physicians
  (Germany), 183–184, 191
Federal Association of Sickness Funds
  (Germany), 189 (fig.), 190, 191
Federal Commission for Analyses,
  Products, and Devices
  (Switzerland), 234

Federal Commission for Medical
    Benefits and Basic Principles
    (Switzerland), 234
Federal Department of Home Affairs
    (FDHA/Switzerland), 231–232,
    234, 250
Federal Drug Commission
    (Switzerland), 234, 250, 251 (fig.)
Federal Health Insurance Law, 1994
    (LAMal/Switzerland), 231, 232,
    234–235, 240, 357
Federal Institute for Pharmaceuticals
    and Medical Devices (Germany),
    188, 189 (fig.)
Federal Insurance Authority
    (Germany), 175
Federal Joint Commission (Germany),
    172, 173, 180, 181–182, 189, 189 (fig.),
    190, 191
Federal Law on Accident Insurance
    (LAA/Switzerland), 236
Federal Law on Disability Insurance
    (LAI/Switzerland), 236, 240
Federal Law on Sickness and
    Accident Insurance, 1911 (LAMA/
    Switzerland), 231
Federal Law on the Supervision of
    Mandatory Health Insurance
    (LSAMal/Switzerland), 236
Federal Law on Therapeutic Products,
    2002 (HMG/Switzerland), 250
Federal Medicaid Assistance
    Percentage (United States FMAP),
    27–28, 63
Federal Office of Public Health (FOPH/
    Switzerland), 230, 231–232, 236,
    240, 248–249, 250–252, 252 (fig.),
    259
Federal Trade Commission (United
    States), 2
Federally Qualified Health Clinics
    (FQHCs/United States), 36
fee-for-service payments
    Australia, 275, 280
    Canada, 65, 67, 68, 68 (fig.), 69, 70,
        71, 80

China, 326, 336–337, 338
France, 153–154, 167, 373
Germany, 182 (fig.), 184
issues with, 372–373, 374, 386
Netherlands, 208, 209 (fig.)
Norway, 121–122, 123, 124 (fig.), 125,
    140, 142
Switzerland, 244, 247, 249, 259
Taiwan, 309, 310, 310 (fig.), 311,
    311 (fig.), 312
United Kingdom, 96
United States, 32–35, 51
Financial Conduct Authority (United
    Kingdom), 91
financing comparisons, 362–363,
    364 (table), 365
    limiting health care spending,
        369–370, 371 (table)
    long-term care, 368–369
    progressive-regressive dimension,
        365–366
    vulnerable groups described, 366
    vulnerable groups protection,
        366–368
financing health care (Australia),
    269–275, 270 (fig.)
    long-term care, 273
    Medicare/PBS, 270 (fig.), 271–272
    out-of-pocket costs/safety nets,
        274–275
    private supplemental insurance,
        270 (fig.), 272–273
    public health/preventive care,
        273
financing health care (Canada), 61–65,
    62 (fig.)
    insurance plans (Territorial/
        Medicare), 61–63, 62 (fig.)
    pharmaceuticals, 59
financing health care (China), 332–336,
    333 (fig.)
    long-term care, 335
    private health insurance, 335
    public health, 335–336
    public/statutory health insurance,
        332, 333 (fig.), 334–335

financing health care (France), 148–151,
149 (fig.)
long-term care, 150
public health, 150–151
SHI, 148–149, 149 (fig.)
voluntary health insurance (VHI),
149–150
financing health care (Germany),
175–179, 176 (fig.)
long-term care, 178–179
out-of-pocket expenditures, 176–177,
177 (fig.)
private health insurance, 177–178
public health, 179
SHI, 173, 175–177, 176 (fig.)
financing health care (Netherlands),
202–206, 203 (fig.)
long-term care, 205–206
out-of-pocket costs, 206
private supplementary insurance
(VHI), 205
statutory health insurance for
curative care, 204–205
financing health care (Norway),
118–121, 119 (fig.)
long-term care, 120
private supplemental insurance, 120
public health, 120–121
public health insurance, 119–120,
119 (fig.)
financing health care (Switzerland),
236–241, 237 (fig.)
cost sharing, 239
long-term care, 239–240
mandatory basic health insurance,
237–238, 237 (fig.)
mental health, 241
public health, 240–241
voluntary private supplemental
insurance, 238
financing health care (Taiwan),
306–309, 307 (fig.)
global budgeting, 307 (fig.), 309
private health insurance, 308
public health insurance/NHI,
307–308, 307 (fig.)

financing health care (United
Kingdom), 88, 91–95, 92 (fig.)
cost sharing, 93–94
"dementia tax," 95
financing health care (United States),
24 (fig.), 26–30
costs/control, 28–29, 50–52
employer-sponsored insurance,
26–27
individual plans, 28
long-term care, 29–30
Massachusetts example, 29
Medicaid, 24 (fig.), 27–28
Medicare, 24 (fig.), 27
rising costs, 21
First Nations/Inuit benefits (Canada),
60
Flexner Report/consequences (United
States), 19
Food and Drug Administration
(China), 341
Food and Drug Administration (FDA/
Taiwan), 317 (fig.), 318
Food and Drug Administration (FDA/
United States), 2, 43–44, 45,
45 (fig.), 46, 74, 106, 218, 288,
381–382
Foundation for Patient Safety
(Switzerland), 248–249
France, health care, 143
challenges, 143, 167–168
coverage, 145–148, 145 (fig.)
delivery, 156–159
financing, 148–151, 149 (fig.)
fragmentation, 143, 158, 167
history, 143–145
human resources, 164–167
payment, 151–156, 152 (fig.), 153 (fig.)
pharmaceuticals, 160–164, 161 (fig.)
population size, 145 (fig.)
World War II effects, 144
See also specific components/individuals
Franco-Prussian War, 170
Fraser, Malcolm, 264
Freed, Gary, 274
"Friendly Societies" (Australia), 262

General Medical Services (GMS/ United Kingdom) contracts, 97–98, 98 (fig.), 99, 109
General Practitioners Society of Australia, 264
George, David Lloyd, 84
German Hospital Federation, 179–180
German National Association of Statutory Health Insurance Physicians (KBV), 16
Germany, health care, 169, 172–173, 175–176
challenges, 193–196
coverage, 145, 173–174, 174 (fig.)
delivery, 157, 185–188
financing, 175–179, 176 (fig.)
history, 143, 170–173
human resources, 192–193
payment, 179–185, 180 (fig.), 182 (fig.)
pharmaceuticals, 188–191, 189 (fig.)
population size, 174 (fig.)
sickness funds, 169, 170–172, 173, 174 (fig.), 175, 176, 176 (fig.), 177, 179–180, 180 (fig.), 181, 182–183, 184, 185, 186, 187, 189 (fig.), 190–191, 193, 194–196
See also specific components/individuals
Government Insurance Scheme (GIS/ China), 325, 327
Grant, Malcom, Sir, 88
Great Depression (United States), early health insurance arrangements, 19–20
Greatest Permissible Gap (GPG), 274

H1N1 influenza outbreak, 322
Hall Commission 1964 (Canada), 59
Hatch, Orrin, 391
Healing of America, The: A Global Quest for Better, Cheaper, and Fairer Health Care (Reid), 13
Health Act, 1999 (United Kingdom), 87
Health and Social Care Act, 2012 (United Kingdom), 88, 101
Health and Wellbeing Boards (United Kingdom), 101, 104

Health Authorities and Health Trusts Act, 2001 (Norway), 117
Health Canada, 74, 78
Health Care Budget (BKZ/ Netherlands), 204, 227
Health Care Prices Act, 1981 (Netherlands), 199
Health Care Structure Act, 1993 (Germany), 171, 173
Health Consumer Powerhouse, 4
health insurance. See coverage/health insurance (specific country)
Health Insurance Act, 1883 (Germany), 170
Health Insurance Act, 1966 (Netherlands), 199, 210
Health Insurance Act, 2006 (ZVW/ Netherlands), 200, 201
health maintenance organizations (HMOs/United States), 34–35, 40, 89
Health Ontario, 66
Health Products and Food Branch (HPFB/Canada), 74
Health Promotion Switzerland, 240–241
Health Reform Law, 2015 (France), 147
Health Systems in Transition (HiT series/ European Observatory on Health Systems and Policies), 13
health technology assessment (HTA) approach (Australia), 267
Health Technology Assessment (HTA/ Norway), 120, 132, 134
Healthcare Resource Groups (HRGs/ United Kingdom), 96
Healthwatch England, 88
High Authority on Health (HAS/ France), 160–161, 161 (fig.), 162
Hill-Burton Act, 1946 (United States), 21
history comparisons/overview
path dependence, 1–2, 359–360
paths to universal health coverage, 358–359

structural decisions/undoing,
  359–360
universal health coverage, 356–358
Hitler, Adolf, 172–173
Hofmeister, Stephan, 16
Home Care Packages Program
  (Australia), 280, 287
home health care
  Australia, 280–281, 287
  Netherlands, 210, 227
  Switzerland, 248
  United States, 39
Homogeneous Group of the Sick
  (France), 151, 152 (fig.)
Hospital at Home (United States), 39
Hospital Benefits Act, 1944 (Australia),
  262
Hospital Benefits Scheme (Australia),
  262
Hospital Compare (United States), 38
Hospital Insurance and Diagnostic
  Services (HIDS) Act, 1957
  (Canada), 56, 57
Hospital Plan for England and Wales, The,
  86
Hospital Purchases HF (Norway), 135
hospitalists, 38
Hospitalization Act, 1947
  (Saskatchewan), 56
hospitals (Australia)
  delivery of health care, 282–284
  hospitalization rates, 282, 283
  payment for health care, 275–278,
    276 (fig.), 278 (fig.)
hospitals (Canada)
  delivery of health care, 70–71
  payment for health care, 66–67,
    66 (fig.), 82
hospitals (China)
  delivery of health care, 339–341
  payment for health care, 336,
    337 (fig.), 338 (fig.)
hospitals (France)
  delivery of health care, 157
  payment for health care, 151–153,
    152 (fig.)

hospitals (Germany), 169, 193–194
  delivery of health care, 157, 185–186
  hospitalization rates, 282
  payment for health care, 179–181
hospitals (Netherlands)
  delivery of health care, 211–213
  independent treatment centers
    (ZBCs), 212–213
  payment for health care, 207–208,
    207 (fig.)
hospitals (Norway)
  delivery of health care, 127–128
  payment for health care, 121–122,
    123 (fig.)
hospitals (Switzerland)
  delivery of health care, 246–247, 255
  payment for health care, 232,
    241–243, 242 (fig.)
hospitals (Taiwan)
  delivery of health care, 313–314
  payment for health care, 310,
    310 (fig.)
hospitals (United Kingdom)
  delivery of health care, 101–102
  payment for health care, 96–97,
    97 (fig.)
hospitals (United States)
  delivery of health care, 37–39, 157
  hospitalization rates, 282
  payment for health care, 30–32,
    31 (fig.)
  quality/ratings, 38–39
  readmissions, 38–39
  regulations/accreditation, 38
  trends, 37 (table)
  vertical/horizontal consolidation,
    37–38
Hsiao, Bill, 301, 303
Hurst, Samia, 259

Imperial Committee of Physicians and
  Sickness Funds (Germany), 171
Independent Hospital Pricing
  Authority (IHPA/Australia), 277
Indian Health Services (IHS/United
  States), 23 (fig.), 25

Institute for Quality and Efficiency in
    Health Care (IQWiG/Germany),
    189 (fig.), 190
Institute for Reimbursement in the
    Hospital, 179
Insurance Law on Access to Care, 1986
    (Netherlands), 199
integrated care systems (ICS/United
    Kingdom), 104
Integrated Comprehensive Care
    Project (Ontario), 67
Inuit/First Nations benefits (Canada),
    60
IQVIA, 15

Johns Hopkins Medical School, 19
Johnson, Boris, 95
Johnson, Lyndon, 21
Joint Commission (United States), 2,
    38

Kaiser Permanente, 40, 129
Kennedy, Ted, 391
Kherad, Omar, 257
King's Fund, The (United Kingdom),
    103, 105

Labor Insurance Scheme (LIS/China),
    325, 327
LaRoque, Pierre, 144
Lavis, John, 55
Legatum rankings, 4
Lifetime Health Cover (LHC/Australia),
    268
Local Health Integration Network
    (LHIN/Ontario), 64, 66
long-term care
    Australia, 268–269, 273, 280–281,
        287
    Canada, 64–65, 70, 73, 82
    China, 335, 338, 340, 347, 348, 350
    financing comparisons, 368–369
    France, 150, 156, 159
    Germany, 178–179, 184, 187, 195
    Netherlands, 130, 202, 205–206, 210,
        216–217

Norway, 120, 125, 142
    Switzerland, 239–240, 245, 247–248
    Taiwan, 302–303, 304 (fig.), 305–306,
        312, 315–316, 323, 355, 369
    United Kingdom, 94–95, 100–101,
        104, 113
    United States, 29–30, 35–36, 42,
        53–54, 362
Long Term Care 2.0 (LTC 2.0/Taiwan),
    305–306, 312, 316, 323
Long-Term Care Act (Netherlands),
    202, 205–206, 210
Lyons, Joseph, 262

managed entry agreements (MEAs/
    Netherlands), 221
Mao Zedong, 325, 357
Marchildon, Gregory, 63–64
market forces factor (MFF/United
    Kingdom), 96
Maryland example, payment for
    health care, 32
Massachusetts example, financing
    health care, 29
maximum average potential price
    (MAPP/Canada), 76
May, Theresa, 88, 95
MBS Review Taskforce (Australia), 267
Medibank (Australia), 264, 357
Medicaid (United States)
    ACA, 21–22, 23–24, 366, 393
    auto-enrollment, 389, 393
    Centers for Medicare and Medicaid
        Services (CMS), 22
    coverage, 23, 23 (fig.), 25
    Federal Medicaid Assistance
        Percentage (United States FMAP),
        27–28, 63
    financing health care, 24 (fig.),
        27–28
    history, 21
    long-term care, 29–30
    payments, 32, 33 (fig.)
    pharmaceuticals, 45
Medical Benefits Scheme (Australia),
    263

Medical Care Act, 1966 (MCA/Canada), 57

Medical Review Board (Germany), 184

medical savings accounts (MSAs/ China), 327, 331, 334

Medical Services Advisory Committee (MSAC/Australia) and subcommittees, 267

Medicare Advantage (United States), 22, 26, 27, 40, 364 (fig.), 365, 395, 400

Medicare (Australia), 264–265, 266 (fig.). *See also* Australia, health care

Medicare Benefits Schedule (MBS/ Australia), 266, 274, 277–279

Medicare (Canada), 55–56. *See also* Canada, health care

Medicare Enhanced Primary Care program (Australia), 266–267

Medicare Levy Surcharge (Australia), 268

Medicare Severity Diagnosis Related Groups Systems (MS-DRG/ United States), 30

Medicare (United States)
  Centers for Medicare and Medicaid Services (CMS), 22
  components/parts described, 22–23
  costs/control, 50–51
  coverage, 22–23, 23 (fig.)
  DRGs, 30, 31
  financing health care, 24 (fig.), 27
  history, 21
  hospital penalties, 38–39
  payments, 32–33, 33 (fig.)
  PBMs, 44
  relative value unit (RVU) system, 32–33, 33 (fig.), 182, 243

Medicines Act, 1968 (United Kingdom), 106

Medicines Act (EU), 218

Medicines and Healthcare products Regulatory Agency (MHRA/ United Kingdom), 106, 107 (fig.)

Medicines Evaluation Board (Netherlands), 218

Medigap program, 147, 364 (fig.), 365, 396

Mental Health Act/Commission (United Kingdom), 87, 103

mental health care
  Australia, 283, 286–287
  Canada, 72–73, 82
  challenges, 12
  China, 340, 349
  comparisons, 379–380
  France, 155, 158–159
  Germany, 187
  Netherlands, 216, 402
  Norway, 125, 129–130, 130
  Switzerland, 241, 245–246, 247, 258–259
  Taiwan, 315, 322
  United Kingdom, 86, 87, 95, 100, 103–104
  United States, 41–42

Mental Health Investment Standard (MHIS/United Kingdom), 95

Menzies, Robert, 263, 264

Ministry for Health and Welfare (Taiwan), 303, 305, 308, 309, 315, 316, 317 (fig.), 318, 320, 322

Ministry of Health and Care Services (Norway), 117, 120, 121, 125, 131, 135, 141, 142, 369–370

Ministry of Health (France), 148, 151–152, 152 (fig.), 154, 155, 164, 165, 166

Ministry of Health (Germany), 179, 186

Ministry of Health (MOH/China), 326, 327

Ministry of Health, Welfare, and Sport (Netherlands), 204, 211, 218–219, 220, 221, 382

Ministry of Human Resources and Social Security (MoHRSS/China), 335, 338

Municipalities Health Services Act, 1982 (Norway), 116

Murray, Richard, 103–104, 105

Mutualité Sociale Agricole (MSA/
    France), 146
My Aged Care system/Assessment
    Team (Australia), 280, 287

NAFTA (North American Free Trade
    Agreement), 77–78
National Aboriginal and Torres Strait
    Islander Health Plan (Australia),
    266
National Academy of Medicine
    (United States), 10–11, 394
National Association for Quality
    Improvement in Hospitals and
    Clinics (ANQ/Switzerland), 249
National Cost Studies with Common
    Methodology (France), 151
National Disability Insurance Agency
    (NDIA/Australia), 269
National Disability Insurance Scheme
    (NDIS/Australia), 269, 273
National Efficient Cost (Australia), 277
National Efficient Price (NEP/
    Australia), 277
National Health Act, 1953 (Australia),
    263
National Health Care Institute (ZIN/
    Netherlands), 204–205, 206
National Health Commission (NHC/
    China), 329, 336, 341
National Health Insurance (NHI/
    Taiwan), 302, 361. See also Taiwan,
    health care
National Health Insurance
    Administration (NHIA/Taiwan),
    303, 313, 314, 318, 319, 321–322
National Health Insurance Fund for
    Salaried Workers/General Fund
    (CNAMTS/France), 146
National Health Service (NHS/United
    Kingdom), 84–89. See also United
    Kingdom, health care
National Health Service Act, 1946
    (United Kingdom), 85, 357
National Health Service Act, 1948
    (Australia), 263

National Health Service (Scotland/
    Ireland) acts, 1947/1948, 85
National Health Service and
    Community Care Act, 1990
    (United Kingdom), 86
National Health Service
    Reorganization Act, 1973 (United
    Kingdom), 86
National Institute for (Health and)
    Care Excellence (NICE/United
    Kingdom), 87, 89, 105, 106, 107
    (fig.), 132
National Insurance Act (United
    Kingdom), 84
National Insurance Scheme (NIS/
    Norway), 116–117, 388. See also
    Norway, health care
National Program for Mental Health
    (Norway), 129
National Reimbursement Drug List
    (NRDL/China), 341–342
National System for the Introduction
    of New Health Technologies
    (Norway), 120
National Union of Health Insurance
    Funds (UNCAM/France), 154, 162,
    373
National Weighted Activity Unit
    (NWAU/Australia), 277
Netherlands, health care, 197–198,
    200
    care example, 197–198
    challenges, 224–228
    coverage, 201–202, 201 (fig.)
    delivery, 211–217
    financing, 202–206, 203 (fig.)
    history, 198–200
    human resources, 222–224
    payment, 206–211, 207 (fig.),
        209 (fig.)
    pharmaceuticals, 218–222, 219 (fig.)
    population size, 201 (fig.)
    World War II and, 198–199
    See also specific components/individuals
Netherlands Medical Association
    (NMG), 198

New Cooperative Medical Scheme (NCMS/China), 327, 328–329, 330, 334, 349
new diagnostic and treatment methods (NUB/Germany) payments, 180
New Drug Submission (NDS/Canada), 74
New Methods system (Norway), 132, 134
NHS England, 88, 89, 90, 92 (fig.), 97 (fig.), 98, 101, 102, 104
NHS Improvement (United Kingdom), 96–97, 102
NIS/Norway. See National Insurance Scheme (NIS/Norway)
Nixon, Richard, 21
North American Free Trade Agreement (NAFTA) and pharmaceuticals, 77–78
Norway
   population, 118 (fig.)
   social safety net, 116
Norway, health care
   challenges, 115–116, 138–142
   coverage, 118, 118 (fig.)
   delivery, 126–130
   as divided/issues, 117, 133–134, 138–139
   financing, 118–121, 119 (fig.)
   history, 116–117
   human resources, 136–138
   payment, 121–126, 123 (fig.), 124 (fig.)
   pharmaceuticals, 131–136, 131 (fig.)
   See also National Insurance Scheme
Norway, Health System Review (European Observatory on Health Systems and Policies), 17
Norwegian Health Economics Administration (HELFO), 117, 119 (fig.), 120, 123, 124, 124 (fig.), 133
Norwegian Medical Association, 122–123, 125
Norwegian Medicines Agency (NoMA), 131–132, 134, 135
Notification of Compliance (NOC/Canada), 74

nurses
   Australia, 295
   Canada, 80–81
   China, 346
   France, 166–167
   Germany, 193
   Netherlands, 223–224
   Norway, 137–138
   Switzerland, 254
   Taiwan, 320–321
   United Kingdom, 110
   United States, 49–50, 53
Nursing and Midwifery Council (NMC/United Kingdom), 110
Nursing Home Compare (United States), 43

Obama, Barack, 21
OECD (Organisation for Economic Co-operation and Development) described, 14, 15
One-child policy/consequences (China), 335, 340, 347, 350
Ontario Drug Benefit, 59–60
Ontario Health Insurance Program (OHIP/+), 59–60, 64
Ontario Health Premium, 62
Ontario Medical Association, 69
Ontario Quality-Based Procedure program, 67
Ontario's Disability Support Program, 60
Organisation for Economic Co-operation and Development (OECD) described, 14, 15
Original Medicare Safety Net (OMSN/Australia), 274
Overall Hospital Quality "star rating system" (United States), 38

pan-Canadian Pharmaceutical Alliance (pCPA), 75, 75 (fig.), 76–77, 81
Patented Medicines Prices Review Board (PMPRB/Canada), 74–76, 77–78

Patients' Rights Act, 1999 (Norway), 117
payment comparisons, 370, 374–375
  alignment/coordination, 370, 372–373
  innovation, 374–375
  simplicity for patients/providers,
    373–374
payment for health care (Australia),
    275–281, 276 (fig.), 278 (fig.),
    279 (fig.)
  fee-for-service, 275, 280
  home health care, 280–281
  long-term care providers, 280–281
  physicians, 278–280, 279 (fig.)
  private hospitals, 276, 277–278,
    278 (fig.)
  public hospitals, 275–277, 276 (fig.)
payment for health care (Canada),
    65–70, 66 (fig.), 68 (fig.)
  alternative payment methods, 65,
    67, 68–69, 68 (fig.), 82
  complementary/alternative
    medicine, 70
  fee-for-service payments, 65, 67, 68,
    68 (fig.), 69, 70, 71, 80
  hospitals, 66–67, 66 (fig.), 82
  long-term care, 70
  physicians, 68–69, 68 (fig.)
  preventive medicine, 70
payment for health care (China),
    336–338, 337 (fig.), 338 (fig.)
  ambulatory care institutions,
    336–337
  complementary/alternative, 338
  fee-for-service payments, 326,
    336–337, 338
  hospitals, 336, 337 (fig.), 338 (fig.)
  long-term care, 338
  physicians, 337–338, 338 (fig.)
  public health/preventive medicine,
    338
payment for health care (France),
    151–156, 152 (fig.), 153 (fig.)
  alternative payment models, 154, 167
  "balance billing," 147, 148, 154, 373
  complementary/alternative
    medicine, 156

DRGs, 151, 152, 152 (fig.), 155, 167
fee-for-service, 153–154, 167, 373
hospitals, 151–153, 152 (fig.)
long-term care, 156
mental health care, 155
physicians, ambulatory/office-
    based, 153–155, 153 (fig.)
preventive medicine, 156
payment for health care (Germany),
    179–185, 180 (fig.), 182 (fig.)
  complementary/alternative
    medicine, 184
  DRGs, 172, 179–180, 181
  fee-for-service, 182 (fig.), 184
  hospitals, 179–181
  long-term care, 184
  physicians, ambulatory/office-
    based, 181–184, 182 (fig.)
  preventive medicine, 185
  SHI, 181–182, 182 (fig.), 183, 184
payment for health care (Netherlands),
    206–211, 207 (fig.), 209 (fig.)
  alternative payment methods,
    208–209, 211, 400
  care groups, 211
  chronic conditions care, 208–209
  Diagnosis Treatment Combinations
    (DBCs), 208, 209, 211
  fee-for-service, 208, 209 (fig.)
  hospitals, 207–208, 207 (fig.)
  long-term care/home health
    providers, 210
  negotiations/selective contracting,
    210–211
  pay-for-performance, 209
  physicians, 208–209, 208–210,
    209 (fig.)
payment for health care (Norway),
    121–126, 123 (fig.), 124 (fig.)
  alternative payment models,
    124 (fig.), 125, 140, 142
  complementary/alternative
    medicine, 125–126
  fee-for-service payments, 121–122,
    123, 124 (fig.), 125, 140, 142
  hospitals, 121–122, 123 (fig.)

long-term care, 125
mental health, 125
out-of-pocket payments, 126
preventive care, 126
primary care general practitioners,
    123–125, 124 (fig.)
specialists, 122–123, 123 (fig.),
    124 (fig.)
payment for health care (Switzerland),
    241–246, 242 (fig.), 244 (fig.)
ambulatory physicians, 243–245,
    244 (fig.)
DRGs, 232, 241, 242, 242 (fig.), 243
fee-for-service, 244, 247, 249, 259
hospitals, 232, 241–243, 242 (fig.)
long-term care, 245
mental health, 245–246
payment for health care (Taiwan),
    310–313, 310 (fig.), 311 (fig.)
chronic diseases, 312
complementary/alternative
    medicine, 312
DRGs, 302, 310, 310 (fig.)
fee-for-service, 309, 310, 310 (fig.),
    311, 311 (fig.), 312
hospitals, 310, 310 (fig.)
long-term care, 312
out-of-pocket payments, 311–312,
    311 (fig.)
physicians, 311, 311 (fig.)
public health/preventive medicine,
    313
payment for health care (United
    Kingdom), 95–101, 97 (fig.),
    98 (fig.)
alternative payment models, 96,
    97 (fig.)
DRGs, 372
fee-for-service payments, 96
hospitals, 96–97, 97 (fig.)
long-term care, 100–101
mental health, 100
Payment by Results (PBR), 96,
    97 (fig.)
physicians, 97–100, 98 (fig.)
public health, 101
payment for health care (United
    States), 30–36, 31 (fig.), 33 (fig.)
alternative payment models, 8, 32,
    34, 386, 400
to ambulatory/office-based
    physicians, 32–35, 33 (fig.)
charge master rate, 31
Disproportionate Share Hospital
    (DSH) payments, 31
DRGs, 30–32
fee-for-service payments, 32, 34, 51
to hospitals, 30–32, 31 (fig.)
indirect medical education (IME)
    payments, 31–32
long-term care, 35–36
Maryland exception, 32
Medicare Severity Diagnosis Related
    Groups Systems (MS-DRG), 30
preventive medicine, 36
relative value unit (RVU) system,
    32–33
Pensioner Medical Service Act, 1953
    (Australia), 263
per-member-per-month (PMPM) fee
    (United States), 35
Personal Medical Record (France), 157
Personal Medical Services (PMS/
    United Kingdom) contracts, 98,
    98 (fig.)
Personalized Allowance for Autonomy
    (France), 150
Pharmaceutical Act, 1976 (Germany),
    188
Pharmaceutical Benefit Review (PBR/
    Taiwan), 317 (fig.), 318–319
Pharmaceutical Benefits Act, 1944
    (Australia), 262
Pharmaceutical Benefits Advisory
    Committee (PBAC/Australia), 263,
    267, 289–290, 289 (fig.), 293
Pharmaceutical Benefits program
    (Australia), 263
Pharmaceutical Benefits Scheme (PBS/
    Australia), 132, 262, 263, 266, 270
    (fig.), 271, 286, 288, 293
Pharmaceutical Prices Law (EU), 218

Pharmaceutical Reimbursement
　System (GVS), 218–220, 219 (fig.)
pharmaceuticals comparisons,
　381–382, 384
　costs, 10
　reference pricing, 383, 403
　value-based pricing/cost-
　　effectiveness analysis (CEA), 383,
　　403
pharmaceuticals (Australia)
　coverage determination, 288–290,
　　289 (fig.)
　market, 288
　physician prescriptions regulations,
　　293
　prices paid by patients, 293
　prices/reimbursement regulation,
　　290–293
pharmaceuticals (Canada)
　absence of universal coverage/
　　history, 55–56, 57, 58–59, 81
　CHA, 57
　coverage determination, 74
　financing, 59
　generics, 77, 78–79
　market, 74
　NAFTA, 77–78
　National Forum on Health/debate,
　　59
　off-label use, 78
　patient prices, 79
　physician prescriptions regulations,
　　78–79
　price regulation, 74–79, 75 (fig.),
　　81–82
　provinces, 57–58, 59–61
pharmaceuticals (China)
　coverage determination, 341–342
　market, 341
　physician prescriptions regulation,
　　343–344
　price regulation, 342 (fig.), 343–344
　prices paid by patients, 344
pharmaceuticals (France)
　coverage determination, 160–161
　drugs ratings, 160–161

generics, 162, 163
market, 160
physician prescriptions regulation,
　163–164
price regulation, 161–163, 161 (fig.)
prices paid by patients, 164
pharmaceuticals (Germany)
　coverage determination, 188–189
　market, 188
　physician prescriptions regulation,
　　191
　price regulation, 189–191, 189 (fig.)
　prices paid by patients, 191
pharmaceuticals (Netherlands),
　218–222
　access, coverage, price setting,
　　218–221, 219 (fig.)
　market, 218
　"preferred medicine" policy, 221
　prescriptions regulation/bulk
　　purchasing, 221
　prices paid by patients, 232
pharmaceuticals (Norway)
　generics, 135
　market/coverage determination,
　　131–133, 131 (fig.)
　medication compliance for patients,
　　136
　physician prescriptions regulation,
　　135
　price regulation, 134–135
　prices paid by patients, 135–136
　primary/specialist care division,
　　133–134
pharmaceuticals (Switzerland)
　generic pricing, 252
　market, 250
　market access/coverage
　　determination, 250–252, 251 (fig.)
　physician prescriptions regulation,
　　252
　prices paid by patients, 252–253
pharmaceuticals (Taiwan)
　coverage determination/price
　　regulation, 317 (fig.), 318–319
　market, 317–318

physician prescriptions regulation, 319

prices paid by patients, 319

pharmaceuticals (United Kingdom)
generics, 107
market, 106–107, 107 (fig.)
prices paid by patients, 108
types, 106

pharmaceuticals (United States)
buy-and-bill system, 46
coverage determination, 43–44
generics, 43, 44, 46, 47, 47 (table)
market, 43
off-label use, 45–46
physician prescriptions regulation, 45–46
price/regulation, 44–45, 45 (fig.), 51
prices paid by patients, 46–47, 47 (table)

Pharmacy Act, 2001 (Norway), 136

pharmacy benefit management companies (PBMs/United States), 44

Physician Integrated Networks (Manitoba)

physicians (Australia), 294–295
delivery of health care, 284–286
payment for health care, 278–280, 279 (fig.)
prescriptions regulation, 293

physicians (Canada)
payment for health care, 68–69, 68 (fig.)
prescriptions regulations, 78–79
primary care physicians, 65, 69, 71, 72, 79, 80, 82
strike (1960s), 57

physicians (China), 343–346
barefoot doctors, 325, 326, 345, 357
delivery of health care, 339–340
payment for health care, 337–338, 338 (fig.)
prescriptions regulation, 343–344

physicians (France), 164–166
delivery of health care, 158

payment for health care, 153–155, 153 (fig.)
prescriptions regulation, 163–164

physicians (Germany), 192–193
delivery of health care (Germany), 186–187
payment for health care, 181–184, 182 (fig.)
prescriptions regulation, 191

physicians (Netherlands), 222–223
payment for health care, 208–209, 208–210, 209 (fig.)
prescriptions regulation, 221

physicians (Norway), 136–137
delivery of health care, 128–129
payment for health care, 122–125, 123 (fig.), 124 (fig.)
prescriptions regulation, 135
strike (2016), 122–123

physicians (Switzerland), 253–254
delivery of health care, 247
payment for health care, 243–245, 244 (fig.)
prescriptions regulation, 252

physicians (Taiwan), 320
burnout, 314, 322, 379
delivery of health care, 314–315
payment for health care, 311, 311 (fig.)
prescriptions regulation, 319

physicians (United Kingdom), 47–49, 108–110
creation of nationalized health care system, 85
delivery of health care, 102
"enhanced services," 98
payment for health care, 97–100, 98 (fig.)

physicians (United States)
burnout, 49, 53
hospital consolidations, 37, 38
payment for health care, 32–35, 33 (fig.)
prescriptions regulation, 45–46
statistics on, 47–48, 49

Physicians Services Agreement (Ontario), 69

Po-Chang, Lee, 301, 309
Poor Law (United Kingdom), 84
Powell, Enoch, 86
preventive care. *See* public health/
    preventive care
Primary Care Networks (Alberta), 71
Primary Care Networks (PCNs/United
    Kingdom), 100
primary care trusts (PCTs/United
    Kingdom), 87, 88
Primary Health Networks (PHNs/
    Australia), 285
prior authorization requirements
    (United States), 397
Private Health Insurance
    Administration Council (PHIAC/
    Australia), 273
Prudential Regulation Authority
    (United Kingdom), 91
Public Accounts Committee (United
    Kingdom), 105–106
Public Drug Insurance Plan (PDIP/
    Quebec), 60
Public Health England, 101
public health/preventive care
    Australia, 273, 288
    Canada, 65, 70, 73
    China, 335–336, 338, 341
    France, 146, 150–151, 156, 159,
        167–168
    Germany, 179, 185, 188
    Netherlands, 217
    Norway, 120–121, 126, 130
    Switzerland, 240–241, 248
    Taiwan, 313, 316
    United Kingdom, 95, 101, 104
    United States, 36, 43

quality-adjusted life year (QALY), 106,
    107, 132–133, 291, 383
Quality and Outcomes Framework
    (QOF/United Kingdom), 99,
    112–113
quantitative assessments, 14–15
Quebec, Chaoulli v. (2005), 60–61

ranking countries on health care. *See*
    comparing countries on health
    care
Regime Social des Indépendants (RSI/
    France), 146
Regional Association of Statutory
    Health Insurance Physicians
    (Germany), 171
Regional Care Assessment Center
    (Netherlands), 210
Regional Health Authorities (RHAs/
    Norway), 117, 119 (fig.), 120, 121,
    122, 123 (fig.), 125, 127, 128, 134,
    141
Reid, T. R., 13, 301
Reinhardt, Uwe, 301, 323
Risk Equalization Trust Fund
    (Australia), 270 (fig.), 273
Romand, Jacques-Andres, 246, 257
Rudoler, David, 71–72
Rural Municipality Act, 1916
    (Saskatchewan), 56
Rush, Benjamin, 19

Santesuisse (Switzerland), 236
SARS outbreak, 322, 326
Saskatchewan and Canadian health
    care history, 56, 57
Schakowsky, Jan, 395
Schreve Commission (Netherlands),
    198
Scientific Advisory Board
    (Netherlands), 220
Sickness Act, 1913 (Netherlands), 198
Smarter Medicine (Switzerland), 249
social pooling account (SPA/China),
    333 (fig.), 334
Social Security Finance Act (France),
    154
Social Support Acts (Netherlands),
    202, 206, 210, 217
Sofosbuvir (Sovaldi), 162–163
specialist-owned partnerships (MSBs/
    Netherlands), 209
Spitex (Switzerland), 245, 248

Statutory Health Insurance
    Modernization Act, 2004
    (Germany), 171–172, 173, 174 (fig.),
    175–177, 176 (fig.)
statutory health insurance (SHI)
    scheme (Germany), 173, 174 (fig.),
    175–177, 176 (fig.), 180
Stevens, Simon, 88
strategic health authorities (SHAs/
    United Kingdom), 87, 88
Super Clinic program (Australia), 285
Sustainability and Transformation
    Partnerships (STPs/United
    Kingdom), 88, 104
Swiss Agency for Therapeutic
    Products (Swissmedic), 250
Swiss Inpatient Quality Indicators, 2
    48
Switzerland, health care, 229–230, 232
    challenges, 229–230, 254–260
    coverage, 232–236, 233 (fig.)
    delivery, 246–249
    financing, 236–241, 237 (fig.)
    history, 230–232
    human resources, 253–254
    payment, 241–246, 242 (fig.),
        244 (fig.)
    pharmaceuticals, 250–253, 251 (fig.)
    population size, 233 (fig.)
    See also specific components/individuals

Taiwan Association of Cancer Patients,
    300
Taiwan, health care, 300, 303
    challenges, 321–323
    coverage, 303–306, 304 (fig.)
    delivery, 313–316
    financing, 306–309, 307 (fig.)
    history, 300–303
    human resources, 320–321
    payment, 310–313, 310 (fig.), 311 (fig.)
    pharmaceuticals, 317–319, 317 (fig.)
    population size, 304 (fig.)
    values, 301
    See also specific components/individuals

TARMED (Switzerland), 243–245,
    244 (fig.)
TARPSY (Switzerland), 243
Technology Appraisal Committee
    (TAC), 107
Therapeutic Goods Administration
    (TGA/Australia), 288–289,
    289 (fig.), 290
Therapeutic Products (Canada), 74
township health centers (THCs/
    China), 328
Traditional Chinese Medicine (TCM)
    China, 325, 331, 338, 340–341, 345
    Taiwan, 304, 307 (fig.), 309, 311, 312,
        313, 316, 320, 321, 361
Tricare (United States), 23 (fig.), 25
Trillium Drug Program (TDP/
    Ontario), 60
Truman, Harry S., 20
Trump, Donald, 22, 28, 52, 367
Twain, Mark, 3

Uniform Value Scale (Germany),
    181–182, 184
United Kingdom, health care, 83–84
    challenges, 83–84, 110–114
    coverage, 89–91, 90 (fig.)
    delivery, 101–106
    financing, 88, 91–95, 92 (fig.)
    history, 84–89
    human resources, 108–110
    payment, 95–101, 97 (fig.), 98 (fig.)
    pharmaceuticals, 106–108, 107 (fig.)
    population size, 90 (fig.)
    shortages, 108–109, 110, 111–112
    wait times, 87, 96, 105–106, 112, 127
    See also National Health Service
        (NHS/United Kingdom)
United States, health care
    challenges, 21, 50–54
    comparison conclusions, 4, 6–7, 8,
        355–356, 358, 362, 376, 381, 384,
        385–386
    coverage, 22–26, 23 (table)
    delivery, 36–43, 37 (fig.)

United States, health care (*continued*)
  financing, 24 (fig.), 26–30
  history, 2, 18–22
  human resources, 47–50
  payment, 30–36, 31 (fig.), 33 (fig.)
  pharmaceuticals, 43–47, 45 (fig.),
    47 (table)
  population size, 23 (fig.)
  See also Affordable Care Act
United States National Academy of
    Medicine, 360
Universal Disease Protection Act, 2016
    (PUMA/France), 145
Universal Health Coverage Act, 2000
    (CMU/France), 145
University of Michigan Medical
    School, 19
Urban and Rural Resident Basic
    Medical Insurance (URRBMI/
    China), 329, 330–331, 331 (fig.),
    333 (fig.), 334, 338, 341
Urban Employee Basic Medical
    Insurance (UEBMI/China),
    33 (fig.), 327, 329, 330, 331, 331 (fig.),
    332, 334, 338, 341
Urban Resident Basic Medical
    Insurance (URBMI/China), 327,
    328, 329, 330, 334, 349

Value-Based Healthcare Center of
    Europe, 216
Value-Based Healthcare Prize, 216

vision care
  ACA (United States), 391
  Australia, 266
  Canada, 58, 60, 61, 64, 362
  China, 331
  France, 146, 147, 168
  Netherlands, 201 (fig.), 202
  Norway, 120, 138, 142
  Switzerland, 234, 235, 239
  Taiwan, 303–304, 361
  United Kingdom, 90
  United States, 26, 391
Visiting Medical Officers (VMOs/
    Australia), 279–280
Voluntary Scheme for Branded
    Medicines Pricing and Access
    (VPAS/United Kingdom), 107

wait times comparisons, 378–379
Whitlam, Gough, 264
Wilhelm, I, Kaiser, 170
World Health Organization (WHO), 3,
    360–361
World Health Report 2000 (WHO), 3–4,
    6, 9

Youth Act (Netherlands), 210

ABOUT THE AUTHOR

Stephen Zipp

Ezekiel J. Emanuel is the Vice Provost for Global Initiatives, the Diane v.S. Levy and Robert M. Levy University Professor, and Co-Director of the Health-care Transformation Institute at the University of Pennsylvania. He also serves as the Special Advisor to the Director-General of the World Health Organization. From January 2009 to January 2011 he served as Special Advisor for Health Policy to the Director of the Office of Management and Budget in the White House. From 1997 to 2011 he was chair of the Department of Bioethics at the National Institutes of Health. He is also a breast oncologist.

He is a member of the National Academy of Medicine and the American Association of Arts and Sciences, and he won the Dan David Prize for medical ethics in 2019.

Dr. Emanuel has written and edited 14 books and over 300 articles and is the world's most cited bioethicist. He contributes many articles to the *Atlantic*, the *New York Times*, the *Wall Street Journal*, and the *Washington Post*, among other publications. He co-hosts the podcast *Making the Call* and appears regularly on television news programs, including as co-host of the MSNBC series *A Special Edition of The Last Word: Life in the Time of Coronavirus*.

PublicAffairs is a publishing house founded in 1997. It is a tribute to the standards, values, and flair of three persons who have served as mentors to countless reporters, writers, editors, and book people of all kinds, including me.

I. F. Stone, proprietor of *I. F. Stone's Weekly*, combined a commitment to the First Amendment with entrepreneurial zeal and reporting skill and became one of the great independent journalists in American history. At the age of eighty, Izzy published *The Trial of Socrates*, which was a national bestseller. He wrote the book after he taught himself ancient Greek.

Benjamin C. Bradlee was for nearly thirty years the charismatic editorial leader of *The Washington Post*. It was Ben who gave the *Post* the range and courage to pursue such historic issues as Watergate. He supported his reporters with a tenacity that made them fearless and it is no accident that so many became authors of influential, best-selling books.

Robert L. Bernstein, the chief executive of Random House for more than a quarter century, guided one of the nation's premier publishing houses. Bob was personally responsible for many books of political dissent and argument that challenged tyranny around the globe. He is also the founder and longtime chair of Human Rights Watch, one of the most respected human rights organizations in the world.

•   •   •

For fifty years, the banner of Public Affairs Press was carried by its owner Morris B. Schnapper, who published Gandhi, Nasser, Toynbee, Truman, and about 1,500 other authors. In 1983, Schnapper was described by *The Washington Post* as "a redoubtable gadfly." His legacy will endure in the books to come.

Peter Osnos, *Founder*